Handbook of Biologics for Rheumatological Disorders

Neeraj Jain • Lalit Duggal
Editors

Handbook of Biologics for Rheumatological Disorders

Springer

Editors
Neeraj Jain
Sir Ganga Ram Hospital
New Delhi, India

Lalit Duggal
Sir Ganga Ram Hospital
New Delhi, India

ISBN 978-981-16-7199-9 ISBN 978-981-16-7200-2 (eBook)
https://doi.org/10.1007/978-981-16-7200-2

This Springer imprint is published by the registered company Springer Nature Singapore Pte Ltd.
The registered company address is: 152 Beach Road, #21-01/04 Gateway East, Singapore 189721, Singapore

Preface

It was sheer serendipity, while going through recent chapters and books on rheumatology, written and edited by our brethren, that we decided to embark on this project.

The purpose was to bring out something different, handy, and useful for the beginners as well as for the experienced, in one of the most exciting and happening aspects in rheumatological disorders—the BIOLOGICS. The aforementioned agents have virtually transformed the entire spectrum of approach in managing these often difficult to treat conditions.

From the discovery of MABs (monoclonal antibodies) in 1975, it took about two and a half decades for the approval of the first molecule in rheumatoid arthritis. In the last 10 years or so, there has been an avalanche of sorts of these agents in various fields of rheumatology. The latest kid on the block, the JAK inhibitors, the so-called oral biologics, have been added to the armamentarium.

This treatise is a novel attempt to portray the utility of "on the shelf and in the pipeline" biologics, in common rheumatological diseases. It includes a fascinating introduction to their history, along with a bird's-eye view of their use in the presence of infections, malignancies, their ethical aspects, their off-label use, and the biosimilars, the latter being so very cost relevant in our context. The chapters on biologics in pediatric rheumatologic disorders as well as in osteoarthritis and osteoporosis add value to this book. And finally their usefulness in conditions as varied and diverse as uveitis, sarcoidosis, and the nascent IgG4-related disease will, in all likelihood, complete the major groups where these drugs may be of importance.

It is not to project the biologics as the "be-all and end-all" of treatment in rheumatology. It is a known fact that rheumatologists have to tread very carefully in their use. And except for spondyloarthritis, ANCA-associated vasculitis, and perhaps a few other conditions, their upfront use is not projected and approved at this moment of time.

Contributions from the plethora of pan-India talent, along with a sprinkling of international flavor of erudite scholars, while adding value to this book, will further enrich the knowledge of the readers.

We hope, this one of a kind work, with a virtual catalogue of biologics, is of help to all those looking for a quick reference regarding the practicability of these "wonder drugs" in the field of rheumatology.

New Delhi, India

Neeraj Jain
Lalit Duggal

Contents

About the Editors

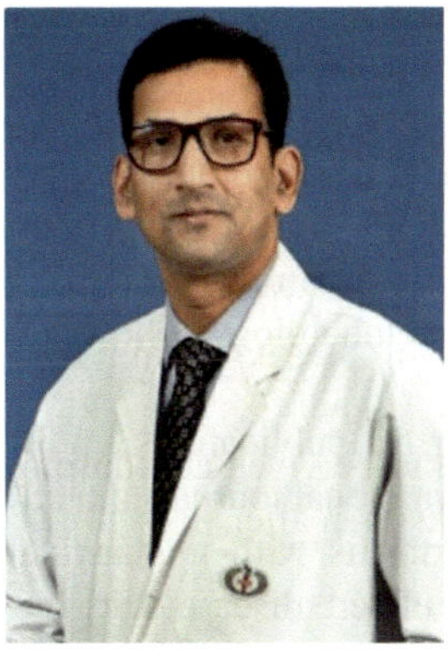

Neeraj Jain is vice-chairman at the Rheumatology and Clinical Immunology Department at Sir Ganga Ram Hospital, New Delhi, India. He is a Professor of GRIPMER, an academic body of Sir Ganga Ram Hospital.

He did his rheumatology training at King Edward Memorial Hospital, Mumbai, India, and Royal National Hospital for Rheumatic Diseases, Bath, UK.

He is a fellow of the Royal College of Physicians of Edinburgh (FRCP), UK, and the American College of Rheumatology (FACR).

He is faculty in the Rheumatology and Clinical Immunology Department at Sir Ganga Ram Hospital, established in 2009.

Dr. Neeraj has more than 30 publications to his credit in both national and international journals. He has contributed several chapters to various books and has peer-reviewed articles in many international rheumatology journals.

He is an active member of the Indian Rheumatology Association (IRA) and Delhi Rheumatology Association. He is a member of the Delhi Rheumatology and Immunology Foundation (DRIF).

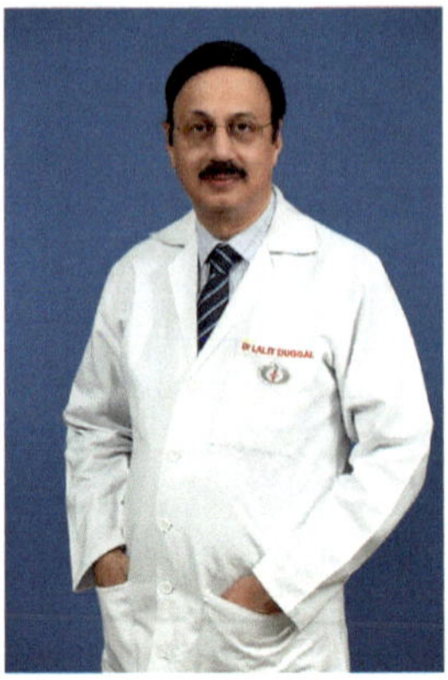

Lalit Duggal is Chairman, Department of Rheumatology and Clinical Immunology at Sir Ganga Ram Hospital, New Delhi, India.

He is a graduate of Armed Forces Medical College Pune and Medicine post-graduate from King George's Medical College Lucknow. He has received Rheumatology training in the USA.

In 2003 he was conferred the fellowship of the Royal College of physicians of Glasgow, and he continues to be actively associated with it as an examiner.

Dr. Duggal has been a temporary advisor to the WHO in 1999.

He has been an active rheumatologist for close to three decades. He is credited with establishing the department of Rheumatology and Clinical immunology at Sir Ganga Ram Hospital in 2009. He was instrumental in initiating the DNB programme in the hospital in 2013 and he also supervises rheumatology fellowship courses in the institution.

Dr. Duggal has more than 50 publications to his credit in both national and international journals including original work in ankle arthritis with mediastinal lymphadenopathy and IgG4-related disease. He has chapters in various rheumatology books and has peer-reviewed articles in international rheumatology journals.

He is an active member and past president of the Delhi Rheumatology Association. He is the founder and president of Delhi Rheumatology and Immunology Foundation (DRIF). This foundation is involved in various social activities including patient and physician education, especially on important dates, such as World arthritis and World lupus days.

A Historical Introduction to the Biological Response Modifier Drugs: The 'Biologicals'

1

Anand N. Malaviya

1.1 Introduction

The real impact of biological drugs in the practice of medicine can hardly be appreciated by today's over-busy young physicians trying to keep up with the increasing workload, spending late hours in the corridors of big-city hospitals. They would not have time to stop to think about how and who was involved in the discovery of 'mabs' and 'cepts', (the biological drugs) that are now available for a wide spectrum of diseases across specialities. These physicians would be least interested in the history of the discovery of these drugs that are nothing short of 'miracles' if there ever was one. Yet the story of the discovery of the biologicals is like a highly engrossing novel with excitements, despair, thrills and ecstasy with an intense ending.

The present-day science is unlike that of the yesteryears. In those good old days, one brilliant mind would get a heavenly inspiration and suddenly discover 'Gravity' (Sir Isac Newton's discovery of gravity), the so-called 'Eureka moment'—a moment of sudden, triumphant discovery, inspiration or insight. The scientific discoveries of modern times are very different and mundane. It usually builds upon a solid foundation of knowledge and newer technologies developed over decades of work involving large teams of scientists in huge laboratories, often with coordination among different centres around the world. The discovery of biologicals has not been

A. N. Malaviya (✉)
Head of the Department of Rheumatology, ISIC Superspeciality Hospital, New Delhi, India

N. Jain, L. Duggal (eds.), *Handbook of Biologics for Rheumatological Disorders*,
https://doi.org/10.1007/978-981-16-7200-2_1

different; with the background knowledge gathered since the late nineteenth century and during the early-middle part of twentieth century, it was only a question of time for these drugs to become available for routine use.

1.2 Historical Background

It is important to note that drugs derived from biological materials (mostly animals) or manufactured in biological systems are not new. The discovery of 'serum therapy' and 'anti-toxin therapy' by Kisato and von Behring in the late nineteenth–early twentieth century for treating diphtheria, tetanus and rabies are still in use [1]. These are also 'biological drugs' (produced in biological systems). Clotting factors and several growth factors (e.g. erythropoietin, colony-stimulating factors; used in haematology and bleeding disorders) are also biologically derived [2]. For that matter, the older generation of insulin was prepared from the pancreas of pigs [3]. In a broader sense, these therapeutic agents have also been 'biologically derived'. Therefore, to clarify what is meant by biological drugs in modern medicine, the National Cancer Institute (NCI, USA) has defined a biological drug as follows 'a substance that is made from a living organism or its products and is used in the prevention, diagnosis or treatment of cancer and other diseases. Biological drugs include antibodies, interleukins (ILs), and vaccines; also called biologic agent and biological agent' [4]. Increasing knowledge of aetiopathology of diseases has often identified a certain molecule that could be central to the pathobiology of a given disease (e.g. tumour necrosis factor-α {TNF-α} in rheumatoid arthritis {RA}). By targeting the putative key pathogenic molecule, theoretically, it could be possible to modify the disease process and ameliorate the disease. With this line of reasoning, biological scientists, mostly working in the field of cancer, started to consider the possibility of developing molecules that would specifically target the most relevant pathogenic molecule and neutralize the same, leading to the recovery from the disease. The most obvious choice for such a therapeutic molecule was a specific antibody that would bind to the pathogenic molecule and neutralize its harmful effects. The prerequisites for such an antibody would be that it is clonal in nature, i.e. all of the same primary, secondary and tertiary structure, same antigenic binding site and same affinity and avidity. Such antibodies were named 'monoclonal antibodies (mAbs)' that are defined as follows: 'an antibody produced by a single clone of cells or cell line and consisting of identical antibody molecules with exactly the same physicochemical and immunological properties'.

1.3 Basic Requirements for Producing Monoclonal Antibodies (MABS) for Therapeutic Use

In decades prior to the development of methods for large commercial-scale production of mAbs, several path-breaking technological advances were made, most of them not necessarily with the intent of producing such antibodies. These included: (1) Identifying the *key pathogenic molecule* for a given disease (if there is one, e.g.

tumour necrosis factor-α (TNF-α, in RA); This would usually require the use of *cell culture to grow the pathological tissue* (e.g. synovial tissue in case of RA) and then study the secreted molecules to identify the putative key pathogenic molecule; (2) Use of *complementary DNA (cDNA) cloning technology* for producing the relevant molecule in pure form (for producing specific monoclonal antibody); (3) Identifying and *isolating the specific antibody-producing cell* that secretes the relevant (specific) antibody; (4) Turning that specific antibody-producing cell into an *immortal self-perpetuating cell line* that would keep producing large amounts of that mAb for times to come.

A brief history of these essential steps and the scientists involved in that work is described below. It must be mentioned that *the example taken is that of RA because historically that was the disease for which the first therapeutic mAb, namely infliximab, was used successfully* [2].

1.3.1 Discovery of Tissue Culture Technique for Studying Biological Systems

Tissue culture and the study of culture supernatants have been the mainstay of understanding cell physiology since the late nineteenth century. The study of synovial tissue using cell culture has, therefore, been the main tool for understanding the pathobiology of RA. It all started with the seminal work of Wilhelm Roux (1885) (a German physician, a student of Rudolf Virchow, with seminal work in experimental embryology who successfully grew medullary plate of an embryonic chicken in the laboratory) [5]. Over the next decades, the technique was perfected by Ross Harrison (an American biologist) and several other biologists culminating in the work of Alexis Carrel (a French surgeon and biologist who won the Nobel Prize in 1912 for pioneering the tissue culture technique). He had worked at the Rockefeller Institute from 1906 to 1927 and had teamed up with Montrose Burrows (1911), a US surgeon and pathologist with special interests in cancer research [6]. *Burrows is credited with the coining of the word 'tissue culture'*. Till the late 1960s, not much was known about the pathobiology of RA except for an exceptionally brilliant work by Vaubel in 1933 on the histopathology of RA synovial tissue [7]. Vaubel is credited with the description of two major classes of cells in the synovium, namely the fibroblast-like synoviocytes (FLS) and the macrophage-like synoviocytes (MLS), the terminology that is still in routine use.

1.3.2 Identifying the *Key Pathogenic Molecule* in RA; Study of the Synovial Tissue and its Molecules in Cell Cultures

Before going into the details of the pathobiology of RA, especially the histopathological abnormalities in the synovial tissue in RA, it would be of interest to describe the prevailing theories of the pathobiology of RA in those early days. At that time (early twentieth century), the debate was between *gum infection* to the *abnormal extracellular matrix* [2]. The term 'collagen disease' (a term used in the past for diseases that are now called systemic immunoinflammatory rheumatic diseases) owes its name to that legacy of 'abnormal extracellular matrix'. Fortunately, the work of Vaubel [7], described below, combined with advances in enzymology, by the early 1970s, the theory of abnormal extracellular matrix was completely demolished [2].

1.3.2.1 Early Studies on Synovial Tissue from RA Patients in Tissue Culture

The seminal work of Jan-Mitchel Dayer from the Faculty of Medicine, University of Geneva, Switzerland, takes precedence over others in the original studies on the synovial tissue from patients with RA. He joined the famous 'Arthritis Unit' headed by Rheumatologist Stephen Krane at Massachusetts General Hospital (MGH, Boston, USA) in the mid-1970s. It was the work of Dayer's team at MGH that paved the way for the modern-day investigation of the pathobiology of RA [8, 9]. Studying the synovial tissue in culture, Dayer and colleagues noted that synovial fibroblasts produced large amounts of collagenase and prostaglandin E2 (PGE2). Their work also showed that physical contact of synovial fibroblasts with the mononuclear cells (monocyte-macrophages {MΦ} that were present in the synovial tissue, albeit in lesser numbers), was essential for this process but only in the early stages of the disease. The same process in the synovial fibroblasts becomes autonomous (a behaviour resembling tumour cells) in those where the disease was more chronic. Using the culture supernatants, these workers purified a small 15 kDa molecule that acted as the sensitizer for the synovial fibroblasts. They named it 'mononuclear-cell factor' (MCF) [8, 9]. In 1979, after chromatographic purification, the same molecule was re-named interleukin-1 (IL-1). Dayer and colleagues also get the credit for analysing the function of the cells in RA synovium. They described the sequence of the activity of the cells as follows: from activated T lymphocytes (TL) → MΦ → synovial fibroblast activation (where direct physical contact of the MΦ was essential) → production of inflammatory cytokines. This paradigm for the pathogenesis of RA holds true till today except for the additional role of B cells producing rheumatoid factor that self-associate and directly stimulate MΦ without the requirement for T cells [10–13].

There were two rather intriguing features of the seminal work done by Dayer's team. Firstly, it seems that this team of workers did not try any method to neutralize MCF for therapeutic purpose. It is likely that at that time (the mid-1970s), the technology was not available to produce any 'agent' (drug, molecules) that could specifically neutralize MCF. The second and more intriguing fact was that they did not report finding tumour necrosis factor-α (TNF-α), which, several years later, was identified as the key driver of inflammation in the synovial tissue (see below). Was this due to some technical issued related to cell culture? The question remains unanswered. Even more intriguing was the fact that years later, when mAb against MCF (i.e. IL-1) became available (by the name anakinra), it did not show much therapeutic effect in RA [14].

1.3.2.2 The Saga of the Discovery of Tumour Necrosis Factor-α (TNF-α) and its Cloning

The credit for the first discovery of a molecule that is now known as TNF-α goes to Carswell et al. [15] working at Memorial Sloan-Kettering Cancer Center, New York. These workers showed that mice primed with substances that induce non-specific reticuloendothelial hyperplasia (mostly activating macrophages non-specifically, substances like BCG, Zymosan, Corynebacteria, several others; in the present-day nomenclature these are called 'adjuvants' that are widely used in experimental immunology) when transplanted with tumours (sarcomas and other transplanted tumours), the tumours showed haemorrhagic necrosis. Thus, the name 'tumour necrosis factor'. This work went totally unnoticed till 1985 when Bruce Beutler and colleagues demonstrated the *role of* TNF-α *in the pathogenesis of diseases* [16]. The work was considered so important that Beutler and Jules A. Hoffmann were awarded Nobel Prize in the year 2011. Beutler had earlier worked in the team of Dayer (mentioned above) and a legendry researcher Anthony Cerami (New York), where these workers had described a lipoprotein lipase-suppressing hormone secreted by endotoxin-induced RAW 264.7 cells (cells are a macrophage-like, Abelson leukaemia virus-transformed cell line derived from BALB/c mice; commonly used model of mouse macrophages for the study of cellular responses to microbes and their products). They had named this molecule '*cachectin*' because the experimental animals developed severe cachexia. Later work demonstrated that TNF-α and cachectin were the same molecules [17–19]. The name cachectin was then dropped, and the molecule came to be known as TNF-α.

Beutler's work that demonstrated the importance of TNF-α in disease pathology had stimulated a lot of work related to this molecule. Scientists, especially the group lead by the famous Cancer specialist at Memorial Sloan-Kettering Centre, New York, Lloyd Old, got together in a small workshop organized by him in December 1994) [2]. This small meeting can be identified as the *beginning of the era of 'biologicals for therapeutic purposes*'. In the conference were present scientists who became famous later on and included, among others, Beutler, Jan Vilček. Bharat Bhushan Aggarwal and several others, some of whom went on to win Nobel Prize (e.g. Beutler). Probably the most notable presentation at that conference was by BB Aggarwal, who presented the cloning and sequencing of the molecule in focus, namely TNF-α [20]. Once purified TNF-α became available, it was easy to produce a specific antibody against it and test it in clinical situations.

1.3.2.3 Discovery of TNF-α as the Key Molecule in the Pathogenesis of Synovitis in a Patient with RA

Ravinder Nath Maini (later Sir Ravinder Nath Maini), an immunologist-rheumatologist, has been working at the Kennedy Institute of Rheumatology, Imperial College, London, since late 1960s. His interest was in understanding rheumatoid arthritis and its immunopathology. He was studying rheumatoid synovial tissue for this purpose. As luck would have it, around the same time, Marc Feldmann (Later Sir Marc Feldmann), a basic scientist, was also working in the same institute and also interested in the abnormalities in the rheumatoid synovium. It was natural that they teamed up to study the pathological abnormalities in the rheumatoid synovium using an advanced tissue culture technique. Their team demonstrated the presence of large amounts of TNF-α along with IL-1 and other cytokines in the supernatants from the rheumatoid synovial culture [21–23]. However, their key finding was that by inhibiting TNF-α using a specific antibody in mice, the whole cascade of inflammatory cytokines (including IL-1) could be inhibited, thus shutting off an inflammatory response in the synovial tissue completely [24]. At that stage, the only issue for them was to obtain a mAb against TNF-α, which could be used therapeutically in humans for conducting a clinical trial in RA [25–28].

1.3.2.4 Identifying and Isolating a Single Antibody-Producing Cell for Producing Monoclonal Antibody: Jerne's 'Haemolytic Plaque Technique' Using Soft Agar-Gel

One of the prerequisites for producing mAb is to identify and then isolate a single antibody-producing cell that would be producing the desired antibody. Even if an animal is injected with a highly purified antigen, the antibodies produced are a heterogeneous family of molecules with different isotypes reacting with different epitopes of the injected antigen. Therefore, it is necessary to identify a single antibody-producing cell that is producing the desired antibody, isolate such a cell, immortalize it with some method and then propagate it in tissue culture where it will continue to produce the same monoclonal antibody over long periods of time without any mutation. Niles Jerne, one of the sharpest minds ever to have worked in the field of immunology (shared the 1984 Nobel Prize with Köhler and Milstein for their work on the important contribution of theory and practice in shaping our understanding of the body's immune system) the first director of the world-famous Basel Institute of Immunology, (Switzerland) had devised a simple technique for identifying single living antibody-producing cell [29] (From 1965 to 1968, while working in the laboratory of Schwartz and Tannenberg in Boston, the author had extensively used Jerne's haemolytic plaque technique in soft agar while studying the lifecycle of antibody-producing cells [30]. Thus, experimentally it became possible to isolate monoclonal anti-TNF-α antibody-producing cells. Some modifications of basically the same technique have since been widely used in laboratories for isolating antibody-producing cells. By the 1970s most immunologists working with antibody and antibody-producing cells (later called B cell-plasma cell line of immune cells) had recognized the urgent need for producing large amounts of antibodies with known specificity. Leading workers in the field in those days were Joseph Sinkovics (M.D. Anderson Hospital and Tumor Institute in Houston Texas, USA) [31, 32], Brigitte Ita Askonas (National Institute of Medical Research, Mill Hill, London) [33] and Norman Klinman (University of Pennsylvania with joint attachment to the Wistar Institute, Philadelphia, USA) [34, 35]. Unfortunately, for various reasons [2] their success was limited; the lifespan of such cells in culture was found to be a few hours to a few days only. Thus, there was a need for some new technology where such an antibody-producing cell could be immortalized in a cell line and exploited for commercial production of the monoclonal antibody.

1.3.2.5 Hybridoma Technology and the Commercial Production of mAbs

César Milstein, an Argentinian biochemist (1927-2002), became a naturalized British citizen in 1958 and joined the Biochemistry Department of Darwin College, University of Cambridge, with a short-term appointment at nearby Medical Research Council (MRC) of UK. Dick Cotton (an Australian Fellow in the laboratory of Milstein in the early 1970s), with help and inspiration from Milstein, developed a technique of *fusing 2 living cells using inactivated Sendai virus* (Sendai virus promoted cell fusion) [2]. For his experiments, Cotton used a variety of mouse myeloma cells (by definition, myeloma cells are monoclonal; all of them produce an exact copy of a single antibody with exactly the same specificity. Such antibodies are called *monoclonal antibodies*). The most exciting aspect of this experiment was that the antibody-producing cellular machinery of the fused cells was fully functional; such cells continued to produce two types of monoclonal antibodies, each of the same original specificity of the two fused cells. Milstein gave the name 'hybridoma' (a hybrid of myeloma cells) to such fused cells. In 1973, Milstein presented his work on 'hybridoma' at the Basel Institute of Immunology (where Niels Jerne was the Director, see above). Georges Köhler, a Ph. D. student at that institute, who was present in the audience, got so inspired by Milstein's work that he joined his research team at Cambridge University, the UK, in 1974. At that stage, Milstein's hybridomas (Potter's mouse myeloma cell line MOPC21) were facing problems that they did not survive long enough in tissue culture. Also, the antibodies being produced were against unknown antigens. At around the same time (the late 1960s), an American Immunologist Norman Klinman at the University of Pennsylvania, with attachment to (nearby) Wistar Institute, was using a technique for producing what he called 'monofocal' antibodies [35]. He used small fragments of spleen from mice injected with a known antigen (sheep red blood cells in this case). He could have been inspired by Jerne's haemolytic plaque in the soft agar gel technique described several years earlier (discussed above). The beauty of Klinman's technique was that by using it, he was able to isolate a single living antibody-producing a cell with known and well-defined specificity (in this case, antibodies against sheep red blood cells). At this advanced stage of the development of cell biology, it was only a question of time for Köhler and Milstein to use an antibody-producing cell (isolated using Klinman's technique) for producing antibody to a defined antigen and fuse it with a mouse myeloma cell using Sendai virus. *They published their successful experiment of having developed a hybridoma that produced a specific monoclonal antibody of desired specificity (in their experiment the antigen was sheep red blood cell)* [36]. *Köhler and Milstein would have suddenly realised that they had developed an antibody-producing cell line that was immortal and capable of producing an endless supply of monoclonal antibodies with known specificity*. Theirs was an epoch-making discovery that opened the doors for producing monoclonal antibodies against any desired antigen by a laboratory-created (man-made) hybridoma. The importance of their discovery was recognized by the Nobel Committee. Köhler and Milstein shared the 1984 Nobel Prize for their work, with Niles Jerne. The rest, as they say, is history! Space does not permit to go into the story of how such an important discovery (hybridoma producing a monoclonal antibody of a known specificity) could not be patented in the United Kingdom. History tells us that Hilary Koprowski, Carlo Croce and Walter Gerhard (Americans) was granted two patents (October 1979 and April 1980) for making mAbs against tumours and influenza virus. It is said that Britain might have lost millions of dollars by not patenting the hybridoma technology in UK [2]. It is of note that Koprowski, working at the Wistar Institute (the famous National Cancer Institute-designated Centre, Philadelphia), co-founded Centocor, one of the earliest biotechnology company for commercial production of mAbs for diagnostics and therapeutics. As discussed below, historically, the first mAb used therapeutically was against anti-TNF-α, infliximab, that was a product of Centocor Laboratory (brand name 'Remicade') [2].

1.3.2.6 TNF-α, Jan Vilček and the Monoclonal Anti-TNF-α

Jan Vilček, originally from (old) Czechoslovakia (under Nazi occupation), had moved over to New York University School of Medicine in 1964. Being a brilliant student from the School of Medicine in Bratislava, he had made a name for himself working with interferons (IFN) [37]. His work at NYU had resulted in the discovery of three forms of IFNs (α, β and the immune interferon, namely IFN-γ). As luck would have it, Vilček was also one of the participants of the famous 1984 workshop organized by Lloyd Old (mentioned earlier), where BB Aggarwal had presented his work on cloning of the TNF-α molecule. Having worked with IFNs for a major part of his scientific career, Vilček wanted to move over to some new exciting area of research. BB Aggarwal's presentation of the cloning of TNF-α molecule drove him to take up research on this molecule. Collaborating with Aggarwal and Genentech Laboratory (Aggarwal was closely associated with it) over the next several years, he made some key discoveries on TNF-α. He showed its property of inducing inflammatory cytokines in different biological systems. He also showed the presence of a specific receptor TNF-α that was widely distributed in different cells and tissues. In short, Vilček's (also that of Bruce Beutler, who showed its role in tissue damage) contributions to the biology of TNF-α and in the development of mAbs against TNF-α, infliximab—the first mAb ever to be therapeutically used in humans, have been immense [37]. He developed a unique relationship with the biotechnology company Centocor (mentioned above), where the academia (his laboratory at NYU) will carry out research while the Centocor will get the patent and exploit the discovery commercially. The work of Cerami and his colleagues on the role of 'cachectin' (TNF-α) in causing cachexia and septic shock has already been mentioned earlier. Cerami's group was keen on trying anti-TNF-α monoclonals to reverse the effect of cachectin (cachexia and septic shock). With Vilček's help, Centocor produced human-mouse chimeric mAb (called cA2) against human TNF in the early 1990s. Unfortunately, when tested in 'sleeping sickness' in cows in Kenya, the results were disastrous; all the animals died [38]. This became a huge stumbling block on any further development on TNF-anti-TNF research for therapeutic use. It was rumoured that with the failure of cA2 in therapeutic experiments, Centocor went into a serious financial crisis. That was exactly the time (1993) when two young immunologists-rheumatologists Ravinder Nath Maini and Marc Feldman from London, approached Centocor to part with some of their cA2 mAb against TNF-α.

1.3.2.7 Maini and Feldmann's First Use of Anti-TNF-α in Human Disease: Rheumatoid Arthritis

The seminal work of Maini, Feldmann and their colleagues in zeroing in on TNF-α as the key cytokine that was shown to drive inflammation in rheumatoid synovium has already been described earlier. Having obtained mAb against TNF-α from Centocor, they systematically proceeded to test it therapeutically in patients with rheumatoid arthritis. In a series of papers on the trial of this mAb (named infliximab, the brand name 'Remicade®') in RA, they are credited with the first-ever use of a mAb in clinical medicine [25–28, 39, 40]. Their discovery paved the way for the development of a huge number of monoclonals for different diseases across all specialities. Mani and Feldmann have since been among the most decorated biological scientists; Maini having bestowed with Crafoord Prize (2000), Albert Lasker Award for Clinical Medical Research (2003), Dr. Paul Janssen Award for Biomedical Research (2008), and Gairdner Foundation International Award (2014). Prof. Marc Feldmann has been honoured with Crafoord Prize (2000), Albert Lasker Award for Clinical Medical Research (2003), EPO European Inventor of the Year Award (2007), Dr. Paul Janssen Award for Biomedical Research (2008), Ernst Schering Prize (2010) and Gairdner Foundation International Award (2014). Finally, for their historic work during 1980s-1990s, culminating in the identification of TNFα as a key cytokine in the pathology of RA, Ravinder Maini and Marc Feldmann were knighted in 2003 and 2010, respectively.

1.4 Conclusion

The history of medicine is full of interesting stories about how the various therapeutic agents were discovered, including the role of serendipity in several such discoveries made in years gone by. In contrast, the discovery of mAbs for therapeutic purposes has been that of decades of hard work by a large number of different scientists working in different laboratories in different countries in different (mostly unrelated) fields of research, mostly carrying out basic research in the field of biology and cell science. But, the final credit must be given to the duo of Sir Ravinder Nath Maini and Sir Marc Feldmann of the Imperial College, Kennedy Institute of Rheumatology, London, for bringing together all the past knowledge, building upon that knowledge and technology and successfully applying it to a human disease (RA) demonstrating its dramatic effect in alleviating signs and symptoms of the disease. No wonder one of the anti-TNF-α drugs (adalimumab) has been among the ten best-selling drugs in the World in 1995 [40].

References

1. Silverstein AM. Emil von Behring: infectious disease, immunology, serum therapy: project MUSE, (review). Bull Hist Med. 2006;80:778–80.
2. Malaviya AN, Mehra NK. A fascinating story of the discovery & development of biologicals for use in clinical medicine. Ind J Med Res. 2018;148:263–78.
3. Quianzon CC, Cheikh I. History of insulin. J Community Hosp Intern Med Perspect. 2012;2 https://doi.org/10.3402/jchimp.v2i2.18701.
4. https://www.cancer.gov/publications/dictionaries/cancer-terms/def/biological-drug
5. Avelar-Gonzalez FJ, Guerrero-Barrera AL. Cell culture: history, development and prospects. Int J Curr Res Acad Rev. 2014;2:188–200.
6. Carrel A, Burrow MT. Cultivation of tissues *in vitro* and its technique. J Exp Med. 1911;13:387–96.
7. Vaubel E. The form and function of synovial cells in tissue cultures: I. morphology of the cells under varying conditions. J Exp Med. 1933;58:63–83.
8. Dayer JM, Graham R, Russell G, Krane SM. Collagenase production by rheumatoid synovial cells: stimulation by a human lymphocyte factor. Science. 1977a;195:181–3.
9. Dayer JM, Robinson DR, Krane SM. Prostaglandin production by rheumatoid synovial cells: stimulation by a factor from human mononuclear cells. J Exp Med. 1977b;145:1399–404.
10. Dayer JM, Bréard J, Chess L, Krane SM. Participation of monocyte-macrophages and lymphocytes in the production of a factor that stimulates collagenase and prostaglandin release by rheumatoid synovial cells. J Clin Invest. 1979a;64:1386–92.
11. Dayer JM, Goldring SR, Robinson DR, Krane SM. Collagenase and prostaglandin in connective tissue destruction: cell-cell and humoral interactions. Bull Schweiz Akad Med Wiss. 1979b;35:329–43.
12. Nardella FA, Dayer JM, Roelke M, Krane SM, Mannik M. Self-associating IgG rheumatoid factors stimulate monocytes to release prostaglandins and mononuclear cell factor that stimulates collagenase and prostaglandin production by synovial cells. Rheumatol Int. 1983;3:183–6.
13. Vey E, Zhang JH, Dayer JM. IFN-gamma and 1,25(OH)2D3 induce on THP-1 cells distinct patterns of cell surface antigen expression, cytokine production, and responsiveness to contact with activated T cells. J Immunol. 1992;149:2040–6.
14. Scott IC, Ibrahim F, Simpson G, Kowalczyk A, White-Alao B, Hassell A, et al. A randomised trial evaluating anakinra in early active rheumatoid arthritis. Clin Exp Rheumatol. 2016;34:88–93.
15. Carswell EA, Old LJ, Kassel RL, Green S, Fiore N, Williamson B. An endotoxin-induced serum factor that causes necrosis of tumours. Proc Natl Acad Sci U S A. 1975;72:3666–70.
16. Beutler B, Milsark IW, Cerami AC. Passive immunization against cachectin/tumour necrosis factor protects mice from lethal effect of endotoxin. Science. 1985c;229:869–71.
17. Beutler B, Greenwald D, Hulmes JD, Chang M, Pan YC, Mathison J, et al. Identity of tumour necrosis factor and the macrophage-secreted factor cachectin. Nature. 1985a;316:552–4.
18. Beutler B, Mahoney J, Le Trang N, Pekala P, Cerami A. Purification of cachectin, a lipoprotein lipase-suppressing hormone secreted by endotoxin-induced RAW 264.7 cells. J Exp Med. 1985b;161:984–95.
19. Dayer JM, Beutler B, Cerami A. Cachectin/tumour necrosis factor stimulates collagenase and prostaglandin E2 production by human synovial cells and dermal fibroblasts. J Exp Med. 1985;162:2163–8.
20. Aggarwal BB, Kohr WJ, Hass PE, Moffat B, Spencer SA, Henzel WJ, et al. Human tumour necrosis factor. Production, purification, and characterization. J Biol Chem. 1985;260:2345–54.
21. Buchan G, Barrett K, Fujita T, Taniguchi T, Maini R, Feldmann M, et al. Detection of activated T cell products in the rheumatoid joint using cDNA probes to interleukin-2 (IL-2) IL-2 receptor and IFN-gamma. Clin Exp Immunol. 1988a;71:295–301.

22. Buchan G, Barrett K, Turner M, Chantry D, Maini RN, Feldmann M, et al. Interleukin-1 and tumour necrosis factor mRNA expression in rheumatoid arthritis: prolonged production of IL-1 alpha. Clin Exp Immunol. 1988b;73:449–55.
23. Feldmann M, Brennan FM, Maini RN. Role of cytokines in rheumatoid arthritis. Annu Rev Immunol. 1996;14:397–440.
24. Brennan FM, Chantry D, Jackson A, Maini R, Feldmann M. Inhibitory effect of TNF alpha antibodies on synovial cell interleukin-1 production in rheumatoid arthritis. Lancet. 1989;2:244–7.
25. Elliott MJ, Maini RN, Feldmann M, Kalden JR, Antoni C, Smolen JS, et al. Randomised double-blind comparison of chimeric monoclonal antibody to tumour necrosis factor alpha (cA2) versus placebo in rheumatoid arthritis. Lancet. 1994a;344:1105–10.
26. Elliott MJ, Maini RN, Feldmann M, Long-Fox A, Charles P, Bijl H, et al. Repeated therapy with monoclonal antibody to tumour necrosis factor alpha (cA2) in patients with rheumatoid arthritis. Lancet. 1994b;344:1125–7.
27. Lipsky PE, van der Heijde DM, St. Clair EW, Furst DE, Breedveld FC, Kalden JR, et al. Infliximab and methotrexate in the treatment of rheumatoid arthritis. Anti-tumour necrosis factor trial in rheumatoid arthritis with a concomitant therapy study group. N Engl J Med. 2000;343:1594–602.
28. Maini RN, Breedveld FC, Kalden JR, Smolen JS, Davis D, Macfarlane JD, et al. Therapeutic efficacy of multiple intravenous infusions of anti-tumour necrosis factor alpha monoclonal antibody combined with low-dose weekly methotrexate in rheumatoid arthritis. Arthritis Rheum. 1998;41:1552–63.
29. Jerne NK, Nordin AA, Henry C. The agar plaque technique for recognizing antibody-producing cells. In: Amos B, Koprowski H, editors. Cell-bound antibodies. Philadelphia: The Wistar Institute Press; 1963. p. 109.
30. Tannenberg WJK, Malaviya AN. The life cycle of antibody-forming cells I. The generation time or 19s hemolytic plaque-forming cells during the primary and secondary responses. J Expl Med. 1968;128:895–925.
31. Sinkovics JG, Drewinko B, Thornell E. Immunoresistant tetraploid lymphoma cells. Lancet. 1970;1:139–40.
32. Sinkovics JG. Discovery of the hybridoma principle in 1968-69 immortalization of the specific antibody-producing cell by fusion with a lymphoma cell. J Med. 1985;16:509–24.
33. Askonas BA, Williamson AR, Wright BEG. Selection of a single antibody-forming cell clone and its propagation in syngeneic mice. Proc Natl Acad Sci U S A. 1970;67:1398–403.
34. Klinman NR, Taylor RB. General methods for the study of cells and serum during the immune response: the response todinitrophenyl in mice. Clin Exp Immunol. 1969;4:473–87.
35. Klinman NR. Antibody with homogeneous antigen binding produced by splenic foci in organ culture. Immunochemistry. 1969;6:757–9.
36. Köhler G, Milstein C. Continuous cultures of fused cells secreting antibody of predefined specificity. Nature. 1975;256:495–7.
37. Vilček J. An interferon-like substance released from tick-borne encephalitis virus-infected chick embryo fibroblast cells. Nature. 1960;187:73–4.
38. Cerami A. The value of failure: the discovery of TNF and its natural inhibitor erythropoietin. J Intern Med. 2011;269:8–15.
39. Elliott MJ, Maini RN, Feldmann M, Long-Fox A, Charles P, Katsikis P, et al. Treatment of rheumatoid arthritis with chimeric monoclonal antibodies to tumor necrosis factor alpha. Arthritis Rheum. 1993;36:1681–90.
40. Monaco C, Nanchahal J, Taylor P, Feldmann M. Anti-TNF therapy: past, present and future. Int Immunol. 2015;27:55–62.

Biologics in Rheumatoid Arthritis

2

Rohini Handa

Case Scenario

A 35-year-old lady with rheumatoid arthritis (RA) of 4 years duration presents to her physician with active disease (CDAI 23). She is on triple drug combination with hydroxychloroquine (200 mg/day), oral methotrexate (15 mg/week) and leflunomide (10 mg/day). Her physician hikes her disease modifying anti rheumatic drug (DMARD) doses to hydroxychloroquine (400 mg/day), subcutaneous methotrexate (25 mg/week) and leflunomide (20 mg/day) and adds low dose prednisolone 5 mg/day. Two months later she reports to him with partial relief: CDAI of 18. She is Cushingoid and wants to stop her corticosteroids. He advises her to take biologics and refers her to a rheumatologist.

2.1 Introduction

The treatment of RA revolves around the use of nonsteroidal anti-inflammatory drugs, corticosteroids, and disease modifying antirheumatic drugs (DMARDs). DMARDs are the anchor drugs used to treat RA with methotrexate deemed the gold standard. DMARDs are currently classified as (Table 2.1):

(a) Synthetic DMARDs (conventional and targeted).
(b) Biologic DMARDs (bio-originators and biosimilars).

R. Handa (✉)
Indraprastha Apollo Hospitals, New Delhi, India

N. Jain, L. Duggal (eds.), *Handbook of Biologics for Rheumatological Disorders*,
https://doi.org/10.1007/978-981-16-7200-2_2

Table 2.1 DMARDs in RA

Synthetic DMARDs	
Conventional—csDMARDs	Methotrexate, Leflunomide, Hydroxychloroquine, Sulfasalazine
Targeted—tsDMARDs	Tofacitinib, Baricitinib, Upadacitinib, Peficitinib, Filgotinib
Biological DMARDs	
Bio-originator DMARDs	Infliximab, Etanercept, Adalimumab, Golimumab, Certolizumab, Rituximab, Tocilizumab, Abatacept, Anakinra, Sarilumab
Biosimilar DMARDs	Infliximab, Etanercept, Adalimumab, Rituximab

2.2 What Are Biologic DMARDs (bDMARDs)?

- Biologic DMARDs are therapeutic agents produced by means of biological (*not chemical*) processes in live-cell systems. The manufacturing usually involves recombinant DNA technology.

2.3 What Are the Types of Biologic DMARDs?

- Biologic DMARDs include monoclonal antibodies (mAbs) and receptor constructs (cepts). Examples of mAbs are infliximab, adalimumab, golimumab, certolizumab, rituximab, etc., while etanercept is the prototype of a receptor construct-fusion protein where the naturally occurring receptor is linked to the immunoglobulin frame. The receptor provides the construct with specificity while the Fc of IgG imparts stability and prolongs half-life.
- The lineage can be ascertained by the name where 'mo' refers to murine, 'xi' to chimeric, 'zu' to humanized and 'mu' to fully human mAbs. For example, infli**xi**mab is a chimeric mAb (75% human and 25% murine), tocili**zu**mab is humanized while adali**mu**mab is fully human.

2.4 What Do bDMARDs Target?

The biologics may target cytokines (both ligands and receptors) or cells. Table 2.2 lists the targets of various FDA-approved biologics and their usual doses in RA.

2.5 When to Initiate Biologics in RA?

Biologics, in general, are initiated in patients who have:

- Inadequate response to csDMARDs in adequate doses (refractory disease).
- Aggressive disease with poor prognostic factors (presence of high titer autoantibodies, high disease activity, early erosions).
- Intolerance to csDMARDs.
- Special situations like RA with corneal melt, rheumatoid vasculitis, some patients with RA-ILD (interstitial lung disease).

Table 2.2 Biologicals for RA

Biologic (Bio-originator)	Target	Route of administration	Usual adult dose	Biosimilar available
Infliximab (Remicade)	TNF	i.v.	In conjunction with methotrexate, 3 mg/kg at 0, 2, and 6 weeks, then every 8 weeks	Yes
Etanercept (Enbrel)	TNF	s.c.	50 mg weekly	Yes
Adalimumab (Humira)	TNF	s.c	40 mg every other week	Yes
Golimumab (Simponi)	TNF	s.c. and i.v.	Subcutaneous: 50 mg once a month. Intravenous: 2 mg/kg infusion over 30 minutes at weeks 0 and 4, and then every 8 weeks	No
Certolizumab (Cimzia)	TNF	s.c.	400 mg initially and at weeks 2 and 4, followed by 200 mg every other week; for maintenance dosing—400 mg every 4 weeks can be considered	No
Tocilizumab (Actemra)	IL-6R	i.v. and s.c.	Intravenous: Recommended starting dose is 4 mg per kg every 4 weeks followed by an increase to 8 mg per kg every 4 weeks based on clinical response. Subcutaneous: 162 mg administered subcutaneously every other week, followed by an increase to every week based on clinical response	No
Sarilumab (Kevzara)	IL-6 R	s.c.	200 mg once every 2 weeks	No
Anakinra (Kineret)	IL-1R	s.c.	100 mg daily	No
Rituximab (MabThera/Rituxan)	CD 20 on B cells	i.v.	The dose for RA in combination with methotrexate is two-1000 mg intravenous infusions separated by 2 weeks (one course) every 24 weeks or based on clinical evaluation, but no sooner than every 16 weeks	Yes

(continued)

Table 2.2 (continued)

Biologic (Bio-originator)	Target	Route of administration	Usual adult dose	Biosimilar available
Abatacept(Orencia)	Selective T cell costimulation modulator	i.v. and s.c.	500–1000 mg intravenous injection (depending on body weight) given initially and at 2 and 4 weeks, then every 4 weeks. Subcutaneous dose is 125 mg once a week	No

TNF Tumor necrosis factor, *IL-6R* Interleukin 6 Receptor, *IL-1R* Interleukin 1 Receptor, *s.c.* subcutaneous, *i.v.* intravenous
Table lists only those biologics that have FDA approval for RA
Doses mentioned are usual adult doses and may need modification in renal disease/liver disease/intercurrent infection. Please refer to the full prescribing information of each drug before use
Subcutaneous rituximab is approved only for hematologic conditions

2.6 How to Initiate Biologics in RA?

- Biologics are initiated only after carrying out screening for infections. The investigations employed include:
  - Hepatitis B surface antigen (HBsAg).
  - Hepatitis B total core antibody (HBcAb).
  - Hepatitis C antibody.
  - HIV screening.
  - Screening for latent tuberculosis (TB).

Screening for latent TB requires Mantoux test, IGRA (interferon-gamma release assays) and chest radiograph (Fig. 2.1)

- Infections including latent TB, if present, should be appropriately treated before commencing biologics.
- It is also recommended that all patients initiating biologic therapy should complete vaccinations for influenza and pneumococcal pneumonia. Herpes zoster vaccination is offered to patients >50 years, depending on availability. Inactivated, adjuvanted, subunit vaccine (Shingrix) is preferred over the earlier live, attenuated vaccine (Zostavax).

These recommendations may vary according to geographic location, national guidelines and resource availability.

2.7 What Do Biologics Achieve in RA?

Biologics help control disease activity in RA in a multitude of ways. They

- Reduce signs and symptoms.
- Improve physical function.

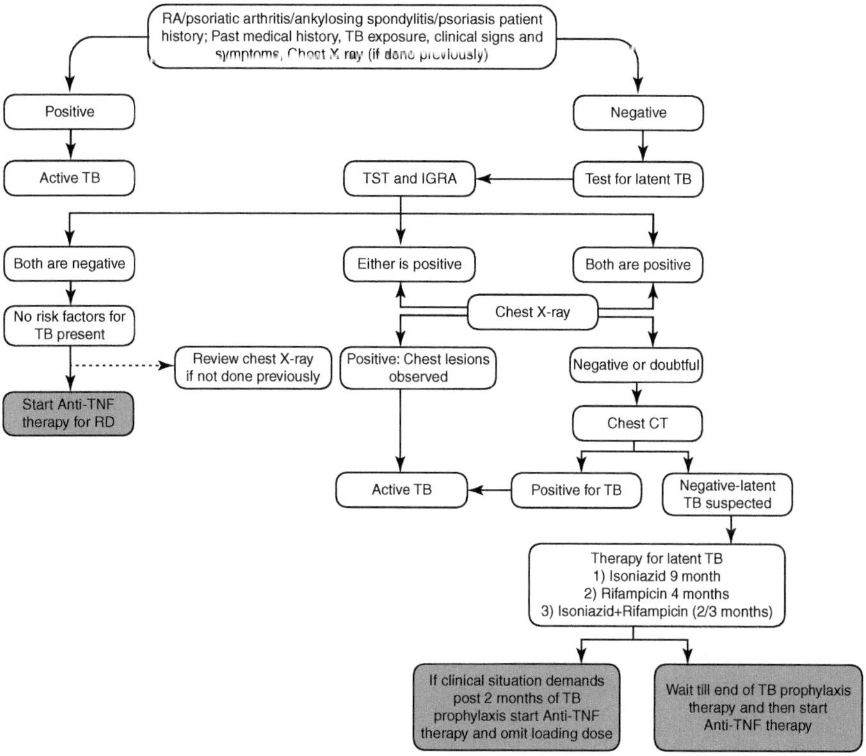

Fig. 2.1 Screening for latent tuberculosis. Reproduced with permission from Handa R, et al. Int J Rheum Dis. 2017; 20:1313–1325

- Enhance the quality of life.
- Inhibit progression of structural damage.

Biologics are superior to methotrexate (MTX) in inhibiting radiographic progression. Trial evidence reveals that the combination of a biologic and MTX inhibits radiographic progression more than either agent alone, reducing both the proportion of patients progressing and the degree of progression of those who do progress.

2.8 Place of Biologics in the Treatment Matrix of RA

- Biologic DMARDs are used primarily after csDMARD failure.
- Methotrexate combination with biologics is preferred over biologic monotherapy. Once sustained remission has been achieved (usually 6 months or even longer), an attempt can be made to de-escalate treatment.
- Should biologics require to be used as monotherapy for reasons of csDMARD intolerance, anti-IL6 agents are preferred (tocilizumab and sarilumab).
- In a typical scenario where a patient is receiving csDMARDs, corticosteroids, and biologics, steroids are the first agents to be withdrawn, followed by biologic DMARDs, and lastly, if remission persists, csDMARD dose can be reduced.

- While several patients can sustain remission with dose reduction of biologic DMARDs, total cessation of bDMARDs is frequently associated with flares (increasing with time since discontinuation). In such a scenario, biologics are re-instituted, and satisfactory control of disease activity can usually be regained.

2.9 Efficacy of Biologics

- Biologics may not work for all patients. In general, the efficacy of biologics in patients failing methotrexate is given by the broad thumb rule of ACR-20/-50/-70 of 60/40/20 percent. That is, ACR 20 response is seen in 60% of such patients, ACR 50 response in 40% patients while ACR 70 response is seen in 20% patients. In patients failing anti-TNFs, the ACR-20/-50/-70 drop further to 50/25/12 percent, respectively.
- Apart from primary non-response, some patients may exhibit partial response or even exhibit worsening disease control with time (secondary non-response). Such situations necessitate a change of drug or increase in dose or frequency of administration.

2.10 What Is Switching of Biologics?

This is required in patients failing a biologic or for reasons of intolerance/adverse effects. If a bDMARD has failed, treatment with another bDMARD or a tsDMARD should be considered. In patients failing one TNFi therapy, biologics with another mechanism of action or another TNFi may be considered.

2.11 Which Biologic for Whom?

- All biologics have roughly the same efficacy and no one agent can be recommended over others for this reason.
- In the absence of biomarkers that predict response, the choice of a biologic is more or less empiric. Patient preference, physician familiarity, drug availability, cost sensibility, and insurer requirements play a role.
- For patients preferring to avoid daycare visits/hospitalization, self-administered subcutaneous injections via pen devices/auto-injectors are preferred. Some drugs like golimumab offer ease of once a month administration, unlike weekly etanercept or fortnightly adalimumab, sarilumab or certolizumab. Rituximab needs to be administered intravenously once in 6 months. For patients with the past history of tuberculosis/latent TB, non-TNF agents like rituximab, tocilizumab, abatacept may be preferred over TNF inhibitors with respect to TB risk.
- Biosimilars may provide a cost advantage.

2.12 Immunogenicity with Biologics

- Repetitive administration of protein-based therapeutics like biologics can induce anti-drug antibodies. Immunogenicity is influenced by drug, disease, and patient characteristics. It may practically translate into decreased serum drug levels, attrition of therapeutic response, adverse events, and treatment discontinuation.
- Concomitant administration of methotrexate or azathioprine may reduce the immunogenicity of biologic DMARDs. Even lower MTX doses like 10 mg/week may suffice when used for this purpose, and higher doses may not be necessary as outlined in the EULAR recommendations.
- As of today, algorithms that integrate therapeutic drug monitoring with immunogenicity and clinical response are not part of routine clinical practice.

2.13 Biologics and Safety Issues

Injection site or infusion reactions, opportunistic infections, and reactivation of TB can be seen with almost all biologics. Drug-induced lupus, psoriasis, demyelinating syndromes may rarely be encountered with TNFi. Rituximab can rarely be associated with hypogammaglobulinemia or progressive multifocal leukoencephalopathy. GI perforation, hypercholesterolemia, and neutropenia have been reported with tocilizumab. Readers are advised to check the full prescribing information provided by various manufacturers for a detailed understanding of adverse effects associated with these agents.

2.14 Biologics in Pregnancy and Breastfeeding

- TNF inhibitors like certolizumab, infliximab, etanercept, adalimumab, golimumab can be continued throughout pregnancy if required. Certolizumab has reduced placental transfer compared with other TNFi. To ensure low/no levels of TNFα inhibitors (TNFi) in cord blood at delivery and if the disease activity permits, etanercept and adalimumab should be avoided in the third trimester and infliximab stopped at 16 weeks because of a theoretical increased infection risk in new-borns. If these drugs are continued later in pregnancy to treat active disease, the live vaccines should be avoided in the infant until 6 months of age.
- Rituximab, anakinra, abatacept, and tocilizumab should be stopped when pregnancy is confirmed.
- Biologics compatible with breastfeeding include the TNFi infliximab, etanercept, adalimumab, golimumab, and certolizumab. The ACR conditionally recommends the use of rituximab, abatacept, tocilizumab during lactation, if required.
- Males wishing to father a child can continue biologics.

2.15 Biologics Versus Targeted Synthetic DMARDs

Biologics are complex protein molecules that need parenteral administration. These entail a complicated manufacturing process that adds to the high cost of these drugs. In contrast, tsDMARDs have a much lower molecular weight, are easier to manufacture and are given orally. These target intracellular signaling pathways. The efficacy is nearly similar.

2.16 Bio-Originators and Biosimilars

- The spiraling costs of bDMARDs in developed countries, limited access in resource-constrained countries and expiry of patent periods have stimulated interest in Biosimilars. A biosimilar is a bio-therapeutic product similar in terms of quality, safety, and efficacy to an already licensed reference bio-therapeutic product.
- Unlike bio-originator DMARDs that require demonstration of clinical efficacy and safety for each indication, extrapolation to other indications is permitted in the case of biosimilars.
- Recommendations regarding switching from bio-originator DMARDs to biosimilars or vice versa and substitution/interchangeability are continuously evolving.

2.17 Future Prospects

Intense efforts are underway to identify which biologic would work best in what patient. This precision medicine is likely to incorporate a multiomic approach using information from the genome, epigenome, transcriptome, proteome, metabolome, and microbiome of the RA patient. Stratification and better delineation of the clinical, immunological, and molecular phenotype of RA hold the key to the inevitable shift from 'protocol driven' treatments of *today* to 'individualized protocols' of *tomorrow*!

Further Reading

1. Lau CS, Chia F, Dans L, Harrison A, Hsieh TY, Jain R, Jung SM, Kishimoto M, Kumar A, Leong KP, Li Z, Lichauco JJ, Louthrenoo W, Luo SF, Mu R, Nash P, Ng CT, Suryana B, Wijaya LK, Yeap SS. 2018 update of the APLAR recommendations for treatment of rheumatoid arthritis. Int J Rheum Dis. 2019;22:357–75.
2. Smolen JS, Landewé RBM, Bijlsma JWJ, Burmester GR, Dougados M, Kerschbaumer A, McInnes IB, Sepriano A, van Vollenhoven RF, de Wit M, Aletaha D, Aringer M, Askling J, Balsa A, Boers M, den Broeder AA, Buch MH, Buttgereit F, Caporali R, Cardiel MH, De Cock D, Codreanu C, Cutolo M, Edwards CJ, van Eijk-Hustings Y, Emery P, Finckh A, Gossec L, Gottenberg JE, Hetland ML, Huizinga TWJ, Koloumas M, Li Z, Mariette X, Müller-Ladner

U, Mysler EF, da Silva JAP, Poór G, Pope JE, Rubbert-Roth A, Ruyssen-Witrand A, Saag KG, Strangfeld A, Takeuchi T, Voshaar M, Westhovens R, van der Heijde D. EULAR recommendations for the management of rheumatoid arthritis with synthetic and biological disease-modifying antirheumatic drugs: 2019 update. Ann Rheum Dis. 2020;79:685–99.

3. Singh JA, Saag KG, Bridges SL Jr, Akl EA, Bannuru RR, Sullivan MC, Vaysbrot E, McNaughton C, Osani M, Shmerling RH, Curtis JR, Furst DE, Parks D, Kavanaugh A, O'Dell J, King C, Leong A, Matteson EL, Schousboe JT, Drevlow B, Ginsberg S, Grober J, St Clair EW, Tindall E, Miller AS, McAlindon T, American College of Rheumatology. 2015 American College of Rheumatology guideline for the treatment of rheumatoid arthritis. Arthritis Care Res. 2016;68:1–25.
4. Handa R, Upadhyaya S, Kapoor S, Jois R, Pandey BD, Bhatnagar AK, Khanna A, Goyal V, Kumar K. Tuberculosis and biologics in rheumatology: a special situation. Int J Rheum Dis. 2017;20:1313–25.
5. Furer V, Rondaan C, Heijstek MW, Agmon-Levin N, van Assen S, Bijl M, Breedveld FC, D'Amelio R, Dougados M, Kapetanovic MC, van Laar JM, de Thurah A, Landewé RB, Molto A, Müller-Ladner U, Schreiber K, Smolar L, Walker J, Warnatz K, Wulffraat NM, Elkayam O. 2019 update of EULAR recommendations for vaccination in adult patients with autoimmune inflammatory rheumatic diseases. Ann Rheum Dis. 2020;79:39–52.
6. Micu MC, Ostensen M, Villiger PM, Micu R, Ionescu R. Safety of anti-rheumatic drugs in men trying to conceive: a systematic review and analysis of published evidence. Semin Arthritis Rheum. 2018;48:343–55.
7. Sammaritano LR, Bermas BL, Chakravarty EE, Chambers C, Clowse MEB, Lockshin MD, Marder W, Guyatt G, Branch DW, Buyon J, Christopher-Stine L, Crow-Hercher R, Cush J, Druzin M, Kavanaugh A, Laskin CA, Plante L, Salmon J, Simard J, Somers EC, Steen V, Tedeschi SK, Vinet E, White CW, Yazdany J, Barbhaiya M, Bettendorf B, Eudy A, Jayatilleke A, Shah AA, Sullivan N, Tarter LL, Birru Talabi M, Turgunbaev M, Turner A, D'Anci KE. 2020 American College of Rheumatology guideline for the management of reproductive health in rheumatic and musculoskeletal diseases. Arthritis Rheumatol. 2020;72:529–56.
8. Flint J, Panchal S, Hurrell A, van de Venne M, Gayed M, Schreiber K, Arthanari S, Cunningham J, Flanders L, Moore L, Crossley A, Purushotham N, Desai A, Piper M, Nisar M, Khamashta M, Williams D, Gordon C, Giles I, BSR and BHPR Standards, Guidelines and Audit Working Group. BSR and BHPR guideline on prescribing drugs in pregnancy and breastfeeding-part I: standard and biologic disease modifying anti-rheumatic drugs and corticosteroids. Rheumatology (Oxford). 2016;55:1693–7.

Biologics in Spondyloarthritis

3

Bimlesh Dhar Pandey

3.1 Introduction

Biological disease-modifying antirheumatic drugs (bDMARDs) have changed the physicians' therapeutic approach to Spondyloarthritis (SpA) since their advent. They are the single most effective treatment option by a distance for axial SpA (axSpA), where the science of rheumatology had found itself limited until a couple of decades back. Apart from their numero uno position in the management of Ankylosing Spondylitis (AS), they are also very effective for treating peripheral SpA (pSpA), as well as non-radiographic axSpA (nr-axSpA). The following text shall provide an overview of the various bDMARDs and their applications in SpA.

3.2 Overarching Principles for Use of Biologicals in Spondyloarthritis

- A chronic triggering of inflammation in genetically predisposed individuals takes place in SpA. Studies have shown that control of inflammation at the very earliest provides the best chance to prevent the ensuing bone formation and the resultant ankylosis. It gives the patients the best chance to maintain function and prevent deformity [1].
- Research over the years had already implicated the dysregulation of cytokine production as the key process driving the inflammation in SpA. With further studies, the cytokines began to be identified. Then came the evidence of involvement of the Interleukin (IL)-23/IL-17 axis. With the above knowledge at hand, tumor necrosis factor-alpha inhibitors (TNFi) and IL-17inhibitors (IL-17i) and

B. D. Pandey (✉)
Fortis Hospital, Noida, Uttar Pradesh, India

N. Jain, L. Duggal (eds.), *Handbook of Biologics for Rheumatological Disorders*,
https://doi.org/10.1007/978-981-16-7200-2_3

IL-12/23i were developed and were found to be effective in blocking the cascade of inflammation in SpA.
- The guidelines for prescribing bDMARDs in SpA in different countries have minor variations, but they are generally recommended in moderate to severe disease not responding to the conventional drugs.
- In axSpA, bDMARDs are recommended where a trial of nonsteroidal anti-inflammatory drugs (NSAIDs) fails to produce a response or these agents are not tolerated. In psoriatic and non-psoriatic peripheral SpA, bDMARDs are recommended where conventional DMARDs have failed or are not tolerated.
- Apart from high axial or peripheral skeletal disease activity, another indication for the institution of bDMARD therapy is severe eye, skin, or intestinal inflammation, which might be organ threatening.
- Although the primary consideration is to provide the best care possible, the cost is of concern when using biologicals. It is for this reason, that EULAR recommends that the choice of bDMARD may be driven by cost where similar outcomes can be expected with the agents under consideration [2].
- Studies have shown that both NSAIDs and TNFi are more effective in patients with shorter disease duration, thus it would be prudent to conclude that early treatment with bDMARDs is likely to result in better outcomes.

3.3 Biological Agents Approved for Spondyloarthritis

The US Food and Drug Administration (USFDA) approved TNFi for the treatment of AS include infliximab (IFX), etanercept (ETN), adalimumab (ADA), certolizumab pegol (CZP), golimumab (GOL), Secukinumab (SEC), and Ixekizumab are IL-17i approved by the agency for AS [3].

3.3.1 Infliximab in Spondyloarthritis

- IFX is a chimeric mouse–human monoclonal antibody. It binds soluble as well as transmembrane TNF alpha.
- Ankylosing Spondylitis Study for the Evaluation of Recombinant Infliximab Therapy (ASSERT) was the landmark trial that established the efficacy of IFX in AS. The drug was found to be effective as early as within 2 weeks of initiation and continued to be effective during the 24 weeks of the study [4].
- The drug has a half-life of 9 days and is recommended to be given at a dose of 5 mg per kg at 0, 2, and 6 weeks, and then every 6 weeks thereafter.

3.3.2 Etanercept in Spondyloarthritis

- ETN is a fusion protein that binds to soluble TNF and lymphotoxin alpha. Studies have shown that the molecule has very low immunogenicity.

- A randomized controlled trial in 2003 found ETN highly effective in AS with improvements in the patient-reported measures, acute phase reactants as well as function. The safety was comparable to the drug's trials in rheumatoid arthritis (RA) and psoriatic arthritis (PsA) [5].
- The drug has a half-life of 4 days and is recommended to be given at a dose of 25 mg twice a week. Studies have also shown 50 mg once a week to be effective as well.

3.3.3 Adalimumab in Spondyloarthritis

- ADA is a human monoclonal antibody that binds soluble as well as transmembrane TNF alpha.
- The ABILITY-1 trial showed that ADA was effective in the treatment of nr-axSpA. The ABILITY-2 trial showed the molecule's efficacy in non-psoriatic peripheral SpA [6, 7].
- ADA has a half-life of 14 days and is recommended to be given at a dose of 40 mg every other week.

3.3.4 Certolizumab Pegol in Spondyloarthritis

- CZP is a Fab fragment of a humanized anti-TNF antibody fused to polyethylene glycol, that binds TNF alpha.
- The RAPID-axSpA and RAPID-PsA studies found CZP efficacious in axSpA and PsA. The patients showed improvement in the extraarticular domains of PsA as well, including skin disease, nail disease, enthesitis, and dactylitis [8, 9].
- The drug has a half-life of 14 days and is recommended to be given at a dose of 400 mg at 1, 2, and 4 weeks, and thereafter at 200 mg fortnightly or 400 mg every 4 weeks.

3.3.5 Golimumab in Spondyloarthritis

- GOL is a human monoclonal antibody that binds soluble as well as transmembrane TNF alpha.
- The results of the GO-RAISE study published in 2008 showed the efficacy and safety of GOL in the treatment of AS in 2008 [10].
- GOL has a half-life of 14 days and is recommended to be given at a dose of 50 or 100 mg every month.

3.3.6 Secukinumab and Ixekizumabin Spondyloarthritis

- SEC is a human monoclonal antibody against interleukin-17A.
- The MEASURE1 and MEASURE2 trials showed the efficacy of SEC in patients with active AS. The studies showed the efficacy of a 150-mg dose with a loading dose in the first 4 weeks [11].
- SEC has a half-life of 27 days and is recommended to be given at a dose of 150 mg at 0, 1, 2, 3, and 4 weeks and then every 4 weeks for SpA.
- Ixekizumab is another IL-17i approved for use in AS. It has a half-life of 13 days and it is used at a dose of 160 mg at dose 0 and then 80 mg every 4 weeks.

3.3.7 Ustekinumab in Spondyloarthritis

- Ustekinumab is a human IL-12 and IL-23 antagonist approved for use in psoriasis, psoriatic arthritis, and Crohn's disease.
- It has a half-life of 20–39 days and is recommended to be given at a dose of 45 mg at 0 and 4 weeks and then every 12 weeks for PsA.

3.4 Biologics in Various Spondyloarthritides

While there is a unifying concept to the SpA family, the differences that exist in various diseases and manifestations of the family translate into a need for customizing the bDMARD therapy. A summary of where different biological agents are effective is given in Table 3.1.

3.4.1 Axial Spondyloarthritis

- AxSpA includes radiographic (r-axSpA) and non-radiographic (nr-axSpA) diseases. The initial approvals for use of bDMARDs in axSpA came only for r-axSpA. The efficacy was also found higher in this subgroup. It was, however, later recognized to be due to a higher degree of certainty of diagnosis in r-axSpA compared to nr-axSpA.
- Biological DMARDs are the cornerstone of therapy for active, moderate to severe axSpA. Younger age, shorter duration of disease, elevated acute phase reactants, HLA-B27 positivity, and inflammation on MRI are predictors of good response to bDMARDs [12].
- Studies have failed to show any significant differences between various biological agents used for the treatment of axSpA. The choice of agent is hence driven by extraarticular manifestations (EAMs), comorbidities, cost, and local availability.
- The newer studies have shown that TNFi and IL-17i reduce radiographic progression. But since the structural damage in axSpA is heterogeneous and is appreciable only over a longer term, it is not a useful tool to guide optimization of bDMARD therapy or switching from one agent to another.

Table 3.1 Biological agents in spondyloarthritis

Drug	Dose	Effective in			
		AxSpA	PsA	IBD	Uveitis
Non-monoclonal antibody tumor necrosis factor alpha inhibitors					
Etanercept	25 mg twice a week	✓	✓		
Monoclonal antibody tumor necrosis factor alpha inhibitors					
Infliximab	5 mg per kg at 0, 2, and 6 weeks, and then every 6 weeks thereafter	✓	✓	✓	✓
Adalimumab	40 mg every 2 weeks	✓	✓	✓	✓
Golimumab	50 or 100 mg every month	✓	✓	✓	✓
Interleukin 17A inhibitor					
Secukinumab	150 mg at 0, 1, 2, 3, 4 weeks, and then every 4 weeks 300 mg dose is used for psoriasis	✓	✓		
Interleukin 12/23 inhibitor					
Ustekinumab	45 mg at 0 and 4 weeks and then every 12 weeks for PsA A 90 mg dose is used above 100 kg weight A weight-based initial intravenous dose followed by 90 mg subcutaneous every 8 weeks starting 8 weeks after the initial infusion is used for Crohn's disease		✓	✓	

axSpA axial spondyloarthritis, *PsA* psoriatic arthritis, *IBD* inflammatory bowel disease

- The recommendations are to start patients with axSpA on NSAIDs and evaluate after 2–4 weeks. Then bDMARD therapy is initiated in those patients who do not respond or are intolerant to NSAIDs. TNFi are the first choice bDMARDs in axSpA and the current recommendations prefer IL17i over targeted synthetic DMARDs (tsDMARDs) as next line agents [2, 13].

3.4.2 Non-psoriatic Peripheral Spondyloarthritis

- In non-psoriatic peripheral SpA (pSpA), conventional DMARDs like methotrexate, sulfasalazine, and leflunomide are used where NSAIDs or local glucocorticoid injections do not work. In patients who fail to respond or are intolerant to these agents, bDMARDs are initiated [14].
- The CRESPA trial with golimumab showed the efficacy of this TNFi in pSpA and demonstrated that a drug-free remission was achievable in nearly 50 percent of these patients.
- The ABILITY-2 trial and the study by Paramarta et al. established the efficacy of Adalimumab in pSpA. These studies were the first to demonstrate the concept of early treatment in pSpA [7, 15].

3.4.3 Psoriatic Arthritis

- The choice of therapy in PsA is guided by the extents of axial involvement, peripheral joint involvement, skin disease, and other EAMs like enthesitis and dactylitis.
- In predominantly axial disease not responding to NSAIDs, bDMARDs are started with the usual practice being to start with a TNFi [16].
- NSAIDs or glucocorticoids are first used in mono or oligoarthritis and enthesitis, and then bDMARDs are instituted in non-responders.
- In PsA patients with predominant polyarthritis, the usual practice is to start with conventional DMARDs and then move to bDMARDs if needed.
- However, recent recommendations do provide the option to use upfront bDMARDs in those with severe arthritis and/or severe skin disease [17].
- Rapid progression, erosions, elevated APRs, and active PsA at multiple sites are considered hallmarks of severe arthritis.
- A PASI score of over 12, involvement of more than 5–10% body surface area (BSA) or physical or mental impairment (even in absence of high PASI or more than 5–10% BSA involvement) are considered to indicate severe psoriasis.
- TNFi, IL-17i, and IL-12/23i have all been found to be effective in PsA. IL-12/23i agents are not used in axial disease.
- TNFi are effective in skin and nail diseases but they paradoxically increase the lesions in some patients. IL-17i and Il12/23i are the preferred agents in patients with severe psoriasis.
- When a patient with PsA does not respond to one bDMARD, it is recommended to switch to another agent of the same class or an agent of another class.

3.5 Extraarticular Manifestations and Choice of Biologicals in SpA

- Even in absence of high skeletal disease activity in a patient with SpA, early bDMARD therapy may be warranted because of active inflammatory bowel disease (IBD). Among the TNFi, monoclonal antibody TNFi, e.g., adalimumab and infliximab are preferred over agents like etanercept in patients with IBD [18]. IL-17i are not preferred in patients with IBD. IL-12/23i on the other hand are preferred agents, particularly for Crohn's disease [18].
- In patients with recurrent uveitis, monoclonal antibody TNFi are preferred over other TNFi and non-TNFibDMARDs.
- All the available bDMARDs can be used in patients with enthesitis and dactylitis refractory to NSAIDs and/or local glucocorticoid injections. Tofacitinib and Apremilast are other options in enthesitis refractory to the first-line therapy [16].
- TNFi are effective in AA amyloidosis and also reduce the risk of cardiovascular manifestations and atherosclerotic cardiovascular disease associated with SpA. However, they are best avoided in patients with pre-existing heart failure [19, 20].

3.6 Summary

- Biological disease-modifying anti-rheumatic drugs are effective options for the management of spondyloarthritis.
- Choosing the best-suited agent based on the disease manifestations and other coexisting or comorbid conditions results in better outcomes.
- Early initiation of biological agents in spondyloarthritis has the potential to minimize damage and halt structural progression.

References

1. Furst DE, Louie JS. Targeting inflammatory pathways in axial spondyloarthritis. Arthritis Res Ther. 2019;21:135.
2. van der Heijde D, Ramiro S, Landewé R, Baraliakos X, Van den Bosch F, Sepriano A, et al. 2016 update of the ASAS-EULAR management recommendations for axial spondyloarthritis. Ann Rheum Dis. 2017;76:978–91.
3. Spondyloarthritis. https://www.rheumatology.org/I-Am-A/Patient-Caregiver/Diseases-Conditions/Spondyloarthritis. Accessed 14 Jun 2021.
4. van der Heijde D, Dijkmans B, Geusens P, Sieper J, DeWoody K, Williamson P, et al. Efficacy and safety of infliximab in patients with ankylosing spondylitis: results of a randomized, placebo-controlled trial (ASSERT). Arthritis Rheum. 2005;52:582–91.
5. Davis JC, Heijde DVD, Braun J, Dougados M, Cush J, Clegg DO, et al. Recombinant human tumor necrosis factor receptor (etanercept) for treating ankylosing spondylitis: a randomized, controlled trial. Arthritis Rheum. 2003;48:3230–6.
6. Sieper J, van der Heijde D, Dougados M, Mease PJ, Maksymowych WP, Brown MA, et al. Efficacy and safety of adalimumab in patients with non-radiographic axial spondyloarthritis: results of a randomised placebo-controlled trial (ABILITY-1). Ann Rheum Dis. 2013;72:815–22.
7. Mease P, Sieper J, Van den Bosch F, Rahman P, Karunaratne PM, Pangan AL. Randomized controlled trial of adalimumab in patients with nonpsoriatic peripheral spondyloarthritis. Arthritis Rheumatol. 2015;67:914–23.
8. Landewé R, Braun J, Deodhar A, Dougados M, Maksymowych WP, Mease PJ, et al. Efficacy of certolizumab pegol on signs and symptoms of axial spondyloarthritis including ankylosing spondylitis: 24-week results of a double-blind randomised placebo-controlled phase 3 study. Ann Rheum Dis. 2014;73:39–47.
9. Mease PJ, Fleischmann R, Deodhar AA, Wollenhaupt J, Khraishi M, Kielar D, et al. Effect of certolizumab pegol on signs and symptoms in patients with psoriatic arthritis: 24-week results of a phase 3 double-blind randomised placebo-controlled study (RAPID-PsA). Ann Rheum Dis. 2014;73:48–55.
10. Inman RD, Davis JC, Heijde DVD, Diekman L, Sieper J, Kim SI, et al. Efficacy and safety of golimumab in patients with ankylosing spondylitis: results of a randomized, double-blind, placebo-controlled, phase III trial. Arthritis Rheum. 2008;58:3402–12.
11. Baeten D, Sieper J, Braun J, Baraliakos X, Dougados M, Emery P, et al. Secukinumab, an interleukin-17A inhibitor, in ankylosing spondylitis. N Engl J Med. 2015;373(26):2534–48. https://doi.org/10.1056/NEJMoa1505066.
12. Fragoulis GE, Siebert S. Treatment strategies in axial spondyloarthritis: what, when and how? Rheumatology. 2020;59:iv79–89.
13. Ward MM, Deodhar A, Gensler LS, Dubreuil M, Yu D, Khan MA, et al. 2019 update of the American College of Rheumatology/Spondylitis Association of America/Spondyloarthritis

Research and Treatment Network recommendations for the treatment of ankylosing spondylitis and non-radiographic axial spondyloarthritis. Arthritis Care Res. 2019;71:1285–99.
14. Carron P, Varkas G, Cypers H, Van Praet L, Elewaut D, Van den Bosch F, et al. Anti-TNF-induced remission in very early peripheral spondyloarthritis: the CRESPA study. Ann Rheum Dis. 2017;76:1389–95.
15. Paramarta JE, De Rycke L, Heijda TF, Ambarus CA, Vos K, Dinant HJ, et al. Efficacy and safety of adalimumab for the treatment of peripheral arthritis in spondyloarthritis patients without ankylosing spondylitis or psoriatic arthritis. Ann Rheum Dis. 2013;72:1793–9.
16. Gossec L, Baraliakos X, Kerschbaumer A, de Wit M, McInnes I, Dougados M, et al. EULAR recommendations for the management of psoriatic arthritis with pharmacological therapies: 2019 update. Ann Rheum Dis. 2020;79:700–12.
17. Singh JA, Guyatt G, Ogdie A, Gladman DD, Deal C, Deodhar A, et al. 2018 American College of Rheumatology/National Psoriasis Foundation guideline for the treatment of psoriatic arthritis. Arthritis Care Res. 2019;71:2–29.
18. Bruner V, Atteno M, Spanò A, Scarpa R, Peluso R. Biological therapies for spondyloarthritis. Ther Adv Musculoskelet Dis. 2014;6:92–101.
19. Kobak S, Oksel F, Kabasakal Y, Doganavsargil E. Ankylosing spondylitis-related secondary amyloidosis responded well to etanercept: a report of three patients. Clin Rheumatol. 2007;26:2191–4.
20. Di Minno MND, Iervolino S, Peluso R, Scarpa R, Di Minno G. CaRRDs study group. Carotid intima-media thickness in psoriatic arthritis: differences between tumor necrosis factor-α blockers and traditional disease-modifying antirheumatic drugs. Arterioscler Thromb Vasc Biol. 2011;31:705–12.

Biologics in Psoriatic Arthritis

4

Rahul Sahu, Arvind Ganapati, and Ashish Jacob Mathew

4.1 Introduction

Psoriatic arthritis (PsA) is a complex, immune-mediated disease with varied clinical features, including peripheral arthritis, axial disease, enthesitis, dactylitis, skin and nail disease [1, 2]. Treatment of PsA has witnessed a sea change over the past two decades. Extra-articular manifestations including uveitis and inflammatory bowel disease (IBD), and comorbidities like obesity, metabolic disease and depression play critical roles in treatment selection. Therapies in PsA warrant tailoring to target the affected domains based on shared decision-making between the treating physicians and patients [3]. There has been a swift and continuing expansion of biologic (b) disease-modifying anti-rheumatic drugs (DMARDs) in the treatment armamentarium of patients with PsA. Significant responses in all the relevant clinical domains, coupled with the ability to inhibit progressive structural damage in the joints, have yielded bDMARDs a clear edge over the conventional (c) DMARDs in most patients with PsA.

R. Sahu
Department of Internal Medicine, People's College of Medical Sciences and Research, Bhopal, India

A. Ganapati
Department of Clinical Immunology and Rheumatology, Christian Medical College, Vellore, India

A. J. Mathew (✉)
Department of Clinical Immunology and Rheumatology, Christian Medical College, Vellore, India

Copenhagen Center for Arthritis Research, Center for Rheumatology and Spine Diseases, Copenhagen University Hospital, Rigshospitalet Glostrup, Copenhagen, Denmark
e-mail: mathewaj@cmcvellore.ac.in

N. Jain, L. Duggal (eds.), *Handbook of Biologics for Rheumatological Disorders*,
https://doi.org/10.1007/978-981-16-7200-2_4

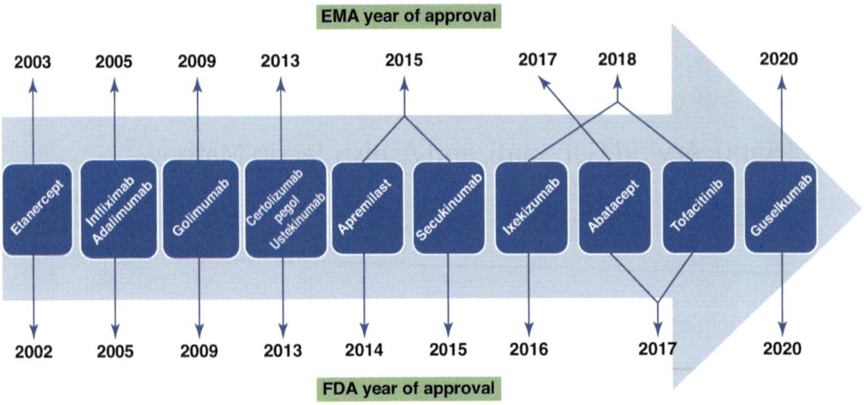

Fig. 4.1 Timeline of United States Food and Drug Administration (USFDA) and the European Medicines Agency (EMA) approval of bDMARDs and tsDMARDs in psoriatic arthritis

The bDMARDs approved by the United States Food and Drug Administration (USFDA) and the European Medicines Agency (EMA) for the treatment of PsA fall in the following groups—tumor necrosis factor inhibitors (TNFi), interleukin (IL)-17 inhibitors, IL-12/23 inhibitors, p19 subunit of IL-23 inhibitors, and T cell co-stimulatory blockade agent [4, 5]. Targeted synthetic (ts) DMARDs, including phosphodiesterase 4 (PDE-4) inhibitor (apremilast) and Janus kinase (JAK) inhibitor (tofacitinib) have also been approved for the treatment of PsA, and novel JAK and tyrosine kinase (TYK) inhibitors are on the anvil [6]. The bDMARDs and tsDMARDs being used in the treatment of PsA are discussed in this chapter (Fig. 4.1).

4.2 Tumor Necrosis Factor Inhibitors (TNFi)

Tumor necrosis factor (TNF) is an inflammatory cytokine with pleiotropic effects, known to play a central role in the immunopathogenesis of psoriatic disease, sustaining inflammation in both Th1 and Th17 pathways and causing articular damage [7]. TNFi are large protein monoclonal antibodies (mAB) directed against TNF.

4.2.1 Approved TNFi in the Treatment of PsA

- Etanercept (ETN), infliximab (IFX), adalimumab (ADA), certolizumab pegol (CZP), and golimumab (GOL) are the TNFi approved by the US FDA and EMA for use in PsA (Table 4.1) [8].
- For axial PsA both the group for research and assessment of psoriasis and psoriatic arthritis (GRAPPA) and the European alliance of associations for rheumatology (EULAR) recommend initiation of therapy with TNFi as the preferred choice (except in conditions with significant psoriasis) after the failure of non-

Table 4.1 Targeted csDMARDs approved for the treatment of psoriatic arthritis

Molecules	Pharmacological structure	Route	Dosage	Adverse effects
Etanercept	Genetically engineered soluble TNF receptor p75-IgG1 fusion protein	SC	50 mg/week	Infusion or injection site reactions, infections including opportunistic infections like tuberculosis, malignancies (skin cancer, lymphoma), demyelinating conditions, congestive heart failure, hepatitis, drug-induced lupus, paradoxical psoriasis, generation of anti-nuclear antibodies, anti-double stranded DNA (DsDNA), and antidrug antibodies (ADA)
Infliximab	Full-length, bivalent, chimeric monoclonal antibody (mAb) against TNF-α	IV	5 mg/kg at weeks 0, 2, and 6 and every 6–8 weeks	
Adalimumab	Full-length, bivalent, fully human anti-TNF-α mAb	SC	40 mg every 2 weeks	
Certolizumab pegol	Humanized, monovalent Fab1 fragment of antiTNF-α mAb	SC	400 mg at 0, 2, and 4 weeks and then 200 mg every 2 weeks	
Golimumab	Full-length, bivalent, fully human IgG1k anti-TNF-α mAb	SC	50 mg/month	
		IV	2 mg/kg at 0, 4, and every 8 weeks (approved in pediatric PsA > 2 years of age)	
Secukinumab	Fully human IgG1 anti IL-17A mAb	SC	For plaque psoriasis (PsO) - 300 mg loading dose at weeks 0,1,2,3 and 4 followed by 300 mg every 4 weeks. For some patients 150 mg may be acceptable instead of 300 mg For patients with PsA with coexistent moderate to severe plaque psoriasis, same dose as above. For other patients of PsA, with a loading dose - 150 mg at weeks 0,1,2,3 and 4, followed by every 4 weeks thereafter. Without a loading dose - 150 mg every 4 weeks If the patient continues to have active disease, to consider switching the dose to 300 mg	Injection site reactions, Nasopharyngitis, upper respiratory tract infections, sinusitis, skin, and mucocutaneous candidiasis
Ixekizumab	Humanized anti-IL-17A mAb	SC	*For PsO*-160 mg once, followed by 80 mg at weeks 2, 4, 6, 8, 10, and 12, and then 80 mg every 4 weeks *For PsA*-160 mg once, followed by 80 mg every 4 weeks	

(continued)

Table 4.1 (continued)

Molecules	Pharmacological structure	Route	Dosage	Adverse effects
Ustekinumab	Monoclonal IgG1 antibody against p40 subunit of IL-12/IL-23	SC	45 mg at weeks 0, 4, and then every 12 weeks 90 mg if >100 kg	Nasopharyngitis, upper respiratory tract infection, headache, fatigue
Guselkumab	Fully human monoclonal antibody against p19 subunit of IL-23	SC	100 mg at weeks 0, 4, and then every 8 weeks	Upper respiratory tract infections, headache, injection site reactions, bronchitis, diarrhea, tinea, and herpes simplex infections
Abatacept	Fusion protein of fc r IgG1 + extracellular domain of CTLA-4	IV/SC	IV dosing <60 kg—500 mg 60–100 kg—750 mg >100 kg—1000 mg 0, 2, and 4 weeks after the first infusion and every 4 weeks SC—125 mg once a week	Headache, upper respiratory tract infection, nasopharyngitis, and nausea
Tofacitinib	Selective inhibitor of JAK 1 and JAK 3	Oral	5 mg twice daily	
Apremilast	Phosphodiesterase-4 inhibitor	Oral	30 mg twice daily	

csDMARD conventional synthetic disease-modifying anti-rheumatic drugs, *SC* subcutaneous, *IV* intravenous steroidal anti-inflammatory drugs. TNFi has also been endorsed along with other bDMARDs for peripheral arthritis and enthesitis [3, 9].

4.2.2 Effectiveness of TNFi on PsA Domains

- Data from clinical trials have shown the efficacy of TNFi in all the domains of psoriatic disease [10–19]. An ACR-50 response of around 50% is reported for peripheral joint symptoms in most clinical trials.
- An observational study evaluating the effectiveness of ETN on axial PsA demonstrated significant improvement in the Bath ankylosing spondylitis disease activity index (BASDAI), Bath ankylosing spondylitis function index (BASFI) and Bath ankylosing spondylitis metrology index (BASMI) at week 52 compared to placebo [20]. Pooled real-life registries have noted ACR20/50/70 responses with TNFi to be 53%/38%/22%, respectively, at 6 months [21].
- A meta-analysis on the evidence available from randomized controlled trials (RCTs) on enthesitis and dactylitis noted an enthesitis resolution pooled relative risk (RR) of 1.75 (95% CI: 0.96–3.21) and dactylitis resolution pooled RR of 1.53 (95% CI: 1.01–2.31), with TNFi at week 12–14 [22].
- Yet another meta-analysis of RCTs of PsA to examine the effect of TNFi on radiographic progression of disease demonstrated 84.5% of the 584 PsA patients not developing radiographic progression at treatment week 24 compared to 68.6% of the 526 patients who received placebo (OR 2.68; 95% CI 1.99–3.6), without significant heterogeneity [23]. Patients with PsA on TNFi have significant lower risk of adverse cardiovascular events (Relative risk 0.67; 95% CI 0.52–0.88; $p = 0.03$) compared to MTX [24].

4.2.3 Persistence of Treatment with TNFi in PsA Patients

- Switching between TNFis is well recognized in the event of inefficiency or toxicity. However, in the NOR-DMARD registry data from Norway, 95 of the 439 patients identified as switchers demonstrated a significantly poorer ACR 50 response of 22.5% as compared to 40% in non-switchers [25].
- Data from the British Society for Rheumatology Biologics Register (BSRBR) demonstrates persistence estimates of 53%, 60%, and 48% for the first, second and third TNFi at 5 years, respectively, in PsA patients. Better 5-year persistence was noted with ADA or ETN compared to IFX [26]. Nevertheless, real-world evidence demonstrates a consistent drop in the proportion of patients continuing with TNFi after switching following the failure of the first drug [27, 28].
- In a large registry data from 12 European countries (EuroSpA) on 14,261 patients, the median 12-month retention rate of TNFi was 77% [21]. Methotrexate (MTX) discontinuation occurs sooner in patients with PsA. However, concomitant use of MTX is associated with lower rates of TNFi discontinuation in PsA [29]. Presence of comorbidities is associated with shorter TNFi persistence [30].

4.2.4 Adverse Events with TNFi in Patients with PsA

- TNFis have a higher risk of serious infections requiring hospitalization following administration as compared to other newer agents in biologic naïve PsA patients. However, in biologic-experienced PsA patients, no difference has been shown across the groups [31]. The risk seems to be 3–4 times higher for IFX and ADA as compared to ETN [32].
- Adequate screening for latent tuberculosis along with prophylaxis against reactivation of tuberculosis for those who test positive should be strongly considered for patients in endemic regions before initiating TNFi [33].
- A 1.5 to 3.4 times higher risk of neuroinflammatory events has been observed with TNFi [34]. Reactivation of chronic hepatitis B is yet another serious matter with TNFi. In the absence of antiviral prophylactic agents, up to 60% of patients receiving TNFi for any indication can develop a reactivation. However, effective antiviral prophylaxis with drugs like Entecavir significantly lowers the risk of reactivation [35, 36]. The possibility of a paradoxical adverse event, mostly psoriasis, should be recognized in patients with PsA on TNFi [37].

4.2.5 Dose Reduction and Withdrawal of TNFi in PsA

A rapid recurrence of PsA is observed in a significant proportion of patients following discontinuation of TNFi, with males demonstrating a higher risk of losing remission [38]. Interestingly, TNFi dose reduction to one-third for at least 6 months in a study led to maintenance in the reduced dose of TNFi for a mean of 1 year in 60% of PsA patients [39].

4.3 Interleukin-17 (IL-17) Inhibitors

The IL-17 superfamily comprises six structurally related cytokines (IL-17 A-F). IL-17A, the most potent pro-inflammatory cytokine in this family, can exist as a homodimer or heterodimer with IL-17F [40]. IL-17A is well recognized to have key contributions in both bone erosions and bone formation, which are hallmarks of PsA [41]. Targeting the Th17 pathway by IL-17 inhibitors has proven effective in all domains of psoriatic disease and in preventing radiographic progression.

4.3.1 IL-17 Inhibitors in the Treatment of Psoriatic Disease

- SEC is a fully human IgG1κ mAB that selectively binds and neutralizes IL-17A. IXE is a humanized IgG4 mAB directed against IL-17A. It neutralizes both IL-17A homodimers and IL-17A/F heterodimers.
- SEC and IXE are US FDA and EMA-approved IL-17 inhibitors for the treatment of PsA. Brodalumab (BRO), a recombinant, fully human IgG2 mAB that binds

to the IL-17 receptor subunit A has been approved by the US FDA for use in moderate to severe plaque psoriasis.

- Bimekizumab, a potential novel therapeutic approach, is an IgG1κ humanized mAb that acts by dual neutralization of IL-17A and IL-17F.

4.3.2 Efficacy of IL-17 Inhibitors in Psoriatic Arthritis

4.3.2.1 Peripheral Joint Outcome

- SEC has demonstrated effectiveness in TNFi naïve and TNFi inadequate responders alike, with better responses in the former. Rapid and clinically meaningful improvements in peripheral joints were shown in the FUTURE clinical trials, with ACR20/50/70 responses at week 24 of around 50%/32%/17%, respectively [42, 43].
- Radiographic progression was significantly inhibited at week 24 in FUTURE 1, with improvements in both erosion and joint space narrowing. This effect was sustained through 52 weeks of therapy [42]. FUTURE 5 study furthermore concluded that subcutaneous SEC loading regardless of the dose demonstrated benefit while aiming for faster and higher levels of response in joint and skin endpoints [44]. Long-term 5-year efficacy data of the FUTURE 2 study demonstrated ACR 20 responses in 74% and 70% in the 300 mg and 150 mg therapy arms, respectively [45].
- In a head-to-head trial (EXCEED) comparing SEC and ADA as the first line biologicals, at week 52, 67% of patients on SEC and 62% of patients on ADA achieved the primary endpoint. SEC did not meet statistical significance for superiority versus ADA in this trial [46].
- IXE is an effective IL-17 inhibitor for moderate to severe PsA, including those previously exposed to csDMARD and TNFi. The SPIRIT-P1 study evaluated two dosing regimens of IXE (80 mg every 2 weeks and 80 mg every 4 weeks) with ADA 40 mg as the reference arm. The primary endpoint of ACR-20 response at week 24 was achieved by 62% and 58% in the 2 weekly and 4 weekly groups, respectively, compared to 30% in the placebo group [47]. Radiographic progression was minimal, especially in those patients who maintained IXE from the initiation through 52 weeks [48].
- The SPIRIT-P2 study evaluated IXE in PsA patients previously exposed to TNFi. The primary endpoint was achieved by IXE in all groups compared to placebo [49]. A head-to-head comparison of the efficacy of IXE and ADA in biological naïve PsA patients met the primary outcome of IXE being superior to ADA for ACR50 response at week 24, with 36% of the patients on IXE and 28% on ADA achieving the primary outcome [50].
- Two phase III clinical trials (AMVISION-1 and AMVISION-2) for BRO at doses of 140 mg and 210 mg with subcutaneous administration bi-weekly were conducted in patients with active PsA following safety concerns related to suicidal ideations in phase II trials. The primary endpoint, ACR20 response at 16 weeks, was achieved by 39.5% and 50.9% in the BRO 140 mg arm in

AMVISION-1 and AMVISION-2 studies, respectively compared to 16% in the placebo arm; and ACR 20 response at 16 weeks in the BRO 210 mg group was achieved by 51.8% and 44.3% in AMVISION-1 and AMVISION-2 studies, respectively compared to 24.8% in the placebo arm. Both studies observed a statistically significant difference between treatment and placebo arms [51].

4.3.2.2 Axial PsA Outcome

- In the primary analysis of the MAXIMISE trial evaluating the efficacy of SEC in axial PsA (axPsA), an ASAS20 response at 12 weeks was met by 63% in the SEC 300 mg group and 66% in the 150 mg group, compared to 31% in the placebo arm [52]. The 52-week analysis of this study demonstrated 75% and 80% of the placebo patients re-randomized at week 12, achieving ASAS20 response rates in the 300 mg and 150 mg groups, respectively. ASAS40 responses at week 52 were 69% and 64% with 300 mg and 150 mg SEC, respectively. Statistical reduction in the Berlin MRI score changes in sacroiliitis was also present at week 12 [53].

4.3.2.3 Enthesitis and Dactylitis Outcome

- Complete resolution of enthesitis and dactylitis was observed with SEC in a significantly greater proportion of patients at week 24 in the FUTURE 1 study. At week 52, dactylitis was resolved in about 90% of the patients, compared to 48% at baseline, and enthesitis had resolved in 80% of patients, compared to 37% at baseline.
- In the FUTURE 2 study, however, changes in dactylitis and enthesitis were not statistically significant, though numerical enhancements in the proportion of patients achieving resolution of enthesitis and dactylitis were observed, compared to the placebo [54].
- A pooled analysis from FUTURE 2 and 3 studies assessing the effect of SEC on the resolution of Leeds Enthesitis Index (LEI) through week 104 observed complete resolution of enthesitis in 65% (300 mg SEC) and 56% (15 mg SEC) of the 466 patients with enthesitis at week 16, compared to 44% in the placebo arm [55].
- The LEI improved over baseline for both groups of IXE in the SPIRIT-P1 study. However, the improvement was not statistically significant compared to the placebo. A posthoc analysis revealed complete resolution of enthesitis at week 24 in about 39% of patients in the 2 weekly group and 43% in the 4 weekly groups of IXE, compared to 19% on placebo, which was statistically significant.
- The improvement in the Leeds dactylitis index (LDI) was statistically significant in both the IXE groups compared to the placebo. The posthoc analysis revealed complete resolution of dactylitis in 75–80% of patients in both the treatment groups, compared to 25% on placebo [47].
- Resolution of enthesitis over six sites and dactylitis at baseline in the brodalumab trials were observed in a significantly higher proportion of patients compared to placebo at weeks 16 and 24 for both doses. Patients on the higher dose of BRO achieved better resolution in dactylitis compared to those on the lower dose [51].

4.3.2.4 Persistence of Treatment with IL-17 Inhibitors in Patients with PsA

In a retrospective analysis from the US administrative claims database, SEC demonstrated lower discontinuation rates (36.5%), higher persistence [mean (SD): 282.8 (117.5) days] and greater adherence compared to TNFi [56].

4.3.2.5 Safety of IL-17 Inhibitors in Patients with PsA

- Long-term safety data of IL-17 inhibitors have been assessed from clinical trials and real-life settings. A concern with IL-17 inhibition is the possible exacerbation of inflammatory bowel disease (IBD). Three cases of new-onset IBD were noted among 1003 patients with PsA in various clinical trials. Nonetheless, the use of IL-17 inhibitors should be avoided in patients with known IBD or with a strong family history of IBD.
- A pooled long-term safety data from SEC clinical trials showed exposure-adjusted incidence rate per 100 patient-years for serious adverse events to be 7.9, 1.9 for serious infections, 1.5 for candida infections, 1.1 for malignancy, 0.05 for inflammatory bowel disease (IBD), 0.4 for major adverse cardiovascular events (MACE), and 0.1 for uveitis [57].
- Pooled data from 21 clinical trials on IXE across indications of plaque psoriasis, PsA, and axial spondyloarthritis demonstrated incidence rates of 6 for serious adverse events and 0.3 for death among the 1401 patients with PsA. Infections, mostly nasopharyngitis and upper respiratory tract infections, were the most commonly reported adverse events.
- Opportunistic infections, mainly oral and esophageal candidiasis, were reported in patients with PsA with an incidence of 3.9 per 100 patient-years. MACE and malignancies in PsA patients had an incidence of 0.5 per 100 patient-years and 0.3 per 100 patient-years, respectively. Incidence of depression following treatment with IXE was noted in 1.7 per 100 patient-year, with suicidal behavior noted in one patient. The incidence of IBD was higher in de novo cases [58]. Other uncommon adverse events include neutropenia and iritis.
- In the AMVISION trials on BRO, only one case of suicidal ideation was reported among the 318 patients enrolled in the BRO 140 mg group. No such cases were reported in the BRO 210 mg group [51].

4.4 IL-23 Inhibitors

The Th17-Th22-IL23 axis has a central role in the pathogenesis of psoriasis and PsA. Both Th17 and Th22 cells require IL-23 for their expansion and maintenance. IL-23 cytokine is upstream of IL-17 and is important for proliferation of Th17 cells, leading to the production of IL-17 [59]. Th17 and Th22 can have a common as well as contrasting function in the pathogenesis of skin and joint disease [60]. IL-23 shares its p40 subunit with IL-12 and is an important therapeutic target in both psoriasis and PsA. Agents targeting IL-23 are of two types: (A) anti-IL-12/IL-23p40

(Ustekinumab) and (B) anti-IL-23p19 (guselkumab, tildrakizumab, risankizumab, brazikumab, mirikizumab).

4.5 Interleukin-12/Interleukin-23p40 Inhibitor

Ustekinumab (UST), a fully human IgG1k mAB binding to the p40 subunit of IL-23 and IL-12, inhibits both the cytokines. The PSUMMIT1 and PSUMMIT2 phase III clinical trials demonstrated efficacy of UST in PsA. It has been approved for the treatment of active PsA alone or in combination with MTX.

4.5.1 Effectiveness of UST on Axial PsA, Enthesitis, and Dactylitis

- Pooled data from the PSUMMIT1 and two trials were analyzed for spondylitis-related endpoints in TNFi naïve patients at week 24. Mean improvements in neck/back/hip pain were larger in the UST group compared to placebo. Modified BASDAI also showed a similar trend [61].
- In the enthesitis clearance in psoriatic arthritis (ECLIPSA) open-label study comparing UST and TNFi in complete clearance of enthesitis defined by the spondyloarthritis research consortium of Canada (SPARCC) enthesitis index at week 24, 74% of patients on UST and 42% of patients on TNFi achieved the primary endpoint. This is the first study to show the superiority of UST over TNFi in PsA enthesitis [62]. Effect of UST on dactylitis was evaluated as secondary endpoints in the PSUMMIT trials.
- In the PSUMMIT1 study, at week 24, 56.6% in the UST 45 mg group and 55.8% in the UST 90 mg group had residual dactylitis, compared to 76% in the control group. A similar numerical difference in the proportions was seen in PSUMMIT2 data on dactylitis [63, 64]. Evaluation of radiographic changes in the hands and feet of patients enrolled in the PSUMMIT trials demonstrated a significant reduction in progression of erosions and joint space narrowing in the treatment arm compared to the placebo arm at 24 weeks. This reduction was maintained through 52 weeks also [62].

4.5.2 Persistence of Treatment with UST in PsA Patients

- In a longitudinal cohort, 160 PsA patients initiated on UST due to failure of cDMARDs or inadequate response to prior TNFi were evaluated for drug survival at 12 months.
- The global UST survival rate was 74.4%, with biologic-naïve patients demonstrating a significantly higher UST retention rate (87%) compared to the TNFi inadequate responders (68%). Combination with MTX did not affect the drug survival [65].

4.5.3 Safety of UST in PsA Patients

UST is a well-tolerated bDMARD with an overall favourable safety profile. An integrated analysis of UST safety data up to 1 year of follow-up from multiple clinical trials across indications including psoriasis, PsA, and Crohn's disease, including 5884 patients, revealed a low incidence of major adverse cardiovascular events, malignancies, and death [66].

4.6 Interleukin-23p19 Inhibitors

Guselkumab (GUS) is a fully human monoclonal antibody against p19 subunit of IL-23 and binds to it with high specificity and affinity. The results of two phase-3 clinical trials DISCOVER-1 and DISCOVER-2 demonstrated efficacy in different domains of PsA in biologic naïve and inadequate responders [67, 68]. Risankizumab and Tildrakizumab are undergoing phase-3 trials in patients with PsA.

4.6.1 Efficacy of Guselkumab for Peripheral Joint Outcomes in Active PsA

- DISCOVER-1 study included patients with inadequate response to or intolerance to standard treatment. The primary endpoint of ACR20 response at 24 weeks was met for both GUS dosing regimens (59% of patients in every 4 weeks group and 52% of patients in every 8 weeks group) compared with only 22% of patients in the placebo group [67].
- In the DISCOVER-2 study, biologic naïve patients with active PsA were recruited, with the same primary outcome as DISCOVER-1. ACR20 response at 24 weeks was met by 64% of patients in both the GUS dosing regimens, compared with 33% of patients in the placebo group. Furthermore, the four-week GUS regimen at week 24 inhibited the progression of structural damage compared with placebo [68]. The responses were shown to be maintained through 52 weeks in biologic naïve PsA patients [69].

4.6.2 Guselkumab in Axial PsA

- Data from DISCOVER-1 and 2 clinical trials were assessed for efficacy of GUS in patients with imaging-confirmed (consistent with sacroiliitis) axial involvement. Of the 312 patients who presented with axial involvement, 91 received 8 weekly GUS, and 103 received the 4 weekly regimens. BASDAI-50 was achieved by 40.5% and 37.9% of the patients in the 8 weekly and 4 weekly regimens, respectively, as compared with 19% of patients in the placebo arm. A greater proportion of the GUS treated patients also achieved ASDAS responses of inactive disease, major improvement and clinically important improvement compared to the placebo group [70].

4.6.3 Efficacy in Enthesitis and Dactylitis

- In the baseline pooled data across both studies, resolution of enthesitis was observed in patients on both 4 weekly (45%) and 8 weekly (50%) GUS regimens (45%), compared with those on placebo at week 24 (29%).
- Numerically greater improvements in LEI were also observed in both the GUS groups. Similarly, resolution of dactylitis was observed in a significantly higher proportion of patients in both 4 weekly (64%), and 8 weekly (59%) GUS regimens compared to those on placebo (42%).

4.6.4 Safety of Guselkumab in PsA Patients

The overall safety profile of GUS in both clinical trials was good. Infections and MACE were comparable to the placebo group. Transaminitis was reported in 10% of patients on the 4 weekly GUS regimen, compared to 6% in the 8 weekly regimens and 4% in the placebo group. This safety profile was maintained through the 52-week results.

4.7 Co-Stimulation Blockade in PsA

Abatacept (ABA), a co-stimulation modulator, is a fusion protein of the Fc region of immunoglobulin G1 with the extracellular domain of CTLA-4. It binds to CD80/86 and prevents the second signal in the T cell immunological synapse and subsequent activation of T cells. It was approved by the US FDA and EMA in 2017 for treating active PsA in adult patients who are partial/complete non-responders to cDMARDs, not requiring additional systemic therapy for psoriatic skin lesions. In the trial which led to the approval of ABA in PsA (ASTRAEA), PASI 50/75 response rates were only modest and did not differ from placebo [71].

4.8 Small Molecules in PsA

Novel small molecules, including the Janus kinase inhibitors (JAKinib) and the phosphodiesterase 4 inhibitor Apremilast, have been developed over the past decade. Their small and relatively simpler structure makes them easier to be synthesized, bringing down cost compared to the biologics. Furthermore, since these are not protein molecules, they can be administered orally, which improves patient convenience to a great extent, and they do not have the tendency to form antidrug antibodies, unlike biologics.

4.9 Targeting the JAK/STAT Pathway: The JAK Inhibitors

The Janus Kinase-Signal Transducer and Activator of Transcription (JAK-STAT) pathway is a crucial intracellular signaling system for wide range of cytokines and growth factors. The four different types of JAK proteins include JAK1, JAK2, JAK3, and TYK2. Tofacitinib (TOFA) is the only JAKinib that has been approved by the US FDA and EMA for active psoriatic arthritis. However, JAKinibs, including Upadacitinib, Filgotinib, and a novel TYK2 inhibitor, Deucravacitinib, are in the pipeline for regulatory approvals for active PsA.

4.9.1 Tofacitinib (TOFA)

Tofacitinib (TOFA), a selective inhibitor of JAK 1 and JAK 3 is approved for the treatment of active PsA in patients with inadequate response or intolerance to MTX or other csDMARDs. Two phase III clinical trials, OPAL Broaden and OPAL Beyond, confirmed its efficacy in different PsA clinical domains.

4.9.1.1 Efficacy of TOFA on Peripheral and Axial Arthritis

- Both the trials demonstrated superior efficacy of TOFA (both 5 mg and 10 mg twice daily doses) over placebo for peripheral arthritis, with the efficacy maintained or improved at 6 months [72–74].
- The OPAL Balance sub-study showed no clinically meaningful differences in the efficacy between TOFA 5 mg twice daily as a monotherapy and in combination with MTX [75]. A unique finding with TOFA has been its association with rapid and sustained effect on pain in patients with inflammatory arthritis, including PsA. The effect was seen as early as 3 months following treatment [76].
- In the OPAL Broaden study, more than 90% of patients met the criteria for radiographic non-progression after 12 months [77]. In a pooled analysis of the two phase III clinical trial data, in patients diagnosed as having spondylitis by the investigators, changes in BASDAI at 3 months were greater in both TOFA 5 mg and 10 mg twice daily doses, as compared to the placebo ($p < 0.05$). This improvement was maintained in both groups at 6 months [74].

4.9.1.2 Efficacy of TOFA on Enthesitis and Dactylitis

- Mean changes in the LEI scores with TOFA 5 mg and 10 mg were −0.8 and −1.5, respectively, in the OPAL Broaden study and −1.3 in both the groups in the OPAL Beyond study. These changes were not statistically significant compared to the placebo or ADA reference arms.
- Mean changes in the dactylitis severity score with TOFA 5 mg and 10 mg were −3.5 and −5.5, respectively in the OPAL Broaden study, and −5.2 and −5.4, respectively in the OPAL Beyond study [72, 73].

4.9.1.3 Tolerability and Safety Profile of TOFA in Psoriatic Arthritis

- The tolerability profile of TOFA 5 mg twice daily in combination with a csD-MARD has been good in all three major studies. The 3-month incidence of adverse events in OPAL Broaden was 39%, compared to 35% in the placebo arm for TOFA 5 mg twice daily; in OPAL Beyond, it was 55% compared to 44% in the placebo arm. OPAL Balance, which is an open-label, long-term extended study of the patients enrolled in OPAL Broaden and OPAL Beyond clinical trials, reported adverse events in 80% and serious adverse events in 14% of the patients after 3 years [78]. Some signals for low absolute lymphocyte count have been described, though generally being minimal and not related to serious infections. A modest decrease in the lymphocyte counts has been noted in the OPAL Balance data. Transaminitis has been noted in patients on TOFA 5 mg twice daily, though more than thrice the upper limit of normal was rare up to 12 months. No cases with hepatic injury were noted. There is a concern regarding the elevation of lipid levels after 3 months of treatment, maintained over 6 and 12 months of treatment, though that did not translate to increased risk of MACE [79]. The OPAL Balance data noted incidence rates of 1.7% for serious infections, 2.9% for herpes zoster, 0.7% for MACE, and 3.5% for malignancies, including non-melanoma skin cancer [78]. Physicians should be cognizant of the noted risk of thrombosis, which has been flagged as a warning and/or as an adverse drug reaction to JAKinibs. A meta-analysis showed a pooled incidence of 0.68 (95% CI 0.36–1.29), 0.44 (95% CI 0.28–0.7) and 0.59 (95% CI 0.31–1.15) for venous thromboembolism, pulmonary embolism, and deep vein thrombosis, respectively [80]. TOFA is contraindicated in patients with severe hepatic impairment, active tuberculosis, serious or opportunistic infections, those with a low lymphocytic count and in those with high risk for thrombosis.

4.9.2 Upadacitinib (UPA)

Upadacitinib (UPA) selectively inhibits JAK1 over JAK2, JAK3, and TYK2. Two phase III trials have been conducted on active PsA patients with previous inadequate responses to cDMARDs (SELECT-PsA-1) and bDMARDs (SELECT-PsA-2), with good reports of efficacy across all the disease domains [81, 82].

4.9.2.1 Efficacy of UPA on Peripheral and Axial Arthritis

- In both trials, a superior efficacy of UPA for both 15 mg and 30 mg was noted in peripheral arthritis outcomes. SELECT-PsA-1 had ADA 40 mg as a comparator arm. UPA 15 mg was non-inferior to ADA, while UPA 30 mg was found to be superior to ADA for all the ACR response rates. Interestingly, the effect of UPA was noted as early as the second week, significantly more than the effect in the placebo group. The proportion of patients achieving ACR 20 response increased over time for both the doses, with a plateauing observed at week 12 for the 30 mg dose group, while the 15 mg dose group continuing to show the increase till week 20.

- The efficacy of UPA for axPsA symptoms was assessed using pooled data from the two studies for both doses of UPA. Treatment with either dose of UPA resulted in significantly greater improvements in the overall BASDAI and ASDAS-CRP endpoints from the baseline at week 12. A significantly higher percentage of patients on either dose of UPA achieved BASDAI 50, ASDAS inactive disease and ASDAS clinically important improvement responses [83].

4.9.2.2 Efficacy of UPA on Enthesitis and Dactylitis

- Resolution of enthesitis was observed with both the doses of UPA compared to placebo using both the LEI and SPARCC enthesitis indices. At week 12, 39.1% on UPA 15 mg and 48% on UPA 30 mg achieved complete resolution of enthesitis by LEI in the SELECT-PsA-2 study. In the SELECT-PsA-1 study, complete resolution of enthesitis by LEI at 24 weeks was noted in 53.7% and 57.7% in the 15 mg and 30 mg dose groups, respectively and both these groups were statistically significant compared to ADA (47.2%). Resolution of dactylitis at week 12 was noted in 63.6% and 76% in UPA 15 mg and 30 mg dose groups, respectively, both being statistically significant compared to the placebo group in the SELECT-PsA-2 study.

4.9.2.3 Safety of UPA in PsA

- Adverse events were noted to be higher in the 30 mg dose group at week 24 in the 2 phase III trials. Serious adverse events were noted in 5.7% and 8.3% of patients on 15 mg and 30 mg dose groups, respectively. Pneumonia was the most commonly reported serious adverse event. Herpes zoster was reported in eight patients on UPA 30 mg. Hepatic disorders were observed in 8.3% of patients on UPA 30 mg compared to 1.9% of those on UPA 15 mg. MACE and venous thromboembolism were reported in patients with at least one risk factor.

Filgotinib, a selective JAK1 inhibitor, has completed a phase 2 trial (EQUATOR) and was found to be efficacious for the treatment of active PsA [84]. **Deucravacitinib**, with a novel mechanism of selective TYK2 inhibition, is efficacious over placebo at week 16 in patients with active PsA in a phase 2 trial [85]. JAKinibs hold great promise in PsA, with many more drugs being available in the future.

4.10 Phosphodiesterase-4 (PDE4) Inhibitor: Apremilast

PDE4 is an intracellular enzyme that is responsible for the hydrolysis of cyclic adenosine monophosphate (cAMP) into AMP, the intracellular second messenger. Inhibition of PDE4 leads to cAMP-dependent activation of protein kinases and cAMP response element-binding proteins. This, in turn, has a role in inducing the synthesis of IL-10 and the inhibition of pro-inflammatory cytokines. Apremilast

(APR) monotherapy, or in combination with other csDMARDs at the dose of 30 mg twice daily is recommended for the treatment of active PsA in adult patients with inadequate response or intolerance to prior csDMARD therapy.

4.10.1 Efficacy of APR on Peripheral Arthritis

- APR showed consistent clinical efficacy in reducing peripheral arthritis symptoms at the 30 mg twice daily dose in all the phase III clinical trials. The ACR responses, however, were noted to be lower than the TNFi, IL-17 and JAKinibs, and comparable to ustekinumab. The overall efficacy was shown to increase over time in the PALACE 1 extension study. Higher ACR 20 response rates were noted in bio-naïve patients compared to bio-experienced patients or those who failed previously [86]. Long-term efficacy data on APR shows response rates of 67.2%, 44.4%, and 27.4% for ACR20, ACR50 and ACR70, respectively, in the patients continuing to take 30 mg twice daily at 5 years. The mean swollen and tender joint counts improved by 63.3% and 49.8% at week 52, which further increased to 82.3% and 72.7%, respectively at 5 years [87].

4.10.2 Efficacy of APR on Enthesitis and Dactylitis

- Pooled data analysis from PALACE 1, 2, and 3 studies was conducted for the effectiveness of APR on enthesitis and dactylitis through 156 weeks [88]. At 52 weeks, 31% of the patients on APR 30 mg twice daily demonstrated complete resolution of enthesitis, which increased to 55% of the patients at week 156. Long-term effects of APR 30 mg dose schedule on a complete resolution of dactylitis-by-dactylitis count were also good but not statistically significant compared to the placebo. At week 156, mean changes from the baseline were −3.0 in the 30 mg dose schedule group, with about 80% achieving a dactylitis count of 0.

4.10.3 Persistence and Safety of APR in Patients with PsA

- Contraindications to bDMARDs, lack of poor prognostic factors and higher risk of infection are the most frequent reasons for APR prescription. In an Italian study, the 6-month retention rate of APR was 72% [89]. The overall safety profile of APR is favorable to patients at risk of serious infections, in whom other bDMARDs, including JAKinibs, may not be preferable. Gastrointestinal (GI) side effects, though common in the initial weeks, tend to settle gradually. Less than 2% had to discontinue therapy with APR due to GI side effects in the PALACE program. Weight loss is observed in patients on APR at 52 weeks. A weight loss of 2% with APR 30 mg dose schedule was noted at week 24. Depression was noted to be higher in the APR groups compared to placebo, with a rate of <2% in long-term studies.

4.11 Positioning of Targeted DMARDs in the Recommendations for PsA

- There are currently three recommendations for the management of PsA, namely 2019 updated EULAR recommendations, the American College of Rheumatology/ National Psoriasis Foundation (ACR/NPF) 2018 guidelines, and the GRAPPA 2015 recommendations [3, 9, 90].
- *The EULAR recommendations* include biologicals in Phase III of their management algorithm, wherein it is recommended for csDMARD failure in peripheral arthritis and NSAID/local glucocorticoid injection failure in axial disease patients. TNFis or IL-17 inhibitors are recommended in axial disease, and IL-23 inhibitors can be considered in peripheral arthritis only, alongside the other two classes of biological agents. Phase IV of EULAR recommendations deals with biological failures and recommends switching within/between the classes of TNFi or IL-17 inhibitors for axial disease. For biological failure in peripheral predominant disease with arthritis and/or enthesitis, a switch within/between classes of biologicals or switching over to JAK inhibitors/PDE4 inhibitors (in situations where biological/JAK inhibitor therapy is inappropriate) is recommended.
- *The GRAPPA 2015 recommendations* follow two routes for biologicals viz. standard therapeutic route and expedited route. In the standard therapeutic route, bDMARDs (TNFi or IL-17 inhibitors or IL-12/IL-23 inhibitors) are recommended for csDMARD failure in peripheral arthritis and dactylitis, NSAID failure in axial disease and enthesitis. Switching of bDMARD is recommended with failure to initial bDMARD. PDE4 inhibitors can be considered in mild arthritis/ enthesitis/dactylitis except for axial disease. In the expedited route, bDMARDs can be considered in arthritis/axial disease/dactylitis, and also in severe presentations.
- The *ACR/NPF 2018 guidelines* differ from the other two recommendations in their placement of bDMARDs as an upfront conditional choice alongside csDMARDs in treatment naïve active PsA patients, as evidence for these agents is of low quality. Other aspects of the guidelines are fundamentally similar in the above-mentioned recommendations; however, abatacept is also recommended, which is unique to this guideline. Tofacitinib, as per this guideline, is recommended in active PsA following csDMARD/TNFi failure.

4.12 Conclusion

Treatment for patients with PsA should be individualized as per predominant clinical domain affected, other manifestations and comorbid conditions. Widespread pain, patient function, and comorbidities should be considered while deciding therapeutic goals. Various treatment guidelines, as proposed by GRAPPA, EULAR and ACR/NPF may aid rheumatologists in choosing a therapy. Adverse effects of therapies should be monitored regularly, as recommended. Finally, the huge cost of continuous biologic therapy may be a limiting factor for its use in resource-limited settings; hence cost-effective treatment strategies with the use of biosimilars, tapering and withdrawal strategies warrant further study.

References

1. Ritchlin CT, Colbert RA, Gladman DD. Psoriatic arthritis. New Engl J Med. 2017;376:957–70.
2. Coates LC, Helliwell PS. Psoriatic arthritis: start of the art review. Clin Med (Lond). 2017;17:65–70.
3. Coates LC, Kavanaugh A, Mease PJ, Soriano ER, Acosta-Felquer ML, Armstrong AW, et al. Group for research and assessment of psoriasis and psoriatic arthritis 2015 treatment recommendations for psoriatic arthritis. Arthritis Rheum. 2016;68:1060–71.
4. Khanna I, Kozicky O, Fischer H. Use of FDA-approved medications: biologics for psoriatic arthritis in patients at an urban outpatient rheumatology clinic. ACR Open Rheumatol. 2019;12:580–4.
5. Ruyssen-Witrand A, Perry R, Watkins C, Braileanu G, Kumar G, Kiri S, et al. Efficacy and safety of biologics in psoriatic arthritis: a systematic literature review and network meta-analysis. RMD Open. 2020;6:e001117.
6. Gladman DD, Orbai A-M, Gome-Reino J, Chang-Douglass S, Leoncini E, Burton HE, et al. Network meta-analysis of tofacitinib, biologic disease-modifying antirheumatic drugs, and apremilast for the treatment of psoriatic arthritis. Curr Ther Res Clin Exp. 2020;93:100601.
7. Croft M, Siegel RM. Beyond TNF: TNF superfamily cytokines as targets for the treatment of rheumatic diseases. Nat Rev Rheumatol. 2017;13:217–33.
8. Mantravadi S, Ogdie A, Kraft WK. Tumor necrosis factor inhibitors in psoriatic arthritis. Expert Rev Clin Pharmacol. 2017;10:899–910.
9. Gossec L, Baraliakos X, Kershchbaumer A, de Wit M, McInnes I, Dougados M, et al. EULAR recommendations for the management of psoriatic arthritis with pharmacological therapies: 2019 update. Ann Rheum Dis. 2020;79:680–2.
10. Mease PJ, Goffe BS, Metz J, VanderStoep A, Finck B, Burge DJ. Etanercept in the treatment of psoriatic arthritis and psoriasis: a randomised trial. Lancet. 2000;356:385–90.
11. Mease PJ, Gladman DD, Collier DH, Ritchlin CT, Helliwell PS, Liu L, et al. Etanercept and methotrexate as monotherapy or in combination for psoriatic arthritis: primary results from a randomized, controlled phase III trial. Arthritis Rheumatol. 2019;71:1112–24.
12. Antoni CE, Kavanaugh A, Kirkham B, Tutuncu Z, Burmester GR, Schneider U, et al. Sustained benefits of infliximab therapy for dermatologic and articular manifestations of psoriatic arthritis. Arthritis Rheum. 2005;52:1227–36.
13. Antoni C, Krueger GG, de Vlam K, Birbara C, Beutler A, Guzzo C, et al. Infliximab improves signs and symptoms of psoriatic arthritis: results of the IMPACT 2 trial. Ann Rheum Dis. 2005;64:1150–7.
14. Mease PJ, Gladman DD, Ritchlin CT, Ruderman EM, Steinfeld SD, Choy EHS, et al. Adalimumab for the treatment of patients with moderately to severely active psoriatic arthritis. Arthritis Rheum. 2005;52:3279–89.
15. Genovese MC, Mease PJ, Thomson GTD, Kivitz AJ, Perdok RJ, Weinberg MA, et al. Safety and efficacy of adalimumab in treatment of patients with psoriatic arthritis who had failed disease modifying antirheumatic drug therapy. J Rheumatol. 2007;34:1040–50.
16. Kavanaugh A, McInnes I, Mease P, Krueger GG, Gladman D, Gomez-Reino J, et al. Golimumab, a new human tumor necrosis factor alpha antibody, administered every four weeks as a subcutaneous injection in psoriatic arthritis. Arthritis Rheum. 2009;60:976–86.
17. Mease PJ, Fleischmann R, Deodhar AA, Wollenhaupt J, Khraishi M, Kielar D, et al. Effect of certolizumab pegol on signs and symptoms in patients with psoriatic arthritis: 24-week results

of a phase 3 double-blind randomised placebo-controlled study (RAPID-PsA). Ann Rheum Dis. 2014;73:48–55.
18. Kavanaugh A, Husni ME, Harrison DD, Kim L, Lo KH, Leu JH, et al. Safety and efficacy of intravenous golimumab in patients with active psoriatic arthritis. Results through week twenty-four of the GO-VIBRANT study. Arthritis Rheum. 2017;69:2151–61.
19. Vieira-Sousa E, Alves P, Rodrigues AM, Teixeira F, Tavares-Costa J, Bernardo A, et al. GO-DACT: a phase 3b randomised, double-blind, placebo-controlled trial of golimumab plus methotrexate (MTX) versus placebo plus MTX in improving dactylitis in MTX-naïve patients with psoriatic arthritis. Ann Rheum Dis. 2020;79:490–8.
20. Lubrano E, Spadaro A, Marchesoni A, Olivieri I, Scarpa R, D'Angelo S, et al. The effectiveness of a biologic agent on axial manifestations of psoriatic arthritis. A twelve months observational study in a group of patients treated with etanercept. Clin Exp Rheumatol. 2011;29:80–4.
21. Brahe CH, Ørnbjerg LM, Jacobsson L, Nissen MJ, Kristianslund EK, Mann H, et al. Retention and response rates in 14261 PsA patients started TNF inhibitor treatment – results from 12 countries in EuroSpA. Rheumatology. 2020;59:1640–50.
22. Mourad A, Gniadecki R. Treatment of dactylitis and enthesitis in psoriatic arthritis with biologic agents: a systematic review and meta-analysis. J Rheumatol. 2020;47:59–65.
23. Goulabchand R, Mouterde G, Barnetche T, Lukas C, Morel J, Combe B. Effect of tumor necrosis factor blockers on radiographic progression of psoriatic arthritis: a systematic review and meta-analysis of randomized controlled trials. Ann Rheum Dis. 2014;73:414–9.
24. Yang Z, Lin N, Li L, Li Y. The effect of TNF inhibitors on cardiovascular events in psoriasis and psoriatic arthritis: an updated meta-analysis. Clin Rev Allergy Immunol. 2016;51:240–7.
25. Fagerli KM, Lie E, van der Heijde D, Heiberg MS, Kalstad S, Rødevand E, et al. Switching between TNF inhibitors in psoriatic arthritis: data from the NOR-DMARD study. Ann Rheum Dis. 2013;72:1840–4.
26. Fagerli KM, Kearsley-Fleet L, Watson KD, Packham J, BSRBR-RA Contributors Group, Symmons DPM, et al. Long-term persistence of TNF-inhibitor treatment in patients with psoriatic arthritis. Data from the British society for rheumatology biologics register. RMD Open. 2018;4:e000596.
27. Clunie G, McInnes IB, Barkham N, Marzo-Ortega H, Patel Y, Gough A, et al. Long-term effectiveness of tumor necrosis factor-α inhibitor treatment for psoriatic arthritis in the UK: a multicentre retrospective study. Rheumatol Adv Pract. 2018;2:rky042.
28. Vieira-Sousa E, Eusèbio M, Ávila-Ribeiro P, Khmelinskii N, Cruz-Machado R, Rocha TM, et al. Real-world long-term effectiveness of tumor necrosis factor inhibitors in psoriatic arthritis patients from the rheumatic diseases Portuguese register. J Rheumatol. 2020;47:690–700.
29. George MD, Baker JF, Ogdie A. Comparative persistence on methotrexate and TNF inhibitors in rheumatoid arthritis, psoriatic arthritis, and ankylosing spondylitis. J Rheumatol. 2020;47:826–34.
30. Ballegaard C, Højgaard P, Dreyer L, Cordtz R, Jørgensen TS, Skougaard M, et al. Impact of comorbidities on tumor necrosis factor inhibitor therapy in psoriatic arthritis: a population-based study. Arthritis Care Res. 2018;70:592–9.
31. Li X, Andersen KM, Chang H-Y, Curtis JR, Alexander GC. Comparative risk of serious infections among real-world users of biologics for psoriasis or psoriatic arthritis. Ann Rheum Dis. 2020;79:285–91.
32. Cantini F, Niccoli L, Goletti D. Adalimumab, etanercept, infliximab, and the risk of tuberculosis: data from clinical trials, national registries, and postmarketing surveillance. J Rheumatol. 2014;91:47–55.
33. Handa R, Upadhyaya S, Kapoor S, Jois R, Pandey BD, Bhatnagar AK, et al. Tubercuosis and biologics in rheumatology: a special situation. Int J Rheum Dis. 2017;20:1313–25.
34. Kopp TI, Delcoigne B, Arkema EV, Jacobsen RK, Magyari M, Ibfelt EH, et al. Risk of neuroinflammatory events in arthritis patients treated with tumor necrosis factor alpha inhibitors: a collaborative population-based cohort study from Denmark and Sweden. Ann Rheum Dis. 2020;79:566–72.

35. Chiu Y-M, Chen D-Y. Infection risk in patients undergoing treatment for inflammatory arthritis: non-biologics versus biologics. Exp Rev Clin Immunol. 2020;16:207–28.
36. Lin T-C, Yoshida K, Tedeschi SK, de Abreu MM, Hashemi N, Solomon DH. Risk of hepatitis B reactivation in inflammatory arthritis patients receiving disease modifying anti-rheumatic drugs (DMARDs): a systematic review and meta-analysis. Arthritis Care Res. 2018;70:724–31.
37. Li SJ, Perez-Chada LM, Merola JF. TNF inhibitor-induced psoriasis: proposed algorithm for treatment and management. J Psoriasis Psoriatic Arthritis. 2019;4:70–80.
38. Araujo EG, Finzel S, Englbrecht M, Schreiber DA, Faustini F, Hueber A, et al. High incidence of disease recurrence after discontinuation of disease-modifying antirheumatic drug treatment in patients with psoriatic arthritis in remission. Ann Rheum Dis. 2015;74:655–60.
39. Fong W, Holroyd C, Davidson B, Armstrong R, Harvey N, Dennison E, et al. The effectiveness of a real-life dose reduction strategy for TNF inhibitors in ankylosing spondylitis and psoriatic arthritis. Rheumatology. 2016;55:1837–42.
40. Beringer A, Miossec P. Systemic effects of IL-17 in inflammatory arthritis. Nat Rev Rheumatol. 2019;15:491–501.
41. McGonagle D, McInnes IB, Kirkham BW, Sherlock J, Moots R. The role of IL-17A in axial spondyloarthritis and psoriatic arthritis: recent advances and controversies. Ann Rheum Dis. 2019;78:1167–78.
42. Mease PJ, McInnes IB, Kirkham B, Kavanaugh A, Rahman P, van der Heijde D, et al. Secukinumab inhibition of interleukin-17A in patients with psoriatic arthritis. N Engl J Med. 2015;373:1329–39.
43. McInnes IB, Mease PJ, Kirkham B, Kavanaugh A, Ritchlin CT, Rahman P, et al. Secukinumab, a human anti-interleukin-17A monoclonal antibody, in patients with psoriatic arthritis (FUTURE 2): a randomised, double-blind, placebo-controlled, phase 3 trial. Lancet. 2015;386:1137–46.
44. Mease P, van der Heijde D, Landewé R, Mpofu S, Rahman P, Tahir H, et al. Secukinumab improves active psoriatic arthritis symptoms and inhibits radiographic progression: primary results from the randomised, double-blind, phase III FUTURE 5 study. Ann Rheum Dis. 2018;77:890–7.
45. McInnes IB, Mease PJ, Kivitz AJ, Nash P, Rahman P, Rech J, et al. Long-term efficacy and safety of secukinumab in patients with psoriatic arthritis: 5-year (end-of-study) results from the phase 3 FUTURE 2 study. Lancet Rheumatol. 2020;2:e227–35.
46. McInnes IB, Behrens F, Mease PJ, Kavanaugh A, Ritchlin C, Nash P, et al. Secukinumab versus adalimumab for treatment of active psoriatic arthritis (EXCEED): a double-blind, parallel-group, randomised, active-controlled, phase 3b trial. Lancet. 2020;395:1496–505.
47. Mease PJ, van der Heijde D, Ritchlin CT, Okada M, Cuchacovich RS, et al. Ixekizumab, an interleukin-17A specific monoclonal antibody, for the treatment of biologic-naïve patients with active psoriatic arthritis: results from the 24-week randomised, double-blind, placebo-controlled and active (adalimumab)-controlled period of the phase III trial SPIRIT-P1. Ann Rheum Dis. 2017;76:79–87.
48. van der Heijde D, Gladman DD, Kishimoto M, et al. Efficacy and safety of ixekizumab in patients with active psoriatic arthritis: 52-week results from a phase III study (SPIRIT-P1). J Rheumatol. 2018;45:367–77.
49. Nash P, Kirkham B, Okada M, Rahman P, Combe B, Burmester G-R, et al. Ixekizumab for the treatment of patients with active psoriatic arthritis and an inadequate response to tumor necrosis factor inhibitors: results from the 24-week randomised, double-blind, placebo-controlled period of the SPIRIT-P2 phase 3 trial. Lancet. 2017;389:2317–27.
50. Mease PJ, Smolen JS, Behrens F, Nash P, Leage SL, Li L, et al. A head-to-head comparison of the efficacy and safety of ixekizumab and adalimumab in biological-naïve patients with active psoriatic arthritis: 24-week results of a randomised, open-label, blinded-assessor trial. Ann Rheum Dis. 2020;79:123–31.
51. Mease PJ, Helliwell PS, Hjuler KF, Raymond K, McInnes I. Brodalumab in psoriatic arthritis: results from the randomised phase III AMVISION-1 and AMVISION-2 trials. Ann Rheum Dis. 2021;80(2):185–93. https://doi.org/10.1136/annrheumdis-2019-216835.

52. Baraliakos X, Coates L, Gossec L, Jeka S, Mera A, Schulz B, et al. Secukinumab improves axial manifestations in patients with psoriatic arthritis and inadequate response to NSAIDs: primary analysis of phase 3 trial (abstract). Arthritis Rheumatol. 2019;71(suppl 10). https://acrabstracts.org/abstract/secukinumab-improves-axial-manifestations-in-patients-with-psoriatic-arthritis-and-inadequate-response-to-nsaids-primary-analysis-of-phase-3-trial/. Accessed 23 Oct 2021.
53. Baraliakos X, Gossec L, Pournara E, Jeka S, Blanco R, D'angelo S, et al. Secukinumab improves clinical and imaging outcomes in patients with psoriatic arthritis and axial manifestations with inadequate response to NSAIDs: week 52 results from the MAXIMISE trial (abstract). Ann Rheum Dis. 2020;79:35–6.
54. Mease P, McInnes IB. Secukinumab: a new treatment option for psoriatic arthritis. Rheumatol Ther. 2016;3:5–29.
55. Coates LC, Wallman JK, McGonagle D, Schett GA, McInnes IB, Mease PJ, et al. Secukinumab efficacy on resolution of enthesitis in psoriatic arthritis: pooled analysis of two phase 3 studies. Arthritis Res Ther. 2019;21:266.
56. Oelke KR, Chambenoit O, Majjhoo AQ, Gray S, Higgins K, Hur P. Persistence and adherence of biologics in US patients with psoriatic arthritis: analyses from a claims database. J Comp Eff Res. 2019;8:607–21.
57. Deodhar A, Mease PJ, McInnes IB, Baraliakos X, Reich K, Blauvelt A, et al. Long-term safety of secukinumab in patients with moderate-to-severe plaque psoriasis, psoriatic arthritis, and ankylosing spondylitis: integrated pooled clinical trial and post-marketing surveillance data. Arthritis Res Ther. 2019;21:111.
58. Genovese MC, Mysler E, Tomita T, Papp KA, Salvarani C, Schwartzman S, et al. Safety of ixekizumab in adult patients with plaque psoriasis, psoriatic arthritis and axial spondyloarthritis: data from 21 clinical trials. Rheumatology. 2020;59(12):3834–44. https://doi.org/10.1093/rheumatology/keaa189.
59. Sakkas LI, Zafiriou E, Bogdanos DP. Mini review: new treatments in psoriatic arthritis. Focus on the IL-23/17 axis. Front Pharmacol. 2019;10:872.
60. Benham H, Norris P, Goodall J, Wechalekar MD, FitzGerald O, Szentpetery A, et al. Th17 and Th22 cells in psoriatic arthritis and psoriasis. Arthritis Res Ther. 2013;15:R136.
61. Helliwell PS, Gladman DD, Chakravarty SD, Kafka S, Karyekar CS, You Y, et al. Effects of ustekinumab on spondylitis-associated endpoints in TNFi-naïve active psoriatic arthritis patients with physician-reported spondylitis: pooled results from two phase 3, randomised, controlled trials. RMD Open. 2020;6:e001149.
62. Araujo EG, Englbrecht M, Hoepken S, Finzel S, Kampylafka E, Kleyer A, et al. Effects of ustekinumab versus tumor necrosis factor inhibition on enthesitis: results from the enthesial clearance in psoriatic arthritis (ECLIPSA) study. Semin Arthritis Rheum. 2019;48:632–7.
63. McInnes IB, Kavanaugh A, Gottlieb AB, Puig L, Rahman P, Ritchlin C, et al. Efficacy and safety of ustekinumab in patients with active psoriatic arthritis: 1 year results of the phase 3, multicentre, double-blind, placebo-controlled PSUMMIT 1 trial. Lancet. 2013;382:780–9.
64. Ritchlin C, Rahman P, Kavanaugh A, McInnes IB, Puig L, Li S, et al. Efficacy and safety of the anti-IL 12/23 p40 monoclonal antibody, ustekinumab, in patients with active psoriatic arthritis despite conventional non-biological and biological anti-tumor necrosis factor therapy: 6-month and 1-year results of the phase 3, multicentre, double-blind, placebo-controlled, randomised PSUMMIT 2 trial. Ann Rheum Dis. 2014;73:990–9.
65. Iannone F, Santo L, Bucci R, Semeraro A, Carlino G, Paoletti F, et al. Drug survival and effectiveness of ustekinumab in patients with psoriatic arthritis. Real-life data from the biologic Apulian registry (BIOPURE). Clin Rheumatol. 2018;37:667–75.
66. Ghosh S, Gensler LS, Yang Z, Gasink C, Chakravarty SD, Farahi K, et al. Ustekinumab safety in psoriasis, psoriatic arthritis, and Crohn's disease: an integrated analysis of phase I/III clinical development programs. Drug Saf. 2019;42:751–68.
67. Deodhar A, Helliwell PS, Boehncke W-H, Kollmeier AP, Hsia EC, Subramanian RA, et al. Guselkumab in patients with active psoriatic arthritis who were biologic-naïve or had pre-

viously received TNF-α inhibitor treatment (DISCOVER-1): a double-blind, randomised, placebo-controlled phase 3 trial. Lancet. 2020;395:1115–25.
68. Mease PJ, Rahman P, Gottlieb AB, Kollmeier AP, Hsia EC, Xu XL, et al. Guselkumab in biologic-naive patients with active psoriatic arthritis (DISCOVER-2): a double-blind, randomised, placebo-controlled phase 3 trial. Lancet. 2020;395:1126–36.
69. McInnes IB, Rahman P, Gottlieb AB, Hsia EC, Kollmeier AP, Chakravarty SD, et al. Efficacy and safety of guselkumab, an interleukin-23p19-specific monoclonal with psoriatic arthritis previously treated with open-label tofacitinib plus Rheum. 2020; https://doi.org/10.1002/art.41553.
70. Helliwell P, Gladman DD, Poddubnyy D, Mease PJ, Baraliakos X, Kollmeier A, et al. Efficacy of guselkumab, a monoclonal antibody that specifically binds to the p-19 subunit of IL-23, on endpoints related to axial involvement in patients with active PsA with imaging-confirmed sacroiliitis: week-24 results from two phase 3, randomized, double-blind, placebo-controlled studies (abstract). Ann Rheum Dis. 2020;79:36–7.
71. Mease PJ, Gottlieb AB, van der Heijde D, FitzGerald O, Johnsen A, Nys M, et al. Efficacy and safety of abatacept, a T-cell modulator, in a randomised, double-blind, placebo-controlled, phase III study in psoriatic arthritis. Ann Rheum Dis. 2017;76:1550–8.
72. Mease P, Hall S, FitzGerald O, van der Heijde D, Merola JF, Avila-Zapata F, et al. Tofacitinib or adalimumab versus placebo for psoriatic arthritis. N Engl J Med. 2017;377:1537–50.
73. Gladman D, Rigby W, Azevedo VF, Behrens F, Blanco R, Kaszuba A, et al. Tofacitinib for psoriatic arthritis in patients with an inadequate response to TNF inhibitors. N Engl J Med. 2017;377:1525–36.
74. Nash P, Coates LC, Fleischmann R, Papp KA, Gomez-Reino JJ, Kanik KS, et al. Efficacy of tofacitinib for the treatment of psoriatic arthritis: pooled analysis of two phase 3 studies. Rheumatol Ther. 2018;5:567–82.
75. Nash P, Mease PJ, Fleishaker D, Wu J, Coates LC, Behrens F, et al. Tofacitinib as monotherapy following methotrexate withdrawal in patients with psoriatic arthritis previously treated with open-label tofacitinib plus methotrexate: a randomised, placebo-controlled sub-study of OPAL balance. Lancet Rheumatol. 2020; https://doi.org/10.1016/S2665-9913(20)30339-8.
76. Ogdie A, de Vlam K, McInnes IB, Mease PJ, Baer P, Lukic T, et al. Efficacy of tofacitinib in reducing pain in patients with rheumatoid arthritis, psoriatic arthritis or ankylosing spondylitis. RMD Open. 2020;6:e001042.
77. van der Heijde D, Gladman DD, FitzGerald O, Kavanaugh A, Graham D, Wang C, et al. Raiographic progression according to baseline c-reactive protein levels and other risk factors in psoriatic arthritis treated with tofacitinib or adalimumab. J Rheumatol. 2019;46:1089–96.
78. Nash P, Coates LC, Kivitz AJ, Mease PJ, Gladman DD, Covarrubias-Cobos J, et al. Safety and efficacy of tofacitinib in patients with active psoriatic arthritis: interim analysis of OPAL balance, an open-label, long-term extension study. Rheumatol Ther. 2020;7:553–80.
79. Gladman DD, Charles-Schoeman C, McInnes IB, Veale DJ, Thiers B, Nurmohamed M, et al. Changes in lipid levels and incidence of cardiovascular events following tofactinib treatment in patients with psoriatic arthritis: a pooled analysis across phase III and long-term extension studies. Arthritis Care Res. 2019;71:1387–95.
80. Yates M, Mootoo A, Adams M, Bechman K, Rampes S, Patel V, et al. Venous thromboembolism risk with JAK inhibitors: a meta-analysis. Arthritis Rheum. 2020; https://doi.org/10.1002/art.41580.
81. Mease PJ, Lertratanakul A, Anderson JK, Papp K, Van den Bosch F, Tsuji S, et al. Upadacitinib for psoriatic arthritis refractory to biologics: SELECT-PsA 2. Ann Rheum Dis. 2020;80(3):312–20.
82. McInnes I, Anderson J, Magrey M, Merola JF, Liu Y, Kishimoto M, et al. Efficacy and safety of upadacitinib versus placebo and adalimumab in patients with active psoriatic arthritis and inadequate response to non-biologic disease-modifying anti-rheumatic drugs (SELECT-PsA-1): a double-blind, randomized controlled phase 3 trial (abstract). Ann Rheum Dis. 2020;79:16–7.
83. Deodhar A, Ranza R, Ganz F, Gao T, Anderson JK, Östör A. Efficacy and safety of upadacitinib in patients with psoriatic arthritis and axial involvement (abstract). Arthritis Rheumatol.

2020;72(suppl 10). https://acrabstracts.org/abstract/efficacy-and-safety-of-upadacitinib-in-patients-with-psoriatic-arthritis and axial-involvement/. Accessed 15 Dec 2020.
84. Mease P, Coates LC, Helliwell PS, Stanislavchuk M, Rychlewska-Hanczewska A, Dudek A, et al. Efficacy and safety of filgotinib, a selective janus kinase 1 inhibitor, in patients with active psoriatic arthritis (EQUATOR): results from a randomised, placebo-controlled, phase 2 trial. Lancet. 2018;392:2367–77.
85. Mease P, Deodhar A, van der Heijde D, Behrens F, Kivitz A, Kim J, et al. Efficacy and safety of deucravacitinib (BMS-986165), an oral, selective tyrosine kinase 2 inhibitor, in patients with active psoriatic arthritis: results from a phase 2, randomized, double-blind, placebo-controlled trial (abstract). Arthritis Rheumatol. 2020;72(suppl 10). https://acrabstracts.org/abstract/efficacy-and-safety-of-deucravacitinib-bms-986165-an-oral-selective-tyrosine-kinase-2-inhibitor-in-patients-with-active-psoriatic-arthritis-results-from-a-phase-2-randomized-double-blind-plac/. Accessed 15 Dec 2020.
86. Kavanaugh A, Mease PJ, Gomez-Reino JJ, Adebajo AO, Wollenhaupt J, Gladman DD, et al. Longterm (52-week) results of a phase III randomized, controlled trial of apremilast in patients with psoriatic arthritis. J Rheumatol. 2015;42:479–88.
87. Kavanaugh A, Gladman DD, Edwards CJ, Schett G, Guerette B, Delev N, et al. Long-term experience with apremilast in patients with psoriatic arthritis: 5-year results from a PALACE 1-3 pooled analysis. Arthritis Res Ther. 2019;21:118.
88. Gladman DD, Kavanaugh A, Gomez-Reino JJ, Wollenhaupt J, Cutolo M, Schett G, et al. Therapeutic benefit of apremilast on enthesiti and dactylitis in patients with psoriatic arthritis: a pooled analysis of the PALACE 1-3 studies. RMD Open. 2018;4:e000669.
89. Favalli EG, Conti F, Selmi C, Iannone F, Bucci R, D'Onofrio F, et al. Retrospective evaluation of patient profiling and effectiveness of apremilast in an Italian multicentric cohort of psoriatic arthritis patients. Clin Exp Rheumatol. 2020;38:19–26.
90. Singh JA, Guyatt G, Ogdie A, Gladman DD, Deal C, Deodhar A, et al. 2018 American College of Rheumatology/National Psoriasis Foundation guideline for the treatment of psoriatic arthritis. Arthritis Care Res. 2019;71:2–29.

Biologics in Gout

5

Abhishek

Case
A 55-year-old man with tophaceous gout and multiple recurrent mono- and oligo-articular gout flares in the previous 12-months is referred to the rheumatology clinic. He previously experienced hypersensitivity reaction to allopurinol, and deranged liver function tests with febuxostat. His serum urate is 9.1 mg/dL, and eGFR is 30 mL/min. Other comorbidities include staghorn calculi, hypertension, poorly controlled type-1 diabetes, and hyperlipidaemia. You are asked to advise on long-term urate-lowering treatment and management of gout flares.

5.1 Introduction

Xanthine Oxidase inhibitors (e.g. Allopurinol) and uricosuric drugs (e.g. Lesinurad, Sulfinpyrazone, Probenecid, and Benzbromarone) are recommended as first- and second-line drugs, respectively, in the long-term treatment of people with gout and recurrent flares. For the vast majority of patients, gout can be "cured" in a few years if these drugs are taken at doses that reduce the serum urate level to <6 mg/dL in a "treat-to-target" approach. Pegloticase, a biologic urate-lowering drug should be considered when conventional urate-lowering treatments (ULTs) cannot be prescribed due to inefficacy, intolerance, or contraindications (Box 5.1).

Gout flares are treated with low-dose prednisolone, colchicine, and NSAIDs and, these drugs are also used for flare prophylaxis when initiating treat-to-target ULT. However, anti-IL1 biologic agents may be used to prevent or treat gout flares

Abhishek (✉)
University of Nottingham, Nottingham, UK

Nottingham University Hospitals NHS Trust, Nottingham, UK
e-mail: abhishek.abhishek@nottingham.ac.uk

N. Jain, L. Duggal (eds.), *Handbook of Biologics for Rheumatological Disorders*,
https://doi.org/10.1007/978-981-16-7200-2_5

when these drugs are contraindicated (Box 5.1). Prescribers should check licenced indications of biologic drugs in their country before using them in the treatment of gout or, discuss with the patient that such use if off-label.

Box 5.1: Indications for the Use of Biologic Agents in the Treatment of Gout According to the 2020 American College of Rheumatology Gout Treatment Guidelines [1]

Indications for Pegloticase

- Failure to achieve serum urate <6 mg/dL despite a maximum tolerated dose of XOI treatment, uricosurics, their combination and other dietary and lifestyle interventions.
- Presence of subcutaneous tophi or frequent gout flares (≥2 flares/year).

Indications for using anti-IL1 agents

- Gout flare unresponsive to colchicine, NSAIDs, and corticosteroids.
- Contraindication or intolerance to the above anti-inflammatory therapies.

Indications for using anti-IL1 agents to prevent gout flares

- Contraindication or intolerance to colchicine, NSAIDs, and corticosteroids.

5.2 Urate Lowering Drugs

5.2.1 Pegloticase

- *Mechanisms of action*: Pegloticase is a mammalian PEGylated recombinant uricase enzyme that breaks down uric acid to more soluble, inert, and readily excreted allantoin. Due to an inactivating mutation in the uricase gene, humans are unable to metabolize uric acid.
- *Dosing*: It should be administered as an intravenous infusion (1 mL of 8 mg/mL Pegloticase diluted in 250 mL 0.9% or 0.45% Saline and administered over at least 2 h) twice a week for 6 months followed by twice weekly or monthly dosing [2, 3]. The diluted solution is stable at 2–8 °C and 20–25 °C for 4 h and the SmPC recommends treatment should be completed within 4 h of dilution.
- FDA approved for the treatment of "refractory gout". It may be used off-label for the initial treatment of people with high urate burden, e.g. multiple large tophi with or without destructive arthropathy.
- *Pre-medication, infusion, and post-infusion management*: Due to high risk of infusion reactions and anaphylaxis, Pegloticase infusions should be preceded by anti-histamines, paracetamol, and corticosteroids. In its replicate clinical trials,

patients were treated with oral fexofenadine, 60 mg the evening before and again before infusion; paracetamol, 1000 mg; and IV hydrocortisone, 200 mg, immediately before infusion [2].

  - Pegloticase should only be administered in healthcare settings with facilities to treat anaphylaxis. The infusion may be stopped and re-started at a lower rate, or the rate of infusion may be slowed if there are infusion reactions. Infusion reactions can occur after completion of infusion, and patients should be monitored for 1–2 h post-infusion.
- *Duration of treatment*: The optimal duration of Pegloticase treatment is not known, and, it is possible that low-dose XOI or uricosuric drugs may be used after initial control of gout using Pegloticase.
- *Efficacy profile*: At the above dose 47% of patients achieved serum urate <6 mg/dL on 80% occasions between months 3 and 6 of treatment and 40% experienced complete resolution of at least one tophus by month 6 [2]. In an open-label extension study, 60% of patients experienced complete resolution of at least one tophus by month 24 and serum urate reduction was maintained [3].

  Immunogenicity to Pegloticase is the primary reason for lack of response. Recently, methotrexate at a dose of 15–25 mg/week with folic acid has been used with Pegloticase to reduce the risk of immunogenicity [4, 5]. This strategy may be used in clinical practice, however, this is an unlicenced indication for methotrexate.
- *Safety profile*: Patients should be fully educated about these risks prior to treatment.
  - *Anaphylaxis*: Was reported in 6.5%* patients treated with Pegloticase in initial clinical trials [2].
  - *Infusion reaction*: Occurred in 26% to 41%* patients receiving Pegloticase at 2 weekly and 4 weekly intervals respectively [2].
  - Delayed-type hypersensitivity reactions have also been reported.

    *Patients in these studies received pre-medications that may have reduced the risk and/or severity of anaphylaxis and infusion reactions.
- Cautions and contraindications:
  - Contraindicated in patients with G6PD deficiency due to the risk of haemolysis and methaemoglobinaemia.
  - Some patients with heart failure experienced exacerbation of this condition when treated with Pegloticase in initial clinical trials. Extreme caution in this group is warranted.
  - Dose adjustments in renal impairment are not required.
  - Serum urate should be checked prior to each infusion, and, an increase in serum urate to >6 mg/dL, especially if present on two consecutive occasions indicates presence of neutralizing antibodies and higher risk of anaphylaxis. Because oral ULTs may blunt this rise in serum urate, concurrent use of these drugs with Pegloticase is not recommended.
  - Consideration should be given to discontinuing Pegloticase should the serum urate rise to >6 mg/dL after initial good response.

- Pegloticase causes impressive reductions in serum urate and consequent crystal mobilization and precipitates gout flares. Thus, gout flare prophylaxis should be started a week before the first infusion of Pegloticase and administered for at least 3 months when initiating treatment.

5.2.2 Rasburicase

This is a recombinant fungal uricase and is used to lower the serum urate in tumour lysis syndrome. It is highly immunogenic and is not used to treat hyperuricaemia in gout due to this.

5.3 Anti-IL1 Agents

The 2020 ACR guidelines conditionally recommend using drugs from this class for treating gout flares in settings where NSAIDs, colchicine, and corticosteroids cannot be used.

5.3.1 Anakinra

- *Mechanism of action*: Anti-IL1 receptor antagonist.
- *Dosing*: 100 mg by subcutaneous injection daily for 3–5 days.
- Reported to be effective in the treatment of gout flares unresponsive to conventional anti-inflammatory agents in case series and case reports.
- A double-blind placebo-controlled non-inferiority trial reported no difference in efficacy between a 5-day course of anakinra and conventional anti-inflammatory drugs in the treatment of gout flares [6].
- Based on trial data, Anakinra cannot be recommended over other inexpensive medicines such as colchicine, corticosteroids, and NSAIDs. However, Anakinra may be used when these drugs are contraindicated or not tolerated as it is non-inferior to these drugs in the treatment of gout flares.
- As anakinra is an anti-IL-1 blocking agent, it increases the risk of infections.
- Anakinra is not licenced in the USA or Europe for either treatment or prevention of gout flares and, use for this indication remains off-licence.

5.3.2 Rilonacept

- *Mechanism of action*: Rilonacept is a fully human, recombinant, soluble decoy receptor protein engineered from human IL-1 receptors and IgG1Fc that binds IL-1α and IL-1β, thus preventing their activation of cell surface receptors [7].
- *Dosing*: For treatment of gout flares: 320 mg/week [7]; For prevention of gout flares when initiating ULT: 160 or 320 mg loading dose followed by 80 or

160 mg/week. Lower dosages appear to be as effective in preventing gout flares as the higher dosages [8, 9].

- Rilonacept was not better than NSAID in treating gout flares and should not be used in place of first-line drugs to treat gout flares [7].
- Rilonacept was more effective than placebo in preventing gout flares over a 16-week period for patients initiated on Allopurinol 300 mg/day. The mean number of gout flares were 0.21 and 0.34, 0.29 and 0.35, and 1.06 and 1.23 for rilonacept 160 mg/week, rilonacept 80 mg/week, and placebo, respectively, in phase-III clinical trials [8, 9].
- Rilonacept is not licenced in the USA or Europe for either treatment or prevention of gout flares and any such use remains off-licence.

5.3.3 Canakinumab

- *Mechanism of action*: Canakinumab is a fully human anti-IL-1β monoclonal antibody [10].
- *Dosing*: For treating gout flares: 150 mg administered by subcutaneous injection; for preventing gout flares: ≥50 mg administered by subcutaneous injection [11].
- Canakinumab 150 mg subcutaneous injection was more effective than triamcinolone 40 mg intramuscular injection in the treatment of gout flare, with more rapid improvement in daily pain score (mean difference of 8.1 points by 24 h and 10.7 points by 72 h of treatment on a 0–100 mm Visual Analogue Scale for pain), and significantly lower CRP at 72 h and 1 week [10].
- However, it is extremely expensive, and its use is associated with cytopenia and serious infections requiring hospitalization in phase III clinical trials [10].
- Patients treated with canakinumab 150 mg subcutaneous injection were significantly less likely to experience another gout flare (Hazard Ratio (95%CI) 0.44 (0.32–0.60)) in the next 24 weeks than those treated with triamcinolone 40 mg intramuscular injection [10].
- In a dose ranging study, a single dose of at least 50 mg Canakinumab was more effective than colchicine 0.5 mg/day in preventing gout flares over a 16-week period in patients initiated on allopurinol. Forty-five percent patients treated with colchicine experienced at least 1 gout flare while 15–19% patients treated with at least 50 mg Canakinumab experienced at least one gout flare. Twenty-seven percent patients treated with 25 mg Canakinumab experienced at least one gout flare [11].
- Canakinumab is licenced by the EMEA for the symptomatic treatment of adults with frequent gout flares (>2 flares in the previous 12 months) in whom NSAIDs and colchicine are contraindicated, not tolerated, or do not provide an adequate response, and in whom repeated courses of corticosteroids are not appropriate. It is not approved by the FDA for the treatment of gout.
- Canakinumab is not licenced for the prophylaxis of gout flares when initiating ULT by either EMEA or FDA.

5.4 Summary

Biologic drugs provide the last chance for an improvement in quality of life for patients with difficult to treat gout and should be considered as a therapeutic option. Their use is limited by availability, cost, and restricted licenced indications.

References

1. FitzGerald JD, Dalbeth N, Mikuls T, et al. 2020 American College of Rheumatology guideline for the management of gout. Arthritis Care Res. 2020;72(6):744–60. https://doi.org/10.1002/acr.24180.
2. Sundy JS, Baraf HS, Yood RA, et al. Efficacy and tolerability of pegloticase for the treatment of chronic gout in patients refractory to conventional treatment: two randomized controlled trials. JAMA. 2011;306(7):711–20. https://doi.org/10.1001/jama.2011.1169.
3. Becker MA, Baraf HS, Yood RA, et al. Long-term safety of pegloticase in chronic gout refractory to conventional treatment. Ann Rheum Dis. 2013;72(9):1469–74. https://doi.org/10.1136/annrheumdis-2012-201795.
4. Botson JK, Tesser JRP, Bennett R, et al. Pegloticase in combination with methotrexate in patients with uncontrolled gout: a multicenter, open-label study (MIRROR). J Rheumatol. 2021;48(5):767–74. https://doi.org/10.3899/jrheum.200460.
5. Albert JA, Hosey T, LaMoreaux B. Increased efficacy and tolerability of pegloticase in patients with uncontrolled gout co-treated with methotrexate: a retrospective study. Rheumatol Ther. 2020;7(3):639–48. https://doi.org/10.1007/s40744-020-00222-7.
6. Janssen CA, Oude Voshaar MAH, Vonkeman HE, et al. Anakinra for the treatment of acute gout flares: a randomized, double-blind, placebo-controlled, active-comparator, non-inferiority trial. Rheumatology (Oxford). 2019; https://doi.org/10.1093/rheumatology/key402.
7. Terkeltaub RA, Schumacher HR, Carter JD, et al. Rilonacept in the treatment of acute gouty arthritis: a randomized, controlled clinical trial using indomethacin as the active comparator. Arthritis Res Ther. 2013;15(1):R25. https://doi.org/10.1186/ar4159.
8. Mitha E, Schumacher HR, Fouche L, et al. Rilonacept for gout flare prevention during initiation of uric acid-lowering therapy: results from the PRESURGE-2 international, phase 3, randomized, placebo-controlled trial. Rheumatology (Oxford). 2013;52(7):1285–92. https://doi.org/10.1093/rheumatology/ket114.
9. Schumacher HR Jr, Evans RR, Saag KG, et al. Rilonacept (interleukin-1 trap) for prevention of gout flares during initiation of uric acid-lowering therapy: results from a phase III randomized, double-blind, placebo-controlled, confirmatory efficacy study. Arthritis Care Res. 2012;64(10):1462–70. https://doi.org/10.1002/acr.21690.
10. Schlesinger N, Alten RE, Bardin T, et al. Canakinumab for acute gouty arthritis in patients with limited treatment options: results from two randomised, multicentre, active-controlled, double-blind trials and their initial extensions. Ann Rheum Dis. 2012;71(11):1839–48. https://doi.org/10.1136/annrheumdis-2011-200908.
11. Schlesinger N, Mysler E, Lin HY, et al. Canakinumab reduces the risk of acute gouty arthritis flares during initiation of allopurinol treatment: results of a double-blind, randomised study. Ann Rheum Dis. 2011;70(7):1264–71. https://doi.org/10.1136/ard.2010.144063.

Biologics in Systemic Lupus Erythematosus (SLE) 6

Chi Chiu Mok

6.1 Introduction

- SLE is a multisystemic autoimmune disease with an unpredictable course that consists of periods of remission and flares.
- The pathogenesis of SLE is unclear but multiple genetic, epigenetic, hormonal, and environmental factors are involved.

6.2 Unmet Needs in the Management of SLE

- The major reasons for mortality and morbidities of SLE are uncontrolled (refractory) disease activity (e.g., lupus nephritis [LN]) and therapy-related toxicities (especially glucocorticoids).
- Although survival of SLE has improved substantially, further improvement in recent years is hindered by the relatively slow development of novel therapies.
- Many randomized controlled trials (RCTs) of newer biological/targeted therapies failed to show benefits in SLE, which were related to the immunological and clinical heterogeneity of the disease, issues of study design, limitation of existing assessment tools, and potent background immunosuppression.
- More effective but less toxic therapeutic agents and appropriate patient stratification are needed to improve SLE care.

C. C. Mok (✉)
Department of Medicine, Tuen Mun Hospital, Hong Kong SAR, China

N. Jain, L. Duggal (eds.), *Handbook of Biologics for Rheumatological Disorders*,
https://doi.org/10.1007/978-981-16-7200-2_6

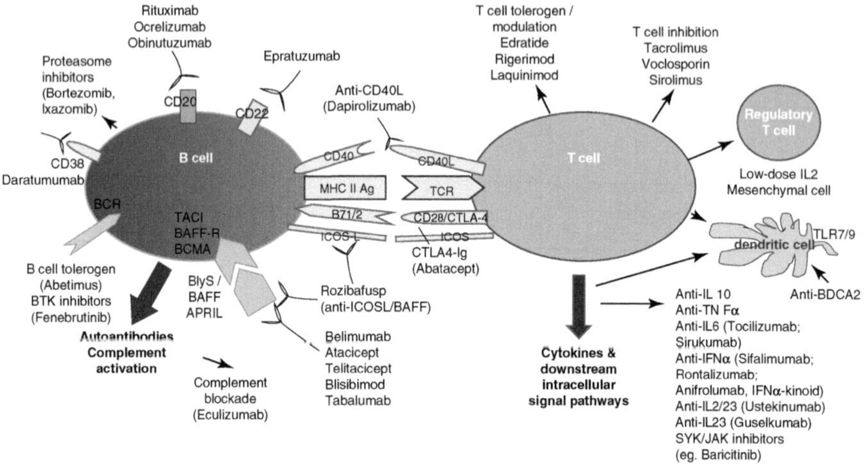

Fig. 6.1 Points of intervention in the immunological pathways of SLE

6.3 Points of Intervention in the Immunological Pathways of SLE (Fig. 6.1)

- Biological/targeted agents interact with cellular receptors, intracellular enzymes and molecules, cytokines, and other proteins to modulate immune activation, autoantibody production, and tissue inflammation (Table 6.1).

6.4 Biological Therapies for SLE

6.4.1 Targeting B Cell Growth and Survival Factors

- B lymphocyte stimulator (BlyS), or B cell-activating factor (BAFF), binds to three surface receptors of B cells (TACI, BCMA, and BAFF-R) and modulates their maturation, survival, proliferation, and immunoglobulin class switching.
- APRIL (a proliferation-inducing ligand), a homolog of BAFF that influences the survival and activation of B cells, binds to TACI and BCMA with a higher affinity compared to BAFF.
- BlyS mRNA and serum levels are increased in SLE patients and correlate with activity scores. Agents have been developed to inhibit BlyS, APRIL, or both (belimumab, tabalumab, blisibimod, and atacicept).

6.4.2 Belimumab

- Two phase 3 RCTs (BLISS-52/76) in seropositive SLE patients with SLEDAI score ≥ 6 and stable treatment were performed [1, 2]. Patients were randomized to intravenous (IV) belimumab or placebo (PBO) in combination with standard of care (SOC) therapies.

Table 6.1 Biologic/targeted agents in SLE trials

Drugs	Nature	Targets and actions	Pivotal studies	Background therapies	Dosage regimens in studies
Belimumab	mAb (H)	Soluble BAFF and prevents its interaction with the BAFF receptors	BLISS-52, BLISS-76, BLISS-SC, BLISS-LN (p3)	SOC	10 mg/kg (IV) every 2 weeks for 3 doses, then every 4 weeks; 200 mg (SC) weekly
Tabalumab	mAb (H)	Soluble and membrane-bound BAFF	ILLUMINATE1/2 (p3)	SOC	120 mg (SC) every 2 weeks
Blisibimod	Fusion protein	Soluble BAFF	CHABLIS-SC1 (p3)	SOC	200 mg (SC) once weekly
Atacicept	Fusion protein	Soluble and membrane-bound BAFF and APRIL	2RCTs (P2/3), ADDRESS II (p3)	SOC	75 mg/150 mg (SC) weekly
Rituximab	mAB (C)	CD20 on B cells, leading to depletion of B cells, from pre-B to memory B stage, with sparing of pro-B cells and plasma cells	EXPLORER, LUNAR (p3)	SOC, HD Pred + MMF	1 g 2-weekly for 2 doses × 2 courses (month 0 and 6)
Ocrelizumab	mAb (H)	CD20 on B cells	BEGIN, BELONG (p3)	HD Pred + MMF or euro-lupus CYC/AZA	IV (400 mg or 1000 mg) every 2 weeks for 2 doses; repeat after 4 months
Obinutuzumab	mAb (H)	CD20 on B cells (more ADCC, less CDC)	NOBILITY (p2)	HD pred + MMF/MPA	IV (1000 mg) infusion on days 1,15, 168, 182
Epratuzumab	mAb (H)	CD22 on B cells, modulate BCR signaling, cellular activation and survival	EMBODY 1/2 (p3)	SOC	IV 600 mg every week or 1200 mg every other week for 4 cycles
Abatacept	Fusion protein	Binds CD80/86 with a higher affinity than CD28, thus inhibits the co-stimulatory signal for T cell activation	RCT (p3), ACCESS (p2)	HD Pred + MMF, HD Pred + euro-lupus CYC/AZA	10 mg/kg or 500-1000 mg depending on body weight

(continued)

Table 6.1 (continued)

Drugs	Nature	Targets and actions	Pivotal studies	Background therapies	Dosage regimens in studies
Dapirolizumab	Fab fragment (H)	CD40L	RCT (p2b)	SOC	IV (6/23/45 mg/kg) every 4 weeks
Sirukumab	mAb (H)	IL-6	RCT (p2)	SOC	IV (10 mg/kg) every 4 weeks
Rontalizumab	mAb (H)	Neutralizes 12 subtypes of IFNα but does not bind to IFNβ or IFNω.	RCT (p2)	Existing therapies stopped except HCQ and Pred	750 mg IV every 4 weeks till week 20, followed by 300 mg SC every 2 weeks till week 22
Sifalimumab	mAb (H)	Binds and neutralizes most subtypes of IFNα	RCT (p2b)	SOC	IV (200/600/1200 mg) on days 1, 15 and 29, then every 28 days
Anifrolumab	mAb (H)	Type I IFN receptor—blocks signaling of type I IFNs, including IFNα, IFNβ, IFNε, IFNκ and IFNω	RCT (p2), 2RCTs (p3)	SOC	IV (150/300 mg) (p2); IV (300 mg) (p3) every 4 weeks
Interferon-α-kinoid	IFNα vaccine	Induces neutralizing antibodies against 13 IFNα subtypes	RCT (p2b)	SOC	Five injections of vaccine at days 0,7,28 and months 3 and 6
Ustekinumab	mAb (H)	IL-12 and IL-23 (p40 subunit)	RCT (p2)	SOC	IV 260-520 mg at week 0, followed by SC 90 mg every 8 weeks
Baricitinib	Jakinib	JAK1/2	RCT (p2)	SOC	2 or 4 mg/day
Fenebrutinib	BTKi	BTK	RCT (p2)	SOC	150 mg or 400 mg/day

mAb monoclonal antibody, *H* fully humanized, *C* chimeric, *BAFF* B cell activation factor, *SOC* standard of care, *p2* phase 2, *p3* phase 3, *RCT* randomized controlled trial, *IV* intravenous, *SC* subcutaneous, *HD* high-dose, *Pred* prednisolone, *MMF* mycophenolate mofetil, *MPA* mycophenolic acid, *CYC* cyclophosphamide, *AZA* azathioprine, *HCQ* hydroxychloroquine, *IL* interleukin, *JAK* Janus kinase, *ADCC* antibody dependent cytotoxicity, *CDC* complement dependent cytotoxicity, *BCR* B cell receptor, *IFN* interferon, *BTKi* Bruton tyrosine kinase inhibitor

- The primary efficacy endpoint was the SRI (SLE responder index)-4 response (improvement in SLEDAI scores ≥4, no worsening of British Isles Lupus Assessment Group [BILAG] [new A or two B flares] and physicians' global assessment [PGA] [increase ≥0.3]). Both trials showed significantly higher SRI-4 rates in belimumab (10 mg/kg) than PBO groups (58% vs 44% in BLISS-52; and 43% vs 34% in BLISS-76). Belimumab was more effective than PBO in the musculoskeletal and mucocutaneous domains of BILAG.

- Patient subsets with SLEDAI ≥10, anti-dsDNA positivity, depressed complements, or steroid use at baseline had higher rates of SRI-4 and other secondary endpoints (severe SLE flares, steroid-sparing effect, improvement in quality of life and fatigue) to belimumab.
- In phase 2/3 trials, the frequencies of adverse events (AEs) and serious AEs (SAEs), including serious infections and cancer, were not higher with belimumab, except for depression and suicide (numerically more common).
- Serious infusion reaction, which might be delayed, was more frequent in belimumab than PBO (0.9% vs 0.4%).
- Extension of the BLISS studies for 8 years in those who were continuously treated with belimumab showed a static yearly incidence of AEs and SAEs [3]. Majority (88%) of patients did not have an increase in SLICC/ACR SLE damage index compared to baseline, indicating low organ damage accrual and a stable safety profile of belimumab.
- Post-marketing experience: Belimumab is most frequently used in refractory musculoskeletal and mucocutaneous manifestations. Clinical improvement and a steroid-sparing effect were achieved in 49–78% of patients.
- Belimumab is not indicated in patients with severe renal or neuropsychiatric (NP) SLE.
- In a RCT (BLISS-SC), SLE patients with SLEDAI ≥8 were randomized to receive weekly subcutaneous (SC) belimumab or PBO in combination with SOC for 52 weeks [4]. Similar to IV belimumab, the SC preparation was associated with a significantly higher SRI-4 response than PBO (61% vs 48%).
- IV belimumab is approved for treatment of adult and pediatric (age ≥5 years) patients with active, autoantibody-positive SLE despite standard therapies. The SC preparation has also been approved in adult patients with the same indications.
- A phase 3 RCT (BLISS-LN) showed that IV belimumab increased the renal response rates at 104 weeks when added to SOC treatment (mycophenolate mofetil [MMF] and glucocorticoids in 74% patients) in patients with LN without increasing the incidence of AEs [5].

6.4.3 Tabalumab

- Two phase 3 RCTs of SC tabalumab in moderate/severe active SLE without serious renal or NP manifestations were published [6, 7].
- The primary efficacy endpoint (SRI-5 response) was met in one study but not in the other, although SAEs and treatment-emergent AEs (TEAEs) were not more common with tabalumab treatment. Further clinical trial of the drug was halted.

6.4.4 Blisibimod

- A phase 3 RCT (CHABLIS-SC1) randomized autoantibody-positive SLE patients with active disease (SLEDAI ≥10) to receive either SC blisibimod or PBO in combination with SOC [8].
- The SRI-6 response (primary outcome) was not significantly different between blisibimod and PBO at week 52 (47% vs 42%).

6.4.5 Atacicept

- A phase 2/3 RCT of atacicept in patients with active LN who were treated with background high-dose steroid and MMF was halted for the development of serious infections [9].
- Another phase 2/3 RCT randomized patients with active SLE (≥1 BILAG A and/or B) to receive two doses of SC atacicept or PBO with a steroid taper [10]. The primary outcome, percentage of patients having a new BILAG A/B flare, was not achieved in the atacicept (75 mg) arm.
- The atacicept 150 mg arm was terminated because of fatal pulmonary infections in two patients. TEAEs (including serious infections) were not different across the three groups.
- Patients with increased serum BlyS and APRIL levels achieved a greater reduction in lupus flares.
- Despite the increased risk of infections with atacicept, a 24-week phase 2b RCT (ADDRESS II) in seropositive SLE patients with active disease (SLEDAI-2K ≥6) despite SOC was repeated [11]. No increase in TEAEs (including serious infections) was demonstrated in users of atacicept (75 mg/150 mg).
- Although the primary SRI-4 endpoint was not met, subgroups of patients with more active disease at baseline (SLEDAI-2K ≥10) or active lupus serology, or both, achieved a significantly higher SRI-4 and SRI-6 rates in the atacicept arms.
- Further studies are necessary in view of the conflicting evidence in efficacy and toxicity.

6.4.6 Targeting B Cell Surface Molecules

6.4.6.1 Rituximab

- Two pivotal RCTs of rituximab in SLE were performed.
- The EXPLORER study randomized patients with moderate/severe extra-renal SLE (≥1 BILAG A or ≥2 BILAG B domains) despite SOC [12] to receive either rituximab or PBO (two courses 6 months apart).
- Clinical responses (major and partial), disease activity scores, flares, and time to flare did not show statistically significant differences between the two groups, although rituximab was not associated with increased rates of AEs and SAEs.
- The LUNAR study included patients with active LN (class III/IV) using a similar protocol [13]. Patients were randomized to receive rituximab or PBO in addition to steroid and MMF.
- At week 52, the primary and secondary endpoints did not show statistically significant differences between the two groups.
- Hypotension, leukopenia, infusion-related reactions, herpes zoster (HZ), and opportunistic infections were more numerically more frequent in patients treated with rituximab.

- Post-marketing experience: 13% SLE patients developed infusion reaction to rituximab (serious in 12% and delayed in 29%). Serious infections: 6.6/100 patient-years.
- Despite benefits not shown in RCTs, rituximab is often used off-label to treat refractory SLE. Clinical response to rituximab was reported in 67–86% of SLE patients with various refractory manifestations such as articular, mucocutaneous, renal, and hematological disease.
- Rituximab (375 mg/m^2 weekly × 4 doses or 1 g 2-weekly × 2 doses) was often administered in combination with steroid and/or cyclophosphamide (CYC), MMF, azathioprine (AZA), and methotrexate (68–76% cases).

6.4.6.2 Ocrelizumab

- A phase 3 double-blind RCT of ocrelizumab in non-renal SLE (BEGIN) was terminated prematurely [14].
- Another RCT (BELONG) [15] recruited patients with active LN (class III/IV) to receive ocrelizumab for two doses or PBO in combination with high-dose steroid and either MMF or Euro-Lupus CYC/AZA.
- This study was also terminated prematurely for an excess rate of serious infections in the ocrelizumab group.
- In patients who completed ≥32 weeks' treatment, the renal response rate of the combined ocrelizumab groups was numerically higher than PBO.

6.4.6.3 Obinutuzumab

- Obinutuzumab is a newer generation anti-CD20 monoclonal antibody that induces greater B cell cytotoxicity than rituximab.
- Results of a phase 2 RCT in patients with class III/IV LN showed superiority of this biologic to PBO when combined with steroid and MMF or mycophenolic acid (MPA) [16].

6.4.6.4 Epratuzumab

- Two phase 3 RCTs (EMBODY 1/2) recruited seropositive SLE patients with moderate/severe activity (SLEDAI-2K ≥6, BILAG ≥1A or ≥2Bs in mucocutaneous, musculoskeletal, or cardiorespiratory domains) despite SOC to receive epratuzumab (two doses) or PBO infusion [17].
- The primary endpoint, BILAG-based combined lupus assessment (BICLA) response rate at week 48, was not significantly different between the epratuzumab and PBO groups.
- AEs and TEAEs were, however, similar across all treatment arms.

6.4.6.5 Daratumumab

- Daratumumab is an anti-CD38 monoclonal antibody that depletes plasma cells.
- A recent report described two SLE patients with refractory disease responding clinically to daratumumab in addition to SOC, with documented depletion of the long-lived plasma cells [18].
- The safety and efficacy of daratumumab in SLE has to be confirmed by further studies.

6.4.7 Targeting Co-Stimulatory Molecules

6.4.7.1 Abatacept

- A phase 2/3 RCT recruited patients with active class III/IV LN to be randomized to IV abatacept (two dosing regimens) or PBO infusion in combination with steroid and MMF [19].
- The primary endpoint, time to complete renal response, was not significantly different in the abatacept group as compared to PBO at week 52.
- However, HZ infection, gastroenteritis, and SAEs were non-significantly more frequent in abatacept users.
- Another phase 2 RCT randomized patients with class III/IV LN (ACCESS) to receive IV abatacept or PBO in combination with high-dose steroid and the Euro-Lupus CYC regimen [20].
- The rate of complete renal response was not significantly higher in the abatacept group at week 24.
- The rates of partial response, AEs and SAEs, and other secondary endpoints were also similar between the two groups.

6.4.7.2 Dapirolizumab

- Despite an earlier study of anti-CD40L monoclonal antibody (ruplizumab) raised the concern of thromboembolism in SLE, a newer anti-CD40L molecule that consists of a Fab fragment conjugated to polyethylene glycol and lacks the Fc portion (dapirolizumab pegol) was tested in moderate/severe nonrenal SLE in a phase 2 trial [21].
- Preliminary results demonstrated safety and greater improvement in multiple endpoints as compared to PBO at week 24. However, a dose response relationship was not observed.

6.4.8 Combination/Sequential Biological Therapies

- Rituximab treatment leads to variable B cell depletion and time to repopulation (particularly memory B cells and plasmablasts), which might contribute to the differential clinical response and lupus flares.
- Rise of BlyS level after rituximab treatment, which may contribute to reduced response and more flare, may be reduced by concomitant belimumab therapy.
- A phase 2a proof-of-concept study (SynBioSe) of combined rituximab and belimumab in refractory SLE has reported safety of the regimen [22]. Three RCTs with similar objectives are ongoing: BLISS-BELIEVE (combined SC belimumab and rituximab vs belimumab ± SOC), CALIBRATE (IV CYC-rituximab with vs without belimumab in LN), and BEAT-LUPUS (SOC + rituximab, followed by belimumab vs PBO 4–8 weeks later).

6.4.9 Targeting Cytokines

6.4.9.1 IL-6

- Elevation of IL-6 was demonstrated in SLE and correlated with disease activity.
- Despite a phase I study showed promise of IL-6 receptor blockade (tocilizumab) in SLE patients with mild/moderate activity [23], a phase 2 proof-of-concept RCT of an anti-IL6 monoclonal antibody (sirukumab) in refractory LN [24] did not demonstrate the anticipated efficacy or safety.

6.4.9.2 Type I Interferons (IFNs)

- In SLE, type I IFNs are produced by plasmacytoid dendritic cells when induced by immune complexes.
- IFNα promotes T cell activation and autoantibody production by B cells.
- Levels of IFN-α, IFN-driven chemokines and expression of IFN-regulated genes increased in SLE patients and correlated with activity score.
- Two monoclonal antibodies (rontalizumab and sifalimumab) that direct against IFNα and one monoclonal antibody against the IFNα receptor (anifrolumab) have been developed.

6.4.9.3 Rontalizumab

- A phase 2 study was conducted in SLE patients with moderate/severe nonrenal disease (≥1 BILAG A or ≥2 BILAG B domains) [25].
- Participants were randomized to receive rontalizumab or PBO. At week 24, the BILAG and SRI response rates were not different between the rontalizumab and PBO groups.
- Although a significant increase in viral or other infectious AEs was not observed with rontalizumab, further development of this biologic was halted.

6.4.9.4 Sifalimumab

- A phase 2 RCT [26] randomized seropositive SLE patients with active disease (SLEDAI of ≥6, ≥1 BILAG A or ≥2 BILAG B, and PGA ≥1) to receive IV sifalimumab or PBO in addition to SOC.
- At week 52, the SRI-4 response rate was significantly higher in the 1200 mg group compared to PBO (60% vs 45%; $p = 0.03$).
- Sin scores (CLASI) and joint counts also improved.
- Patients with baseline high IFN signature responded better to sifalimumab.
- Sifalimumab was generally well-tolerated but HZ reactivation was more common.
- Further trial of this biologic was not pursued.

6.4.9.5 Anifrolumab

- A phase 2b RCT included nonrenal SLE patients with active disease despite SOC [27].
- Participants were randomized to IV anifrolumab or PBO monthly for 48 weeks.

- The SRI-4 response (primary endpoint) and a persistent steroid-sparing effect were met in the anifrolumab group (300 mg) compared to PBO at day 169 (34% vs 18%; $p = 0.01$).
- Achievement of secondary endpoints (SRI-4, reduction in steroid dosage, improvement in skin and joint activity) were also significantly more common in those treated with anifrolumab.
- Improvement in multiple endpoints was more pronounced in patients with high IFN signature.
- AEs were not more common in anifrolumab users except for influenza and HZ infections.
- A phase 3 RCT (TULIP-2) in patients with active SLE (SLEDAI-2K ≥6 and clinical SLEDAI-2K ≥4) receiving SOC therapies showed superiority of IV anifrolumab (300 mg) to PBO in achieving a BICLA response at week 52 (47.8% vs 31.5%; $p = 0.001$) [28].
- Secondary endpoints (glucocorticoid dose reduction, severity of skin disease) were also in favor of anifrolumab.
- However, HZ infection was more frequent in anifrolumab-treated patients (7.2% vs 1.1%).

6.4.9.6 Interferon-α-Kinoid (IFN-K)

- Active immunization of IFN-K generates neutralizing antibodies against 13 subtypes of IFNα.
- A recent phase 2b RCT in ANA positive SLE patients with moderate/severe disease activity (SLEDAI-2 K ≥6 and 1 BILAG A ± 2 BILAG B scores) and positive IFN signature showed that IFN-K was well-tolerated and did not lead to more TEAEs than PBO [29].
- Achievement of a low disease activity state and a steroid-sparing effect was in favor of IFN-K.

6.4.9.7 IL-12/23

- Ustekinumab is a monoclonal antibody targeting IL12/23.
- In a phase 2 RCT, seropositive SLE patients with active disease (SLEDAI-2K ≥6 and 1 BILAG A ± 2 BILAG B) were randomized to receive ustekinumab or PBO in combination with SOC [30].
- The SRI-4 response was significantly higher in the ustekinumab group at week 24 (62% vs 33%; $p = 0.006$).
- Improvement of active joint count was not better but improvement in ≥50% of the skin score (CLASI) was significantly more common with ustekinumab (53% vs 35%; $p = 0.03$).
- The frequency of AEs or infections was similar between ustekinumab and PBO.
- A phase 3 RCT of ustekinumab in SLE (LOTUS) was prematurely terminated for the lack of efficacy on interim analysis.

6.4.10 Targeting Intracellular Pathways

6.4.10.1 JAK Inhibition and Other Small Molecules

- Targeting the downstream intracellular signaling pathways from the type I/II cytokine receptors mediated by the JAK-STAT proteins allows simultaneous suppression of multiple cytokines. A number of Jakinibs have been developed.
- In a phase 2 RCT, SLE patients with active joint/skin disease were randomly assigned to receive baricitinib or PBO in combination with SOC [31].
- At week 24, resolution of skin disease or arthritis was significantly more frequent in the baricitinib 4 mg group (67% vs 53%, $p = 0.04$), and so was the SRI-4 response (64% vs 48%; $p = 0.02$).
- The number of tender joints, but not the severity of skin lesions, was reduced significantly in the baricitinib group.
- Serious infections were nonsignificantly more frequent in the baricitinib 4 mg group (6%) than PBO (1%). Deep vein thrombosis developed in one patient (1%) treated with baricitinib 4 mg.
- Although the effect size of baricitinib in reducing tender joints was small, two further phase 3 RCTs in nonrenal SLE are in progress.
- Bruton's tyrosine kinase (BTK) is a mediator of B-cell receptor and Fc receptor signaling of innate immune cells such as monocytes. A phase 2 RCT of fenebrutinib, a BTK inhibitor, in SLE did not meet the primary endpoint of SRI-4 at week 48 [32]. Another BTK inhibitor, evobrutinib, is being evaluated in SLE (phase 2 RCT).

6.4.10.2 Other Biological Agents and New Molecules

- Lulizumab pegol (anti-CD28), eculizumab (terminal complement inhibitor), anti-IFNγ, voclosporin (a newer generation calcineurin inhibitor), proteasome inhibitors (bortezomib, ixazomib), RNase, edratide, rigerimod, and laquinimod.

6.5 Conclusions

- Despite the futility of many recent trials of biologics in SLE, quest for novel therapies for this disease continues.
- Minimizing the PBO response by reducing background immunosuppression and adoption of organ-specific disease activity indices may better differentiate the treatment effect from PBO.
- Novel endpoints such as low disease activity state and percentage improvement of validated composite indices should be further explored.
- The long-term safety and cost-effectiveness of novel therapeutics in serious or refractory SLE manifestations have to be investigated.

References

1. Navarra SV, Guzmán RM, Gallacher AE, et al. Efficacy and safety of belimumab in patients with active systemic lupus erythematosus: a randomised, placebo-controlled, phase 3 trial. Lancet. 2011;377:721–31.
2. Furie R, Petri M, Zamani O, et al. BLISS-76 Study Group. A phase III, randomized, placebo-controlled study of belimumab, a monoclonal antibody that inhibits B lymphocyte stimulator, in patients with systemic lupus erythematosus. Arthritis Rheum. 2011;63:3918–30.
3. van Vollenhoven RF, Navarra SV, Levy RA, et al. Long-term safety and limited organ damage in patients with systemic lupus erythematosus treated with belimumab: a phase III study extension. Rheumatology (Oxford). 2020;59:281–91.
4. Stohl W, Schwarting A, Okada M, et al. Efficacy and safety of subcutaneous belimumab in systemic lupus erythematosus: a fifty-two-week randomized, double-blind, placebo-controlled study. Arthritis Rheumatol. 2017;69:1016–27.
5. Furie R, Rovin BH, Houssiau F, et al. Two-year, randomized, controlled trial of belimumab in lupus nephritis. N Engl J Med. 2020;383:1117–28.
6. Isenberg DA, Petri M, Kalunian K, et al. Efficacy and safety of subcutaneous tabalumab in patients with systemic lupus erythematosus: results from ILLUMINATE-1, a 52-week, phase III, multicentre, randomised, double-blind, placebo-controlled study. Ann Rheum Dis. 2016;75:323–31.
7. Merrill JT, van Vollenhoven RF, Buyon JP, et al. Efficacy and safety of subcutaneous tabalumab, a monoclonal antibody to B-cell activating factor, in patients with systemic lupus erythematosus: results from ILLUMINATE-2, a 52-week, phase III, multicentre, randomised, double-blind, placebo-controlled study. Ann Rheum Dis. 2016;75:332–40.
8. Merrill JT, Shanahan WR, Scheinberg M, et al. Phase III trial results with blisibimod, a selective inhibitor of B-cell activating factor, in subjects with systemic lupus erythematosus (SLE): results from a randomised, double-blind, placebo-controlled trial. Ann Rheum Dis. 2018;77:883–9.
9. Ginzler EM, Wax S, Rajeswaran A, et al. Atacicept in combination with MMF and corticosteroids in lupus nephritis: results of a prematurely terminated trial. Arthritis Res Ther. 2012;14:R33.
10. Isenberg D, Gordon C, Licu D, et al. Efficacy and safety of atacicept for prevention of flares in patients with moderate-to-severe systemic lupus erythematosus (SLE): 52-week data (APRIL-SLE randomised trial). Ann Rheum Dis. 2015;74:2006–15.
11. Merrill JT, Wallace DJ, Wax S, et al. ADDRESS II investigators. Efficacy and safety of atacicept in patients with systemic lupus erythematosus: results of a twenty-four-week, multicenter, randomized, double-blind, placebo-controlled, parallel-arm, phase IIb study. Arthritis Rheumatol. 2018;70:266–76.
12. Merrill JT, Neuwelt CM, Wallace DJ, et al. Efficacy and safety of rituximab in moderately-to-severely active systemic lupus erythematosus: the randomized, double-blind, phase II/III systemic lupus erythematosus evaluation of rituximab trial. Arthritis Rheum. 2010;62:222–33.
13. Rovin BH, Furie R, Latinis K, et al. LUNAR Investigator Group. Efficacy and safety of rituximab in patients with active proliferative lupus nephritis: the lupus nephritis assessment with rituximab study. Arthritis Rheum. 2012;64:1215–26.
14. Reddy V, Jayne D, Close D, Isenberg D. B-cell depletion in SLE: clinical and trial experience with rituximab and ocrelizumab and implications for study design. Arthritis Res Ther. 2013;15(Suppl 1):S2.
15. Mysler EF, Spindler AJ, Guzman R, et al. Efficacy and safety of ocrelizumab in active proliferative lupus nephritis: results from a randomized, double-blind, phase III study. Arthritis Rheum. 2013;65:2368–79.
16. Furie RA, Aroca G, Cascino MD, et al. B-cell depletion with obinutuzumab for the treatment of proliferative lupus nephritis: a randomised, double-blind, placebo-controlled trial. Ann Rheum Dis. 2021 Oct 6 [in press].

17. Clowse ME, Wallace DJ, Furie RA, et al. Efficacy and safety of epratuzumab in moderately to severely active systemic lupus erythematosus: results from two phase 3, randomized, double-blind, placebo-controlled trials, EMBODY™ 1 and EMBODY™ 2. Arthritis Rheumatol. 2017;69:362–75.
18. Ostendorf L, Burns M, Durek P, et al. Targeting CD38 with daratumumab in refractory systemic lupus erythematosus. N Engl J Med. 2020;383:1149–55.
19. Furie R, Nicholls K, Cheng TT, et al. Efficacy and safety of abatacept in lupus nephritis: a twelve-month, randomized, double-blind study. Arthritis Rheumatol. 2014;66:379–89.
20. ACCESS Trial Group. Treatment of lupus nephritis with abatacept: the abatacept and cyclophosphamide combination efficacy and safety study. Arthritis Rheumatol. 2014;66:3096–104.
21. Furie R, Bruce IN, Dorner T, et al. Efficacy and safety of dapirolizumab pegol in patients with moderately to severely active systemic lupus erythematosus: a randmomised placebo-controlled study. Ann Rheum Dis. 2019;78(Suppl2):A775.
22. Kraaij T, Kamerling SWA, de Rooij ENM, et al. The NET-effect of combining rituximab with belimumab in severe systemic lupus erythematosus. J Autoimmun. 2018;91:45–54.
23. Illei GG, Shirota Y, Yarboro CH, et al. Tocilizumab in systemic lupus erythematosus: data on safety, preliminary efficacy, and impact on circulating plasma cells from an open-label phase I dosage-escalation study. Arthritis Rheum. 2010;62:542–52.
24. Rovin BH, van Vollenhoven RF, Aranow C, et al. A multicenter, randomized, double-blind, placebo-controlled study to evaluate the efficacy and safety of treatment with sirukumab (CNTO 136) in patients with active lupus nephritis. Arthritis Rheumatol. 2016;68:2174–83.
25. Kalunian KC, Merrill JT, Maciuca R, et al. A phase II study of the efficacy and safety of rontalizumab (rhuMAb interferon-α) in patients with systemic lupus erythematosus (ROSE). Ann Rheum Dis. 2016;75:196–202.
26. Khamashta M, Merrill JT, Werth VP, et al. Sifalimumab, an anti-interferon-α monoclonal antibody, in moderate to severe systemic lupus erythematosus: a randomised, double-blind, placebo-controlled study. Ann Rheum Dis. 2016;75:1909–16.
27. Furie R, Khamashta M, Merrill JT, et al. Anifrolumab, an anti-interferon-α receptor monoclonal antibody, in moderate-to-severe systemic lupus erythematosus. Arthritis Rheumatol. 2017;69:376–86.
28. Morand EF, Furie R, Tanaka Y, et al. Trial of anifrolumab in active systemic lupus erythematosus. N Engl J Med. 2020;382:211–21.
29. Houssiau F, Thanou A, Mazur M, et al. IFN-α kinoid in systemic lupus erythematosus: results from a phase IIb, randomised, placebo-controlled study. Ann Rheum Dis. 2020;79:347–55.
30. van Vollenhoven RF, Hahn BH, Tsokos GC, et al. Efficacy and safety of ustekinumab, an IL-12 and IL-23 inhibitor, in patients with active systemic lupus erythematosus: results of a multicentre, double-blind, phase 2, randomised, controlled study. Lancet. 2018;392:1330–9.
31. Wallace DJ, Furie RA, Tanaka Y, et al. Baricitinib for systemic lupus erythematosus: a double-blind, randomised, placebo-controlled, phase 2 trial. Lancet. 2018;392:222–31.
32. Isenberg DA, Furie RA, Jones NS, et al. Efficacy, safety and pharmacodynamic effects of the Bruton's tyrosine kinase inhibitor, fenebrutinib (GDC-0853), in moderate to severe systemic lupus erythematosus in a phase 2 controlled study [abstract]. Ann Rheum Dis. 2020;79(Suppl 1):148.

Biologics in Sjogren's Syndrome

7

Elizabeth Price

7.1 Introduction

Sjögren's syndrome (SS) is a chronic, autoimmune disease of unknown cause for which, to date, there is no known curative nor true disease-modifying treatment. Patients experience widespread dryness, affecting the eyes, mouth, respiratory, gastrointestinal and urogenital tracts. Systemic manifestations, including inflammatory arthritis, skin and haematological disease, neuropathies and lung involvement, are common. Up to 20% have co-existent autoimmune conditions, most commonly thyroid disease but also primary biliary cholangitis, pernicious anaemia and other rheumatic diseases such as scleroderma. There is prominent B-cell lymphoproliferation with a 15 fold increased lifetime risk of B-cell lymphoma compared to the normal population [1–3].

Traditionally the management of SS has focused on conserving, replacing and stimulating secretions. With the increasing understanding of the underlying immunological pathways in rheumatic diseases, the focus is now on effective treatment early in the disease to suppress underlying systemic disease activity with the aim of preventing permanent damage and systemic complications. To date, this approach has not been wholly successful in SS, but progress is being made, and new therapeutic targets are being identified and tested.

7.2 Rationale for Biologics in Sjogren's Syndrome

SS is characterised by a distinctive array of biological and serological abnormalities. Histologically lymphocytic infiltration of exocrine glands, most notably the saliva and lacrimal glands, is a classical finding. Lymphocytic infiltrates can also be

E. Price (✉)
Great Western Hospital NHS FT, Swindon, UK
e-mail: elizabeth.price5@nhs.net

N. Jain, L. Duggal (eds.), *Handbook of Biologics for Rheumatological Disorders*,
https://doi.org/10.1007/978-981-16-7200-2_7

found in other organs, such as the lungs and liver, when they are associated with specific clinical features. SS is also associated with a high prevalence of B-cell lymphoma, with the incidence of this increasing with the length of disease [3]. In early disease, the infiltrates are predominantly CD4+ T cells, which produce pro-inflammatory cytokines, including IFN-gamma, IL-17 and IL-21, causing local inflammation and inducing B-cell activation [4]. In later, more advanced disease B-cells predominate and contribute to the hypergammaglobulinaemia, increased free light chains and beta2-microglobulin and the characteristic anti-Ro and anti-La antibodies [5]. Consequently, either T or B-cells or the cytokines they produce might be considered potential therapeutic targets.

7.3 Rituximab

- Rituximab is a chimaeric anti-CD20 monoclonal initially licenced for the treatment of B-cell lymphoma but now routinely used in rheumatoid arthritis and Systemic lupus erythematosus (SLE). It binds to CD-20 on the surface of mature B-cells leading to cell lysis. Rapid B-cell depletion in seen in the peripheral blood followed by a slow recovery, and levels usually return to normal within 6–12 months post-treatment.
- The inflammatory infiltrates in Sjogren's consist of both T and B-cell infiltrates with B-cells predominating in the germinal centres within the salivary gland, supporting the use of B-cell depleting agents.
- An initial open-label study of rituximab in a small cohort of patients with early SS confirmed effective B-cell depletion and appeared to demonstrate clinical improvement, especially in those with residual glandular function [6] and was followed by a flurry of case reports and small case series reporting successful treatment of systemic complications including lymphoma, immune thrombocytopaenia, cryoglobulinaemia, membranoproliferative glomerulonephritis and neurological disease in patients with SS [6–16].
- Two small randomised controlled trials (RCT's) over 24 and 48 weeks suggested beneficial effects on fatigue [17] and salivary flow rates [18]. However, neither of the subsequent larger Phase III placebo-controlled trials reached their primary endpoint [19, 20], evaluating patient-reported improvements in pain, fatigue and dryness.
- The TEARS study included 120 patients with active disease randomised to either two infusions of Rituximab 2 weeks apart or placebo [19]. This study failed to achieve a significant improvement in visual analogue scale (VAS) measures of dryness, global disease activity, fatigue and pain despite an improvement in salivary flow rates and measurable laboratory response.
- The TRACTISS trial of 133 patients gave two infusions of rituximab at baseline and repeated at 6 months [20]. Again there were no significant improvements in outcomes overall, although the authors noted a small improvement in unstimulated salivary flow rates.

- Two systematic reviews and a meta-analysis of rituximab treatment for Sjogren's [21, 22] concluded that although there was some weak evidence of an improvement in lacrimal gland function, there was no overall evidence of improvement in oral dryness, fatigue or Quality of Life (QoL) and insufficient evidence to support routine use. There is some evidence, however, that it may have a role to play in patients with specific organ manifestations, including interstitial lung disease [23].
- The North American guideline group concluded that there was sufficient evidence to suggest rituximab in those patients for whom conventional therapies, including immunomodulators, had proven insufficient. They recommended that it was considered for those with a range of systemic complications, including vasculitis, severe parotid swelling, inflammatory arthritis, pulmonary disease and peripheral neuropathy [24, 25].
- The most recent European guidelines have suggested Rituximab may be considered for patients with severe, refractory systemic disease, especially those with cryoglobulimaemic vasculitis [26].

7.4 Belimumab

- Treatment with B-cell depleting agents results in up-regulation of B lymphocyte activating factor (BAFF). This may partially explain the disappointing outcome of the rituximab studies [27].
- Belimumab is a fully human monoclonal antibody targeting BAFF and has been trialled and approved for use in SLE. A small open-label study of Belimumab in patients with active SS recruited 30 patients and demonstrated a small but significant improvement in the ESSDAI score from baseline. The effect was most marked in the glandular domain [28]. There are theoretical reasons to support the combination use of rituximab and belimumab and some evidence of efficacy in a single reported case [29, 30].
- Belimumab is currently being studied in combination with rituximab, with the latter being used to induce B-cell depletion and belimumab being utilised to maintain the effect. In the meantime, the European guidelines have suggested Belimumab as rescue therapy in those with severe systemic disease refractory to conventional immunosuppression and rituximab [26].

7.5 Abatacept

- Abatacept blocks the CD28:CD80/CD86 T cell co-stimulatory pathway and is an established safe and effective treatment for RA [31]. An initial open-label pilot study of abatacept in 11 patients with primary SS showed a reduction in glandular inflammation and improvement in salivary flow [32].
- A subsequent open-label proof of concept study in 15 patients found that the drug was well tolerated with improvement in fatigue and health-related quality of life measures. Despite this, there no change in objective measures of glandular function over a 24-week treatment period [33].

- A longer-term open-label prospective observational study of 11 patients on abatacept for 24 months showed small but statistically significant improvements in salivary flow and ESSDAI score but no improvement in fatigue or ocular symptoms or signs [34]. However, a recent randomised double-blind study of abatacept in 80 patients with SS—The ASAP III study—showed no difference in the primary outcome of between-group difference in ESSDAI score at week 24, leading the authors to conclude that they could not recommend abatacept as a treatment for SS [35].

7.6 Anti-CD40 and Anti-CD40 Ligand

- The co-stimulatory molecule CD40 and its ligand have been identified as potential therapeutic targets in SS [36]. CD40 is found on multiple cell types, including B-cells. Interaction between CD40 and its ligand, CD40L, on the surface of both T cells and activated B-cells causes B-cell activation and is instrumental in the germinal centre formation, T cell activation and cytokine release [36].
- An in-vitro study found higher CD40 expression in patients with SS compared to controls, and CD40L staining was noted on infiltrating lymphocytes within their salivary glands [37]. All of this points to a role for CD40-CD40L in SS. Supporting this view lockade of CD40L in mouse models significantly ameliorates autoimmunity [38].
- In early trials in SLE treatment with anti-CD40L reduced levels of dsDNA antibodies, increased complement levels and reduced glomerular inflammation but was associated with an increase in thrombotic events [39].
- Iscalimab (also known as ZF-533) is a fully humanised anti-CD40 monoclonal antibody that blocks CD40. In a phase II placebo-controlled RCT of 44 patients, Iscalimab was shown to be safe and well tolerated with a measurable biological effect on the germinal centre formation and improvements in the ESSDAI and ESSPRI in the treated cohort [40].

7.7 Epratuzumab

- Epratuzumab, a human anti-CD22 monoclonal IgG antibody, was first trialled in an observational study in SS [41]. In this small, open-label study, 16 patients were enrolled to receive up to four infusions of epratuzumab. Reductions of up to 50% were seen in B-cell levels, with just over half of patients achieving a clinical response. Statistically, significant improvements were seen in fatigue and patient and physician global assessments. These findings, combined with those seen in open-label studies in patients with SLE led to the Phase III EMBODY I and II trials investigating the effects of epratuzumab in moderate to severe SLE [42]. Unfortunately, neither showed a benefit for epratuzumab over placebo despite a documented effect on B-cell populations with a median reduction of 30–40% in peripheral B-cell levels.

- A subsequent post hoc analysis looked in detail at the 113 patients who were both anti-Ro positive and had a diagnosis of SS [43]. They noted that this subgroup had a faster reduction in B-cell numbers with evidence of increased B-cell sensitivity and a higher proportion showing a clinical response to treatment without an increase in adverse events. There are currently no ongoing studies of Epratuzumab in either Sjogren's or SLE.

7.8 Anti-TNF Therapy

- Infliximab was initially reported as being beneficial on the basis of two open-label studies [44, 45], but both of these apparently positive studies were subsequently retracted because of evidence that methodological errors had led to the wrong conclusions [46]. A small, open-label study of 15 patients given weekly subcutaneous etanercept showed no improvement in salivary or glandular function, and only four of the 15 reported an improvement in fatigue [47].
- A number of randomised double-blind controlled trials were undertaken in light of the initially positive published results from the open-label studies. These failed to show either clinical or serological improvement with etanercept [48] or infliximab [49]. In light of this, none of the recently published guidelines recommend anti-TNF agents as treatment for primary SS, although they acknowledge that patients with RA or another CTD can safely receive anti-TNF for their associated disease if needed [24, 25].

7.9 JAK and BTK Inhibitors

- Janus kinases (JAKs) are protein tyrosine kinases constitutively bound to cytokine and growth factor receptors. Following cytokine binding, they phosphorylate a tyrosine residue on the receptor, and the resulting conformational change allows binding of signal transducer and activation of transcription (STAT) molecules. Subsequent phosphorylation of the STAT molecules allows them to dimerise and then translocate to the nucleus, where they promote gene transcription [50]. Inhibition of the JAK/STAT pathway suppressed expression of IFN-related genes and BAFF in both a mouse model of SS and human salivary gland epithelial cells in-vitro [51]. There are a number of studies underway looking at JAK inhibitors in SS, but none has reported clinical benefit to date.
- Bruton Tyrosine Kinase (BTK) is a cytoplasmic tyrosine kinase and a member of the Tyrosine-protein kinase (TEC) family. It is selectively expressed on cells of both the adaptive and innate immune system, including B-cells, macrophages, thrombocytes, mast cells and basophils. BTK inhibition has been shown to be effective in B-cell malignancies [52], and interest is growing in its potential use in B-cell driven autoimmune diseases [53]. LOU064 is a novel covalent BTK inhibitor that has shown in-vitro selectivity against relevant kinases with high potency and efficacy in preclinical models of inflammation [54], and Phase II clinical trials are underway.

7.10 Tocilizumab

Tocilizumab is a humanised IgG1 monoclonal antibody against the human interleukin-6 (IL-6) receptor. There were initial case reports of patients with SS responding to treatment with tocilizumab with improvement in salivary and lachrymal flow rates, and reduction of inflammatory infiltrates on minor salivary gland biopsy in one case [55] and improvement in SS associated myelitis in another [56]. A subsequent multi-centre, double-blind RCT of 110 patients failed to show any clinical advantage of tocilizumab compared with placebo over a six-month study period [57].

7.11 Novel Biologics and New Molecules

- There have been preliminary reports of benefit with a number of novel biologics and new molecules but no conclusive trials to date.
- Ianalumab (VAY736) is a monoclonal antibody that both depletes B-cells and blocks BAFF receptors, thus potentially circumventing the amplified BAFF response seen post-B-cell depletion with other agents such as rituximab. A Phase II study in a small cohort of patients demonstrated significant and sustained B-cell depletion with some clinical benefit [58]. A subsequent multi-centre placebo-controlled RCT confirmed clinical efficacy and safety and further analysis is underway [59].
- RSLV-132 is an as yet un-named drug comprising RNase1 fused to the Fc region of IgG1. It promotes digestion of RNA-associated immune complexes reducing Toll-like receptor (TLR) activation. The downstream effect of this is reduced type 1 interferon (IFN), reduced B-cell activation and reduced autoantibody production. In Phase II study RSLV-132 appeared safe and well tolerated. There was no measurable effect on ESSDAI, but there did appear to be a reduction in both physical and mental fatigue in the treatment group [60]. In both of these cases, more studies are needed to confirm clinical benefit.
- Inhibition of T cell B-cell interactions is a potential therapeutic strategy for SS [4]. ALPN-101 is an Fc fusion protein of a human inducible T cell co-stimulator ligand (ICOSL) variant immunoglobulin domain (vIgD™) designed to inhibit simultaneously the CD28 and ICOS co-stimulatory pathways. In-vitro ALPN-101 has been found to suppress a wide variety of pro-inflammatory cytokines released from stimulated PBMCs from both SS patients, and healthy controls and trials are planned [61].
- Another novel agent, MEDI5872, a fully humanised Anti-ICOS Ligand monoclonal antibody, interferes with the inflammatory pathways by binding to ICOSL [62]. In a small placebo-controlled Phase II RCT, a reduction in rheumatoid factor levels was noted in the treatment group, but no change was seen in clinical parameters [62].

7.12 Conclusion

To date, Biologic use in SS has been disappointing. Rituximab showed early promise, but the two largest trials to date failed to reach their primary endpoints, although rituximab is still recommended in those with specific organ-threatening disease. There is ongoing worldwide research into the underlying pathogenesis of SS, and new therapeutic targets are being identified and tested.

References

1. Ramos-Casals M, Solans R, Rosas J, Camps MT, Gil A, Del Pino-Montes J, et al. Primary Sjogren syndrome in Spain: clinical and immunologic expression in 1010 patients. Medicine. 2008;87(4):210–9.
2. Ramos-Casals M, Brito-Zeron P, Solans R, Camps MT, Casanovas A, Sopena B, et al. Systemic involvement in primary Sjogren's syndrome evaluated by the EULAR-SS disease activity index: analysis of 921 Spanish patients (GEAS-SS Registry). Rheumatology (Oxford). 2014;53(2):321–31.
3. Nocturne G, Pontarini E, Bombardieri M, Mariette X. Lymphomas complicating primary Sjögren's syndrome: from autoimmunity to lymphoma. Rheumatology. 2019;60(8):3513–21.
4. Verstappen GM, Kroese FGM, Bootsma H. T cells in primary Sjogren's syndrome: targets for early intervention. Rheumatology (Oxford). 2019;60(7):3088–98.
5. Mielle J, Tison A, Cornec D, Le Pottier L, Daien C, Pers JO. B cells in Sjogren's syndrome: from pathophysiology to therapeutic target. Rheumatology (Oxford). 2019; https://doi.org/10.1093/rheumatology/key332.
6. Pijpe J, van Imhoff GW, Spijkervet FK, Roodenburg JL, Wolbink GJ, Mansour K, et al. Rituximab treatment in patients with primary Sjogren's syndrome: an open-label phase II study. Arthritis Rheum. 2005;52(9):2740–50.
7. Logvinenko OA, Vasil'ev VI, Sedyshev S, Safonova TN, Rodionova EB, Kokosadze NV, et al. Rituximab therapy for systemic manifestations and MALT lymphomas of the parotid gland in Sjogren's disease: preliminary data. Ter Arkh. 2012;84(12):88–96.
8. Iwabuchi T, Kimura Y, Suzuki T, Hayashi H, Fujimoto H, Hashimoto Y, et al. Successful treatment with rituximab in a patient with primary thymic MALT lymphoma complicated with acquired von Willebrand syndrome and Sjogren syndrome. [Rinsho ketsueki] Jpn J Clin Hematol. 2011;52(4):210–5.
9. Seror R, Sordet C, Guillevin L, Hachulla E, Masson C, Ittah M, et al. Tolerance and efficacy of rituximab and changes in serum B cell biomarkers in patients with systemic complications of primary Sjogren's syndrome. Ann Rheum Dis. 2007;66(3):351–7.
10. Seve P, Gachon E, Petiot P, Stankovic K, Charhon A, Broussolle C. Successful treatment with rituximab in a patient with mental nerve neuropathy in primary Sjogren's syndrome. Rheumatol Int. 2007;28(2):175–7.
11. Zhou L, Xin XF, Wu HX. The efficacy and safety of low-dose rituximab in treatment of primary Sjogren's syndrome with thrombocytopenia. Zhonghua Nei Ke Za Zhi. 2012;51(1):37–41.
12. Voulgarelis M, Ziakas PD, Papageorgiou A, Baimpa E, Tzioufas AG, Moutsopoulos HM. Prognosis and outcome of non-Hodgkin lymphoma in primary Sjogren syndrome. Medicine. 2012;91(1):1–9.
13. Mekinian A, Ravaud P, Hatron PY, Larroche C, Leone J, Gombert B, et al. Efficacy of rituximab in primary Sjogren's syndrome with peripheral nervous system involvement: results from the AIR registry. Ann Rheum Dis. 2012;71(1):84–7.

14. Pollard RP, Pijpe J, Bootsma H, Spijkervet FK, Kluin PM, Roodenburg JL, et al. Treatment of mucosa-associated lymphoid tissue lymphoma in Sjogren's syndrome: a retrospective clinical study. J Rheumatol. 2011;38(10):2198–208.
15. Yamout B, El-Hajj T, Barada W, Uthman I. Successful treatment of refractory neuroSjogren with Rituximab. Lupus. 2007;16(7):521–3.
16. Gorson KC, Natarajan N, Ropper AH, Weinstein R. Rituximab treatment in patients with IVIg-dependent immune polyneuropathy: a prospective pilot trial. Muscle Nerve. 2007;35(1):66–9.
17. Dass S, Bowman SJ, Vital EM, Ikeda K, Pease CT, Hamburger J, et al. Reduction of fatigue in Sjogren syndrome with rituximab: results of a randomised, double-blind, placebo-controlled pilot study. Ann Rheum Dis. 2008;67(11):1541–4.
18. Meijer JM, Meiners PM, Vissink A, Spijkervet FK, Abdulahad W, Kamminga N, et al. Effectiveness of rituximab treatment in primary Sjogren's syndrome: a randomized, double-blind, placebo-controlled trial. Arthritis Rheum. 2010;62(4):960–8.
19. Devauchelle-Pensec V, Mariette X, Jousse-Joulin S, Berthelot JM, Perdriger A, Puechal X, et al. Treatment of primary Sjogren syndrome with rituximab: a randomized trial. Ann Intern Med. 2014;160(4):233–42.
20. Bowman SJ, Everett CC, O'Dwyer JL, Emery P, Pitzalis C, Ng WF, et al. Randomized controlled trial of rituximab and cost-effectiveness analysis in treating fatigue and oral dryness in primary Sjogren's syndrome. Arthritis Rheumatol. 2017;69(7):1440–50.
21. Souza FBDV, Porfírio GJM, Andriolo BNG, Albuquerque JVD, Trevisani VFM. Rituximab effectiveness and safety for treating primary Sjögren's syndrome (pSS): systematic review and meta-analysis. PLoS One. 2016;11(3):e0150749-e.
22. Letaief H, Lukas C, Barnetche T, Gaujoux-Viala C, Combe B, Morel J. Efficacy and safety of biological DMARDs modulating B cells in primary Sjogren's syndrome: systematic review and meta-analysis. Joint Bone Spine. 2018;85(1):15–22.
23. Gottenberg JE, Cinquetti G, Larroche C, Combe B, Hachulla E, Meyer O, et al. Efficacy of rituximab in systemic manifestations of primary Sjogren's syndrome: results in 78 patients of the autoImmune and rituximab registry. Ann Rheum Dis. 2013;72(6):1026–31.
24. Vivino FB, Carsons SE, Foulks G, Daniels TE, Parke A, Brennan MT, et al. New treatment guidelines for Sjogren's disease. Rheum Dis Clin N Am. 2016;42(3):531–51.
25. Carsons SE, Vivino FB, Parke A, Carteron N, Sankar V, Brasington R, et al. Treatment guidelines for rheumatologic manifestations of Sjogren's: use of biologics, management of fatigue and inflammatory musculoskeletal pain. Arthritis Care Res. 2017;69(4):517–27.
26. Ramos-Casals M, Brito-Zerón P, Bombardieri S, Bootsma H, De Vita S, Dörner T, et al. EULAR recommendations for the management of Sjögren's syndrome with topical and systemic therapies. Ann Rheum Dis. 2020;79(1):3–18.
27. Pollard RP, Abdulahad WH, Vissink A, Hamza N, Burgerhof JG, Meijer JM, et al. Serum levels of BAFF, but not APRIL, are increased after rituximab treatment in patients with primary Sjogren's syndrome: data from a placebo-controlled clinical trial. Ann Rheum Dis. 2013;72(1):146–8.
28. Mariette X, Seror R, Quartuccio L, Baron G, Salvin S, Fabris M, et al. Efficacy and safety of belimumab in primary Sjogren's syndrome: results of the BELISS open-label phase II study. Ann Rheum Dis. 2015;74(3):526–31.
29. Gandolfo S, De Vita S. Double anti-B cell and anti-BAFF targeting for the treatment of primary Sjogren's syndrome. Clin Exp Rheumatol. 2019;37 Suppl 118(3):199–208.
30. De Vita S, Quartuccio L, Salvin S, Picco L, Scott CA, Rupolo M, et al. Sequential therapy with belimumab followed by rituximab in Sjogren's syndrome associated with B-cell lymphoproliferation and overexpression of BAFF: evidence for long-term efficacy. Clin Exp Rheumatol. 2014;32(4):490–4.
31. Paul D, Fazeli MS, Mintzer L, Duarte L, Gupta K, Ferri L. Comparative efficacy and safety of current therapies for early rheumatoid arthritis: a systematic literature review and network meta-analysis. Clin Exp Rheumatol. 2020;38(5):1008–15.

32. Adler S, Korner M, Forger F, Huscher D, Caversaccio MD, Villiger PM. Evaluation of histologic, serologic, and clinical changes in response to abatacept treatment of primary Sjogren's syndrome: a pilot study. Arthritis Care Res. 2013;65(11):1862–8.
33. Meiners PM, Vissink A, Kroese FG, Spijkervet FK, Smitt-Kamminga NS, Abdulahad WH, et al. Abatacept treatment reduces disease activity in early primary Sjogren's syndrome (open-label proof of concept ASAP study). Ann Rheum Dis. 2014;73(7):1393–6.
34. Machado AC, Dos Santos LC, Fidelix T, Lekwitch I, Soares SB, Gasparini AF, et al. Effectiveness and safety of abatacept for the treatment of patients with primary Sjogren's syndrome. Clin Rheumatol. 2020;39(1):243–8.
35. van Nimwegen JF, Mossel E, van Zuiden GS, Wijnsma RF, Delli K, Stel AJ, et al. Abatacept treatment for patients with early active primary Sjögren's syndrome: a single-Centre, randomised, double-blind, placebo-controlled, phase 3 trial (ASAP-III study). Lancet Rheumatol. 2020;2(3):e153–e63.
36. Jobling K, Ng WF. CD40 as a therapeutic target in Sjogren's syndrome. Expert Rev Clin Immunol. 2018;14(7):535–7.
37. Dimitriou ID, Kapsogeorgou EK, Moutsopoulos HM, Manoussakis MN. CD40 on salivary gland epithelial cells: high constitutive expression by cultured cells from Sjogren's syndrome patients indicating their intrinsic activation. Clin Exp Immunol. 2002;127(2):386–92.
38. Toubi E, Shoenfeld Y. The role of CD40-CD154 interactions in autoimmunity and the benefit of disrupting this pathway. Autoimmunity. 2004;37(6–7):457–64.
39. Sidiropoulos PI, Boumpas DT. Lessons learned from anti-CD40L treatment in systemic lupus erythematosus patients. Lupus. 2004;13(5):391–7.
40. Fisher BZM, Ng WF, Bombardieri M, Posch M, Papas AS, Farag AM, Daikeler T, Bannert B, Kivitz AJ, Carsons SE, Isenberg DA, Barone F, Bowman S, Espie P, Wieczorek G, Moulin P, Floch D, Dupuy C, Ren X, Faerber P, Wright AM, Hockey HU, Rotte M, Rush JS, Gergely P. The novel anti-CD40 monoclonal antibody CFZ533 shows beneficial effects in patients with primary Sjögren's syndrome: a phase IIa double-blind, placebo-controlled randomized trial [abstract]. Arthritis Rheumatol. 2017;69(suppl 10):1784.
41. Steinfeld SD, Tant L, Burmester GR, Teoh NK, Wegener WA, Goldenberg DM, et al. Epratuzumab (humanised anti-CD22 antibody) in primary Sjogren's syndrome: an open-label phase I/II study. Arthritis Res Ther. 2006;8(4):R129.
42. Clowse ME, Wallace DJ, Furie RA, Petri MA, Pike MC, Leszczynski P, et al. Efficacy and safety of Epratuzumab in moderately to severely active systemic lupus erythematosus: results from two phase III randomized, double-blind, placebo-controlled trials. Arthritis Rheumatol. 2017;69(2):362–75.
43. Gottenberg JE, Dorner T, Bootsma H, Devauchelle-Pensec V, Bowman SJ, Mariette X, et al. Efficacy of Epratuzumab, an anti-CD22 monoclonal IgG antibody, in systemic lupus erythematosus patients with associated Sjogren's syndrome: post hoc analyses from the EMBODY trials. Arthritis Rheumatol. 2018;70(5):763–73.
44. Steinfeld SD, Demols P, Appelboom T. Infliximab in primary Sjogren's syndrome: one-year followup. Arthritis Rheum. 2002;46(12):3301–3.
45. Steinfeld SD, Demols P, Salmon I, Kiss R, Appelboom T. Infliximab in patients with primary Sjogren's syndrome: a pilot study. Arthritis Rheum. 2001;44(10):2371–5.
46. Steinfeld SD, Demols P, Salmon I, Kiss R, Appelboom T. Notice of retraction of two articles ("infliximab in patients with primary Sjogren's syndrome: a pilot study" and "infliximab in patients with primary Sjogren's syndrome: one-year followup"). Arthritis Rheum. 2013;65(3):814.
47. Zandbelt MM, de Wilde P, van Damme P, Hoyng CB, van de Putte L, van den Hoogen F. Etanercept in the treatment of patients with primary Sjogren's syndrome: a pilot study. J Rheumatol. 2004;31(1):96–101.
48. Sankar V, Brennan MT, Kok MR, Leakan RA, Smith JA, Manny J, et al. Etanercept in Sjogren's syndrome: a twelve-week randomized, double-blind, placebo-controlled pilot clinical trial. Arthritis Rheum. 2004;50(7):2240–5.

49. Mariette X, Ravaud P, Steinfeld S, Baron G, Goetz J, Hachulla E, et al. Inefficacy of infliximab in primary Sjogren's syndrome: results of the randomized, controlled trial of remicade in primary Sjogren's syndrome (TRIPSS). Arthritis Rheum. 2004;50(4):1270–6.
50. Kelly V, Genovese M. Novel small molecule therapeutics in rheumatoid arthritis. Rheumatology (Oxford). 2013;52(7):1155–62.
51. Lee J, Lee J, Kwok SK, Baek S, Jang SG, Hong SM, et al. JAK-1 inhibition suppresses interferon-induced BAFF production in human salivary gland: potential therapeutic strategy for primary Sjogren's syndrome. Arthritis Rheumatol. 2018;70(12):2057–66.
52. Kim HO. Development of BTK inhibitors for the treatment of B-cell malignancies. Arch Pharm Res. 2019;42(2):171–81.
53. Haselmayer P, Camps M, Liu-Bujalski L, Nguyen N, Morandi F, Head J, et al. Efficacy and pharmacodynamic modeling of the BTK inhibitor evobrutinib in autoimmune disease models. J Immunol (Baltim, MD: 1950). 2019;202(10):2888–906.
54. Bruno Cenni PE, Cabanski M, Jakab A, Funhoff E, Kistowska M, Kinhikar A, Maiolica A, Hirano M, Nuesslein-Hildesheim B, Evans AL, Angst D, Pulz R, Kaul M. LOU064: a highly selective and potent covalent oral BTK inhibitor with promising pharmacodynamic efficacy on B cells for Sjogren's syndrome. Arthritis Rheumatol. 2019;71(suppl 10):2413.
55. Asai S, Okami K, Nakamura N, Ogawa Y, Ohta Y, Ogase Y, et al. The tortoiseshell pattern in one or both sides of the submandibular glands in mucosa-associated lymphoid tissue lymphoma is related to chromosomal aberrations and the disease extent. J Ultrasound Med. 2010;29(1):111–5.
56. Ishikawa Y, Hattori K, Ishikawa J, Fujiwara M, Kita Y. Refractory Sjogren's syndrome myelopathy successfully treated with subcutaneous tocilizumab: a case report. Medicine. 2019;98(27):e16285.
57. Felten RMN, Duffaut P, Saadoun D, Hachulla E, Hatron P, Salliot C, Perdriger A, Morel J, Mekinian A, Vittecoq O, Berthelot J, Dernis E, Le Guern V, Dieudé P, Larroche C, Richez C, Martin T, Zarnitsky C, Blaison G, Kieffer P, Maurier F, Rist S, Cacoub P, Andres E, Chatelus E, Sordet C, Sibilia J, Arnold C, Tawk M, Aberkane O, Seror R, Holterbach L, Mariette X, Gottenberg J. IL-6 receptor inhibition in primary Sjögren syndrome : results from a randomized multicenter academic double blind placebo-controlled trial of tocilizumab in 110 patients [abstract]. Arthritis Rheumatol. 2019;71(suppl 10):1904.
58. Dorner T, Posch MG, Li Y, Petricoul O, Cabanski M, Milojevic JM, et al. Treatment of primary Sjogren's syndrome with ianalumab (VAY736) targeting B cells by BAFF receptor blockade coupled with enhanced, antibody-dependent cellular cytotoxicity. Ann Rheum Dis. 2019;78(5):641–7.
59. Bowman SFR, Dörner T, Mariette X, Papas A, Grader-Beck T, Fisher BA, Barcelos F, De Vita S, Schulze-Koops H, Moots RJ, Junge G, Woznicki J, Sopala M, Luo W-L, Hueber W. Ianalumab (VAY736), a dual mode of action biologic combining BAFF receptor inhibition with B cell depletion, for treatment of primary Sjögren's syndrome: results of an international randomized, placebo controlled dose range finding study in 190 patients [abstract]. Arthritis Rheumatol. 2019;71(suppl 10):L19.
60. Fisher B, Barone F, Jobling K, Gallagher P, Macrae V, Filby A, et al. OP0202 effect of RSLV-132 on fatigue in patients with primary Sjögren's syndrome – results of a phase II randomised, double-blind, placebo-controlled, proof of concept study. Ann Rheum Dis. 2019;78(Suppl 2):177.1.
61. Dillon S, Evans L, Lewis K, Bort S, Rickel E, Yang J, Wolfson M, Susmilch K, Mudri S, Levin S, Bhandari J, Ahmed-Qadri F, Rixon M, Hillson J, Peng S, Swiderek K. ALPN-101, a first-in-class dual ICOS/CD28 antagonist, suppresses key effector mechanisms associated with Sjögren's syndrome [abstract]. Arthritis Rheumatol. 2019;71(suppl 10):2416.
62. Mariette X, Bombardieri M, Alevizos I, Moate R, Sullivan B, Noaiseh G, Kvarnström M, Rees W, Wang L, Illei G. A phase 2a study of MEDI5872 (AMG557), a fully human anti-ICOS ligand monoclonal antibody in patients with primary Sjögren's syndrome [abstract]. Arthritis Rheumatol. 2019;71(suppl 10):2417.

Biologics in Systemic Sclerosis

8

David Roofeh, Alain Lescoat, and Dinesh Khanna

Clinical Vignette:
A 55-year-old female with newly diagnosed diffuse cutaneous systemic sclerosis (dcSSc) presents to your office. Her symptoms of puffy hands began 1 year ago. She is primarily concerned with her rapidly progressive skin thickening and denies dyspnea with exertion or at rest. Physical exam shows a modified Rodnan Skin Score (mRSS) of 20/51. Serological evaluation shows a positive anti-SCL-70 antibody; C-reactive protein is elevated at 1.2 mg/dL. Her spirometry shows a normal total lung capacity, a forced vital capacity percent predicted (FVC%) of 85%, and a diffusion of carbon monoxide (Dlco%) of 80%. High resolution chest CT imaging (HRCT) shows mild interstitial lung disease (ILD) with visual read estimate of 5% fibrosis. Her clinical presentation prompts consideration for a biologic therapy.

8.1 Introduction

Systemic sclerosis (SSc) is an idiopathic autoimmune disease; the pathobiology of this disease involves serological evidence of autoantibody production, vasculopathy, and increased extracellular matrix deposit and fibrosis [1]. Morbidity and mortality of SSc vary based on the extent of cutaneous and visceral organ involvement

D. Roofeh · D. Khanna (✉)
Division of Rheumatology, Department of Internal Medicine, University of Michigan, Ann Arbor, MI, USA
e-mail: khannad@med.umich.edu

A. Lescoat
Univ Rennes, CHU Rennes, Inserm, EHESP, Irset (Institut de Recherche en Santé, Environnement et Travail) – UMR_S 1085, Rennes, France

Department of Internal Medicine and Clinical Immunology, Rennes University Hospital, Rennes, France

N. Jain, L. Duggal (eds.), *Handbook of Biologics for Rheumatological Disorders*, https://doi.org/10.1007/978-981-16-7200-2_8

[2, 3]. In the last three decades, improved phenotyping of patients, clinical trial methodology, and the development of scleroderma centers of excellence have led to improved evaluation and management of the disease [4–6]. Increasing understanding of the immunologic dysregulation in this disease, in the setting of modest benefit of conventional cytotoxic immunosuppressants, provides the impetus for targeted approaches using biologic therapy aiming to marshal treatment options to those unable to tolerate or who are refractory to conventional medications.

8.2 Rationale for Biologics in Systemic Sclerosis

Clinical features of SSc that impact patient quality and quantity of life span several organ systems: cutaneous thickening with resulting joint contractures, calcinosis of the skin, gastrointestinal involvement affecting any portion of the GI tract, cardiac and lung fibrosis, pulmonary arterial hypertension, digital vasculopathy, and scleroderma renal crisis. Organ fibrosis occurs from dysregulated immune responses, such that increased fibroblast activation and trans-differentiation of stromal cells into activated, apoptotic-resistant myofibroblasts that overproduce collagen [7, 8]. Decades of molecular pathophysiology provide rational targeting of key pathways that lead to fibrotic organ damage. Traditional SSc therapies include cytotoxic medications, aiming to impair the activation, migration, or differentiation of immune cells and their mediators. The advent of biologic therapy and targeted small molecule disease-modifying anti-rheumatic drugs aim to achieve the same end, without the limiting side effects associated with cytotoxicity. Specifically, inflammatory/immune and fibrotic pathways have been the target of SSc research, focused on inhibition of T cell activation and production of B cells and their downstream effects, interfering JAK-STAT pathways, and abrogating known pro-fibrotic mediators like TGF-β, IL-6, IL-4, and IL-13. In this overview, we provide evidence for the biologic agents used in the treatment of SSc to achieve low disease activity (Table 8.1).

8.3 Abatacept

- T cells are present in active skin disease in patients with SSc, expressing pro-fibrotic cytokines [26, 27]. Abatacept inhibits a key T cell co-stimulatory pathway, blocking CD28:CD80/CD86 (also called B7-1 and -2), dampening T cell receptor activation. It is approved for the treatment of moderate to severe rheumatoid arthritis [28]. This medication has shown benefit in scleroderma-related disorders like localized scleroderma and morphea profunda [29, 30].
- A small study of ten dcSSc patients (seven on abatacept, three on placebo) demonstrated a significant improvement in mRSS in those on abatacept (−8.6 vs. −2.3) at 24 weeks [31]. The Abatacept Systemic SclErosis Trial (ASSET trial) was a Phase II, 88 patients, multi-center, investigator-initiated, randomized, double-blind, placebo-controlled study evaluating the safety and efficacy of abatacept in patients with early dcSSc [9]. In this population of early dcSSc patients

Table 8.1 Therapies for Systemic Sclerosis by Designated Target

Therapy	Structure	Mechanism of action	Main cellular targets and suspected impact in SSc	Trial/phase	Primary endpoint	Ref.
T-cell targeted						
Abatacept	Fusion protein composed of the Fc region of the immunoglobulin IgG1 fused to the extracellular domain of CTLA-4	Binds to CD80 and CD86 molecules, prevents a co-stimulatory signal, preventing T cell activation.	Abatacept may downregulate the activation of CD4+ Th2 cells that produce pro-fibrotic cytokines and that participate to the activation of both innate and adaptive immunity. Abatacept may down regulate B cell activation and differentiation through its impact on T follicular helpers	NCT02161406/ Phase II (completed)	mRSS	[9–11]
Brentuximab Vedotin	Antibody–drug conjugate: humanized IgG monoclonal antibody directed against CD30 paired with an antimitotic agent monomethyl auristatin E (MMAE)	Binds to the CD30 receptor, is endocytosed, and releases MMAE into the intracellular space disrupting the microtubule network within the cell. This leads to cell cycle arrest and apoptosis.	Brentuximab Vedotin may interfere with Type 2 helper T-cell predominance and high CD30 expression in systemic sclerosis	NCT03222492/ Phase I/II (recruiting)	Proportion of participants who experience at least one Grade 3 or higher adverse event	[12, 13]

(continued)

Table 8.1 (continued)

Therapy	Structure	Mechanism of action	Main cellular targets and suspected impact in SSc	Trial/phase	Primary endpoint	Ref.
B-cell targeted						
Belimumab	Fully humanized IgG1γ monoclonal antibody	Selectively binds to soluble human B lymphocyte stimulator (BLyS) and causes inhibition of BLyS to bind to receptors on B lymphocytes	Belimumab causes inhibition of BLyS, resulting in apoptosis of B lymphocytes, reducing B-cell mediated immunity and autoimmune response	NCT01670565/ Phase II (completed)	mRSS	[14]
				NCT03844061/ Phase II (combination therapy with RTX, see below)	CRISS	
Inebilizumab	Humanized, affinity-optimized, afucosylated IgG1 kappa monoclonal antibody	Binds to the B-cell surface antigen CD-19	Antibody-dependent cell cytotoxicity targeting B cells	NCT00946699/ Phase I (completed)	Safety and tolerability of MEDI-551 in adults with SSc	[15]
Rituximab	Chimeric monoclonal antibody targeting CD20-positive B lymphocytes	Depletes peripheral B cells, impairing humoral autoantibody production, altering cytokine milieu	Rituximab may act by reducing autoantibodies, or independently of autoantibody production.	NCT03844061/ Phase II (ongoing)	CRISS	[16, 17]
				NCT02990286/ NCT01862926/ Phase III (ongoing)	FVC% predicted absolute change in FVC	
				NCT01086540/ Phase II (completed)	Change from baseline in distance walked during a 6-min walk test	
Cytokine targeted						
Rilonacept	Human dimeric fusion protein incorporating extracellular domains of IL-1 receptor and Fc portion of human IgG1	Blocks IL-1 signaling by acting as a soluble decoy receptor preventing its interaction with cell surface receptors	Inhibits IL-1 and its potential role in the fibrosis process	NCT01538719/ Phase I/II (completed)	mRSS and 2G (SSc biomarker)	[18]

Romilkimab	Humanized bi-specific IgG4 antibody	Binds and neutralizes IL-4 and IL-13	Impairs two key Th2 cytokines that play an important role in the pathogenesis of the fibrotic manifestations of SSc	NCT02921971/ Phase II (completed)	mRSS	[19]
Tocilizumab	Humanized monoclonal antibody against the interleukin-6 receptor (IL-6R)	Binds soluble as well as membrane bound interleukin-6 receptors, hindering IL-6 from exerting its pro-inflammatory and pro-fibrotic effects.	Tocilizumab through its direct effects on IL-6 signaling may notably limit the activation of myofibroblasts and may limit the polarization of pro-fibrotic M2 macrophages	NCT01532869/ Phase II (completed)	mRSS	[20, 21]
				NCT02453256/ Phase III (completed)	mRSS	
JAK-STAT pathway targeted						
Tofacitinib	Pyrrolopyrimidine that is pyrrolo[2,3-d]pyrimidine substituted at position 4 by an N-methyl,N-(1-cyanoacetyl-4-methylpiperidin-3-yl) amino moiety	Binds to JAK, the intracellular enzymes involved in signaling pathways affecting hematopoiesis, immunity, and inflammation. Inhibition of these enzymes prevents the activation of the JAK-signal transducers and activators of transcription (STAT) signaling pathway. This decreases production of pro-inflammatory cytokines (IL-6, -7, -15, -21), interferon-alpha and -beta, and may prevent inflammatory cascades and inflammation-induced damage	JAK2 has been shown to be activated in affected skin of SSc patients; inhibiting JAK2 decreases pro-fibrotic effects of TGF-β on fibroblasts.	NCT03274076/ Phase I/II (completed)	Proportion of participants who experience at least one Grade 3 or higher adverse event	[22]

(continued)

Table 8.1 (continued)

Therapy	Structure	Mechanism of action	Main cellular targets and suspected impact in SSc	Trial/phase	Primary endpoint	Ref.
Multi-targeted						
Intravenous Immunoglobulin	Human poly-specific IgG derived from the plasma of thousands of healthy blood donors	Immunomodulatory and antifibrotic effects, hypothesized to neutralize inflammatory cytokines, cause apoptosis of autoreactive B cells, immunoregulate autoantibody production, induce extracellular matrix degradation, and inhibit collagen production by fibroblasts (among other mechanisms)	Hypothesized to decrease collagen deposition, decreased secretion of pro-fibrotic cytokines (IL-4, TGF-B), and inhibition of macrophage recruitment to fibrotic sites	NCT01785056/ Phase II (withdrawn)	Primary endpoint: CRISS Secondary endpoint: mRSS	[23–25]

with active skin disease, the primary endpoint of change from baseline in mRSS at 12 months was not met when compared to placebo (−6.24 ± 1.14 in the treatment arm and −4.49 ± 1.14 in the placebo arm). Patients in the treatment arm did improve in terms of HAQ-DI (health assessment questionnaire-disability index) and the American College of Rheumatology Combined Response Index in Systemic Sclerosis (ACR CRISS) [32]. Importantly, a comparison of treatment and placebo arms in gene expression subsets based on skin biopsy revealed significant changes in the mRSS in those with inflammatory and "normal-like" skin gene expression subsets, but not in those with a fibroproliferative gene expression pattern.
- The ability to use intrinsic skin gene expression subsets to predict response to targeted biological therapy marks a step towards highly personalized, effective treatment in SSc. A key determinant in this medication's role in SSc therapy will depend on the successful targeting of the inflammatory subset in a Phase III trial.

8.4 Brentuximab Vedotin

Patients with SSc have predominant T Helper Type 2 (Th2) cytokine expression with pro-fibrotic IL-4 and IL-13 as putative mediators in disease pathogenesis. Activated Th2 cells also consistently express CD30, which has been found at elevated levels in patients with dcSSc [33]. CD30 protein is increased on certain types of cancer cells and brentuximab vedotin is an antibody–drug conjugate aimed at CD30 with benefit demonstrated for T cell lymphoma. It is approved for use in systemic anaplastic large cell lymphoma and certain cutaneous T-cell lymphomas [12]. This medication is currently being studied in a phase I/II trial (NCT03222492) in early dcSSc [34].

8.5 Belimumab

- Serum levels of B cell activation factor (BAFF) are elevated in SSc patients, correlating with skin involvement, as well as evidence of elevated BAFF mRNA found of SSc skin biopsies [35]. Belimumab is a fully human monoclonal antibody targeting BAFF, causing B lymphocyte apoptosis, decreased activation, and limited autoantibody production. It is approved for treatment-refractory autoantibody-positive systemic lupus erythematosus [36].
- A phase II double-blind randomized control trial of 20 patients compared belimumab with placebo as add-on therapy to mycophenolate mofetil in patients with dcSSc, showing numerically greater reduction in mRSS in the treatment arm but not significantly so [14]. Importantly, serial skin biopsies demonstrated a reduction in gene expression associated with B lymphocytes and fibrosis, consistent with the mechanism of action expected for this medication. NCT03844061 is an ongoing clinical trial, combining rituximab and belimumab compared to standard of care with mycophenolate mofetil in patients with dcSSc [37].

8.6 Inebilizumab

- CD19 is a surface marker of B cells, expressed throughout B cell development. CD19 is overexpressed in SSc patients and participates in B cell activation. Inebilizumab (MEDI-551) is a novel B cell-depleting humanized monoclonal antibody which targets CD19 and exerts its effects notably through an antibody-dependent cellular cytotoxicity. The safety and clinical impact of inebilizumab have been evaluated in patients with either lcSSc or dcSSc. Twenty-eight subjects were enrolled in this phase I, randomized, placebo-controlled, escalating single-dose study, with 24 receiving a single dose of inebilizumab and 4 receiving placebo [15]. Adverse events were recorded in 95.8% of subjects with active therapy and 75% in the placebo group. The majority of these adverse events was considered mild or moderate.
- Two serious adverse events were possibly related to inebilizumab. Numerical impact of inebilizumab on mRSS was observed, as mean mRSS change from baseline to day 85 was −5.4 (±4.2) in the active therapy group, versus +2.3 (±6.1) in the placebo group. These results on skin involvement need to be confirmed in a homogeneous population of well selected SSc patients, especially including early dcSSc.

8.7 Rituximab

- Rituximab is a chimeric monoclonal antibody targeting CD20 that causes B cell depletion; it has indications for use in both oncology (non-Hodgkin's lymphoma, chronic lymphocytic leukemia) and rheumatology (treatment-refractory rheumatoid arthritis, granulomatosis with polyangiitis) [38]. This medication offers increasingly substantive evidence based therapy for SSc [39–42].
- An open-label, randomized, controlled trial of head-to-head rituximab vs. monthly pulse cyclophosphamide in a population of 60 early, treatment-naive, anti-SCL-70+, dcSSc with ILD patients examined the benefit of rituximab on FVC% predicted as its primary endpoint and mRSS as one of its secondary endpoints. Patients in the cyclophosphamide group received 500 mg/m^2 cyclophosphamide IV pulses every 4 weeks for 24 weeks; patients in the rituximab group received two rituximab pulses of 1000 mg at 0 and 15 days. The rituximab arm had improved FVC% at the end of 6 months (improved, 61.3–67.5%) while the cyclophosphamide group did not (59.3–58.1%). Those in the rituximab arm had a significantly reduced mRSS compared to those in the cyclophosphamide arm (−9.67 vs. −5.5, <0.001) [42].
- A recent meta-analysis identified 13 studies analyzing cutaneous response and 12 studies identifying pulmonary function response (a total of 597 participants); their results showed long-term improvement in mRSS and stabilization of the FVC and Dlco [43]. A meta-analysis focusing specifically on rituximab's effect on SSC–ILD, identifying 20 studies examining lung function parameters (a total of 575 participants), found rituximab was not just associated with stabilization, but rather a significant improvement in FVC, DLCO during the first year of treatment [44].

- A recent observational study based on the prospective multi-center EUSTAR (European Scleroderma Trials and Research group) cohort including 254 SSc patients with rituximab and 9575 propensity-score matched patients has highlighted that rituximab was associated with improvement of skin involvement with no significant effect on pulmonary involvement [40]. A dedicated RCT is needed to properly explore the effects of rituximab on skin and lung involvement in SSc. A recent trial investigating the role of rituximab in the treatment of pulmonary arterial hypertension (PAH) (NCT01086540) showed it to be safe and demonstrated promising data warranting further investigation in PAH [45].

8.8 Rilonacept

IL-1β may participate in pathologic fibrosis and myofibroblast differentiation [46]. Rilonacept blocks IL-1 signaling, preventing IL-1's interaction with cell surface receptors. Efficacy and safety of rilonacept were evaluated in a 6 week randomized, double-blind, placebo-controlled trial in patients with dcSSc. Nineteen patients were randomized 2:1 active treatment:placebo in this phase I/II biomarker trial. At week 7, Rilonacept had neither significant effect on the primary endpoint of this study, i.e., skin gene expression as a surrogate marker for mRSS, nor on secondary endpoints such as mean change of mRSS score from baseline [18]. The limited sample size and short duration of this trial may limit conclusions regarding the efficacy of targeting IL-1 signaling in SSc.

8.9 Romilkimab

Romilkimab (SAR156597) is an immunoglobulin-G4 antibody simultaneously targeting IL-4 and IL-13, two key Th2 cytokines that promote the fibrotic manifestations of SSc. The efficacy and tolerance of romilkimab have been assessed in a 24-week, phase II, proof-of-concept study in patients with early dcSSc [19]. The primary endpoint was change in mRSS score from baseline to week 24. Romilkimab demonstrated significant improvement in skin change (least-squares mean (SE) change was −4.76 (0.86) for romilkimab versus −2.45 (0.85) for placebo. These encouraging results from this proof-of-concept study require confirmation in a dedicated phase III trial. The impact of romilkimab on visceral manifestations of SSc such as lung or cardiac involvement is still to be determined.

8.10 Tocilizumab

- IL-6 plays an important role in SSc pathophysiology [47]. Its serum concentrations differ depending on disease duration; early phase dcSSc patients have higher IL-6 than those who have had the disease for over 3 years [48]. Additionally, patients with dcSSc-ILD have higher serum concentrations than those without lung disease

[49]. Tocilizumab is an anti-IL6 receptor monoclonal antibody, preventing IL-6 from binding to the IL-6 receptor and indicated for the treatment of adult patients with rheumatoid arthritis, giant cell arteritis, polyarticular juvenile idiopathic arthritis, and systemic juvenile idiopathic arthritis among others [50]. Two large double-blind randomized control trials (faSScinate study, NCT01532869; focuSSced study, NCT02453256) studied its effect on patients with early, inflammatory dcSSc [20, 21]. Both studies failed to reach statistical significance in terms of their primary endpoint, change in mRSS. Importantly both showed attenuation of the FVC decline over 48 weeks, not seen in the placebo arm.

- Tocilizumab should be considered in early (within 5 years of the first non-Raynaud's phenomenon) dcSSc-ILD with elevated acute-phase reactants and progressive skin disease [6, 51]. This presents an important point of departure from previous thinking, with an aim to prevent decline of lung function before it happens, rather than waiting until patients show clinical symptoms and a functional decline to initiate cytotoxic therapy.

8.11 Tofacitinib

JAK-STAT pathways represent intracellular signaling targets in several autoimmune diseases. SSc patients have increased activation of JAK2 found in dermal fibroblasts on skin biopsy, and inhibition of JAK2 prevented myofibroblasts differentiation and normalized release of collagen in cultured SSc fibroblasts [22]. JAK2 inhibition also limits pro-inflammatory and pro-fibrotic mediators released by macrophages [52]. The pan-JAK inhibitor tofacitinib is indicated for the treatment of adult patients with rheumatoid arthritis, psoriatic arthritis, and ulcerative colitis [53]. It was recently tested in a phase I/II study in early dcSSc, conducted in a double-blind randomized placebo-controlled trial fashion over 6 months; the medication was well-tolerated and had a signal of efficacy in terms of the mRSS and CRISS [54].

8.12 Intravenous Immunoglobulin

Intravenous immunoglobulin modulates the pathological immune responses in those with autoimmune diseases of several disciplines (e.g., rheumatology, hematology, dermatology, and neurology) [23]. IVIG is the collation of pooled serum IgG from blood donors. The purported mechanism includes both the FAB and the FC fragments: neutralizing autoantibodies, inhibiting inflammatory mediators, impairing monocyte/macrophage activation thus impairing key pro-fibrotic pathways, and blocking FC receptors on the surface of B cells [24, 25, 55]. Observational studies have shown significant improvement in skin score reduction, treatment-refractory arthritis, gastrointestinal disease, myopathy, and even lung disease [56–61]. A multi-center, double-blind randomized trial of IVIG in dcSSc failed to show a significant difference in mRSS at 12 weeks, following 400 mg (8 mL)/kg/day for 5 consecutive days (a single course); non-responders (mRSS changed <5 points) received a second round of IVIG, and those receiving two doses were found to have significant improvement at 60 weeks after the first administration compared to one round [62]. Results of a multi-site trial comparing IVIG (2 g/kg/month) vs. placebo for 6 months (NCT01785056) have been completed but is not yet publicly available [63].

8.13 Clinical Practice

At the University of Michigan Scleroderma Program, our clinical practice incorporates biologic therapies based on data from clinical trials and observational studies support the use of IVIG [6]. We utilize IVIG in those who have progressive skin and musculoskeletal worsening (with or without scleroderma myopathy or inflammatory myopathy) in early dcSSc, despite worsening on traditional immunosuppressive therapies. Current data do not support use of other biologics for use for progressive skin involvement but this may due to molecular heterogeneity, as shown in the ASSET trial. For SSc-ILD, we usually initiate traditional immunosuppressive therapies such as mycophenolate mofetil and add rituximab or tocilizumab, if they have progressive disease. The data from a single-center trial on rituximab and two randomized controlled trials in patients with early dcSSc, inflammatory features, high risk of progressive disease with early ILD (as secondary end point) on tocilizumab support use of these therapies in a treatment naïve population. The rituximab data needs to be validated in a double-blind trial. In our practice, in a subset with dcSSc and elevated acute-phase reactants, we initiate tocilizumab in treatment naïve patients although they usually have concomitant inflammatory arthritis since tocilizumab is not approved for SSc-ILD. We also employ biologics for inflammatory polyarthritis, as done in rheumatoid arthritis. Other therapies mentioned above (e.g., belimumab, brentuximab vedotin, rilonacept, inebilizumab, romilkimab) do not have sufficient data to employ in clinical practice.

8.14 Summary

- SSc pathophysiology is multifactorial and no one pathway or therapy is likely to promise a low-disease state [64]. Immunosuppressive treatments fail to provide lasting, disease-modifying properties. These shortcomings may be a combination of challenges in clinical trial design, poor efficacy of medical therapy, limitations to cohort enrichment, dearth of trial outcome measures sensitive enough to detect change, or a combination of all these. Nevertheless, field is moving toward targeted immunological and non-cytotoxic therapies to improve outcomes for this impairing and sometimes deadly disease.
- These newer therapy options are increasingly being understood in the context of three hopeful treatment goals: (1) identifying patients in an early disease state and initiating therapy to prevent advanced disease if the benefit outweighs the risks; (2) secondary prevention in those with clinically impactful disease; and (3)

patients with progressive disease should receive therapy prior to advanced disability or loss of function.

- The modern era of SSc treatment may be understood by considering the vignette at the start of this review. A patient in her mid-50s presenting with early dcSSc-ILD, an mRSS 20/51, and preserved FVC% and Dlco%, with elevated inflammatory markers: her therapy options at one point would include cyclophosphamide or mycophenolate mofetil, typically started based on advancing skin disease or once SSc-ILD has become clinically impactful to the patient (or prior to that if treating advancing skin disease). Recent Food and Drug Administration approval has been given to tocilizumab to slow the rate of decline in pulmonary function in patients with SSc-ILD, based on the results of the faSScinate (NCT01532869) and focuSSced (NCT02453256) trials [65]. In this case, there are data to support the early intervention aimed at attenuating an inflammatory disease state and potentially halting progression to a fibrotic state, preserving lung function [66]. In an alternative scenario, where a SSc-ILD patient with considerably more fibrotic lung disease presents with absence of active skin or musculoskeletal involvement, the recently FDA-approved antifibrotic medication nintedanib has demonstrated efficacy toward goal (2), preservation of lung function without the known side effects of cyclophosphamide or mycophenolate mofetil [67]. The advent of biologic therapy also allows for a patient with SSc-ILD and significant skin disease to consider rituximab therapy, which may be an attractive option when compared to other therapies in terms of side effects (cyclophosphamide with teratogenicity, premature ovarian failure, cytotoxicity) or medical adherence to twice daily therapy (mycophenolate mofetil). Finally, future studies are needed to establish how biologic and newer therapies fit into treatment paradigms to achieve goal (3) for those with progressive or treatment-refractory disease [6]. Understanding of the molecular heterogeneity will aid in targeted therapies for this multisystem disease.

References

1. Denton CP, Khanna D. Systemic sclerosis. Lancet. 2017;390(10103):1685–99.
2. Poudel DR, Jayakumar D, Danve A, Sehra ST, Derk CT. Determinants of mortality in systemic sclerosis: a focused review. Rheumatol Int. 2018;38(10):1847–58.
3. Poudel DR, Derk CT. Mortality and survival in systemic sclerosis. Curr Opin Rheumatol. 2018;30(6):1.
4. Khanna D, et al. Measures of response in clinical trials of systemic sclerosis: the Combined Response Index for Systemic Sclerosis (CRISS) and Outcome Measures in Pulmonary Arterial Hypertension related to Systemic Sclerosis (EPOSS). J Rheumatol. 2009;36(10):2356–61.
5. Khanna D, Merkel PA. Outcome measures in systemic sclerosis: an update on instruments and current research. Curr Rheumatol Rep. 2007;9(2):151–7.
6. Roofeh D, Distler O, Allanore Y, Denton CP, Khanna D. Treatment of systemic sclerosis-associated interstitial lung disease: lessons from clinical trials. J Scleroderma Relat Disord. 2020;5(2S):61–71.
7. Allanore Y, et al. Systemic sclerosis. Nat Rev. 2015;1(April):1–21.

8. Asano Y, Varga J. Rationally-based therapeutic disease modification in systemic sclerosis: novel strategies. Semin Cell Dev Biol. 2020;101:146–60.
9. Khanna D, Spino C, Johnson SR, Chung L. Abatacept in early diffuse cutaneous systemic sclerosis – results of a phase 2 investigator-initiated, multicenter, double-blind randomized placebo-controlled trial. Arthritis Rheumatol. 2019;72(1):125–36.
10. Castellví I, et al. Safety and effectiveness of abatacept in systemic sclerosis: The EUSTAR experience. Semin Arthritis Rheum. 2020.
11. Chung L, et al. Safety and efficacy of abatacept in early diffuse cutaneous systemic sclerosis (ASSET): open-label extension of a phase 2, double-blind randomised trial. Lancet Rheumatol. 2020;2(12):e743–53.
12. Van Der Weyden C, Dickinson M, Whisstock J, Prince HM. Brentuximab vedotin in T-cell lymphoma. Expert Rev Hematol. 2019;12(1):5–19.
13. Higashioka K, et al. Generation of a novel CD30+ B cell subset producing GM-CSF and its possible link to the pathogenesis of systemic sclerosis. Clin Exp Immunol. 2020;201(3):233–43.
14. Gordon JK, et al. Belimumab for the treatment of early diffuse systemic sclerosis: results of a randomized, double-blind, placebo-controlled, pilot trial. Arthritis Rheumatol. 2018;70(2):308–16.
15. Schiopu E, et al. Safety and tolerability of an anti-CD19 monoclonal antibody, MEDI-551, in subjects with systemic sclerosis: a phase I, randomized, placebo-controlled, escalating single-dose study. Arthritis Res Ther. 2016;18(1):1–14.
16. Hasegawa M. B lymphocytes: shedding new light on the pathogenesis of systemic sclerosis. J Dermatol. 2010;37(1):3–10.
17. Schioppo T, Ingegnoli F. Current perspective on rituximab in rheumatic diseases. Drug Des Dev Ther. 2017;11:2891–904.
18. Mantero JC, et al. Randomised, double-blind, placebo-controlled trial of IL1-trap, rilonacept, in systemic sclerosis. A phase I/II biomarker trial. Clin Exp Rheumatol. 2018:146–9.
19. Allanore Y, et al. A randomised, double-blind, placebo-controlled, 24-week, phase II, proof-of-concept study of romilkimab (SAR156597) in early diffuse cutaneous systemic sclerosis. Ann Rheum Dis. 2020:1–8, Epub ahead.
20. Khanna D, et al. Safety and efficacy of subcutaneous tocilizumab in systemic sclerosis: results from the open-label period of a phase II randomised controlled trial (faSScinate). Ann Rheum Dis. 2018;77(2):212–20.
21. Khanna D, Lin CJF, Spotswood H, Siegel J, Denton CP. Safety and efficacy of subcutaneous tocilizumab in systemic sclerosis: results from the open-label period of the phase 3 focuSSced trial. Ann Rheum Dis. 2020;79(1):390.
22. Dees C, et al. JAK-2 as a novel mediator of the profibrotic effects of transforming growth factor β in systemic sclerosis. Arthritis Rheumatol. 2012;64(9):3006–15.
23. Schwab I, Nimmerjahn F. Intravenous immunoglobulin therapy: how does IgG modulate the immune system? Nat Rev Immunol. 2013;13(3):176–89.
24. Cantarini L, et al. Intravenous immunoglobulins (IVIG) in systemic sclerosis: a challenging yet promising future. Immunol Res. 2015;61(3):326–37.
25. Gomes JP, Santos L, Shoenfeld Y. Intravenous immunoglobulin (IVIG) in the vanguard therapy of Systemic Sclerosis. Clin Immunol. 2019;199:25–8.
26. Maehara T, et al. Cytotoxic CD4 + T lymphocytes may induce endothelial cell apoptosis in systemic sclerosis. J Clin Invest. 2020;130(5):2451–64.
27. Zhou Y, et al. The elevated expression of Th17-related cytokines and receptors is associated with skin lesion severity in early systemic sclerosis. Hum Immunol. 2015;76:22–9.
28. Blair HA, Deeks ED. Abatacept: a review in rheumatoid arthritis. Drugs. 2017;77(11):1221–33.
29. Stausbøl-Grøn B, Olesen AB, Deleuran B, Deleuran MS. Abatacept is a promising treatment for patients with disseminated morphea profunda: presentation of two cases. Acta Derm Venereol. 2011;91(6):686–8.
30. Wehner Fage S, Arvesen KB, Olesen AB. Abatacept improves skin-score and reduces lesions in patients with localized scleroderma: a case series. Acta Derm Venereol. 2018;98(4):465–6.

31. Chakravarty EF, Fiorentino D, Bennett D. A pilot study of abatacept for the treatment of patients with diffuse cutaneous systemic sclerosis. Arthritis Rheumatol. 2011;63:707.
32. Khanna D, et al. The American College of Rheumatology provisional composite response index for clinical trials in early diffuse cutaneous systemic sclerosis. Arthritis Rheumatol. 2016;68(2):299–311.
33. Mavilia C, et al. Type 2 helper T-cell predominance and high CD30 expression in systemic sclerosis. Am J Pathol. 1997;151(6):1751–8.
34. Brentuximab Vedotin for Systemic Sclerosis (BRAVOS). ClinicalTrials.gov Identifier: NCT03222492. [Online]. https://clinicaltrials.gov/ct2/show/NCT03222492.
35. Matsushita T, Hasegawa M, Yanaba K, Kodera M, Takehara K, Sato S. Elevated serum BAFF levels in patients with systemic sclerosis: enhanced BAFF signaling in systemic sclerosis B lymphocytes. Arthritis Rheumatol. 2006;54(1):192–201.
36. Blair HA, Duggan ST. Belimumab: a review in systemic lupus erythematosus. Drugs. 2018;78(3):355–66.
37. Belimumab and rituximab combination therapy for the treatment of diffuse cutaneous systemic sclerosis. ClinicalTrials.gov Identifier: NCT03844061. [Online]. https://clinicaltrials.gov/ct2/show/NCT03844061.
38. Rituximab: highlights of prescribing information. [Online]. https://www.accessdata.fda.gov/drugsatfda_docs/label/2018/103705s5450lbl.pdf.
39. Yoshizaki A. Pathogenic roles of B lymphocytes in systemic sclerosis. Immunol Lett. 2018;195(January):76–82.
40. Elhai M, et al. Outcomes of patients with systemic sclerosis treated with rituximab in contemporary practice: a prospective cohort study. Ann Rheum Dis. 2019;78:979–87.
41. Thiebaut M, et al. Efficacy and safety of rituximab in systemic sclerosis: French retrospective study and literature review. Autoimmun Rev. 2018;17(6):582–7.
42. Sircar G, Goswami RP, Sircar D, Ghosh A, Ghosh P. Intravenous cyclophosphamide vs rituximab for the treatment of early diffuse scleroderma lung disease: open label, randomized, controlled trial. Rheumatology. 2018;57(12):2106–13.
43. Tang R, et al. Safety and efficacy of Rituximab in systemic sclerosis: a systematic review and meta-analysis. Int Immunopharmacol. 2020;83(87):106389.
44. Goswami RP, Ray A, Chatterjee M, Mukherjee A, Sircar G, Ghosh P. Rituximab in the treatment of systemic sclerosis–related interstitial lung disease: a systematic review and meta-analysis. Rheumatology. 2020;60(2):557–67.
45. Nicolls M, et al. Safety and E cacy of B-cell depletion with rituximab for the treatment of systemic sclerosis-associated pulmonary arterial hypertension in a multi-center. NIH Clinical Trial. 2019;71(Suppl 10)
46. Artlett CM, Sassi-Gaha S, Rieger JL, Boesteanu AC, Feghali-Bostwick CA, Katsikis PD. The inflammasome activating caspase 1 mediates fibrosis and myofibroblast differentiation in systemic sclerosis. Arthritis Rheum. 2011;63(11):3563–74.
47. Shima Y. The benefits and prospects of interleukin-6 inhibitor on systemic sclerosis. Mod Rheumatol. 2019;29(2):294–301.
48. Hasegawa M, Sato S, Fujimoto M, Kikuchi K, Takehara K. Serum levels of interleukin 6 (IL-6), oncostatin M, soluble IL-6 receptor, and soluble gp130 in patients with systemic sclerosis. J Rheumatol. 1998;25(2):308–13.
49. Scala E, et al. Cytokine and chemokine levels in systemic sclerosis: relationship with cutaneous and internal organ involvement. Clin Exp Immunol. 2004;138(3):540–6.
50. Tocilizumab: highlights of prescribing information. [Online]. https://www.accessdata.fda.gov/drugsatfda_docs/label/2017/125276s114lbl.pdf.
51. Roofeh D, Jaafar S, Vummidi D, Khanna D. Management of systemic sclerosis-associated interstitial lung disease. Curr Opin Rheumatol. 2019;31(3):241–9.
52. Lescoat A, Lelong M, Jeljeli M, et al. Combined anti-fibrotic and anti-inflammatory properties of JAK-inhibitors on macrophages in vitro and in vivo: perspectives for scleroderma-associated interstitial lung disease. Biochem Pharmacol. 2020;178:114103.

53. Tofacitinib: highlights of prescribing information. [Online]. https://www.accessdata.fda.gov/drugsatfda_docs/label/2018/203214s018lbl.pdf.
54. Khanna D, et al. Tofacitinib in early diffuse cutaneous systemic sclerosis—results of phase I/II investigator-initiated, double-blind randomized placebo-controlled trial. Arthritis Rheumatol. 2019;71(10).
55. Lünemann JD, Nimmerjahn F, Dalakas MC. Intravenous immunoglobulin in neurology-mode of action and clinical efficacy. Nat Rev Neurol. 2015;11(2):80–9.
56. Nacci F, et al. Intravenous immunoglobulins improve the function and ameliorate joint involvement in systemic sclerosis: a pilot study. Ann Rheum Dis. 2007;66(7):977–9.
57. Clark KEN, Etomi O, Denton CP, Ong VH, Murray CD. Intravenous immunoglobulin therapy for severe gastrointestinal involvement in systemic sclerosis. Clin Exp Rheumatol. 2015;33:168–70.
58. Raja J, Nihtyanova SI, Murray CD, Denton CP, Ong VH. Sustained benefit from intravenous immunoglobulin therapy for gastrointestinal involvement in systemic sclerosis. Rheumatol (United Kingdom). 2016;55(1):115–9.
59. Poelman CL, Hummers LK, Wigley FM, Anderson C, Boin F, Shah AA. Intravenous immunoglobulin may be an effective therapy for refractory, active diffuse cutaneous systemic sclerosis. J Rheumatol. 2015;42(2):236–42.
60. Sanges S, et al. Intravenous immunoglobulins in systemic sclerosis: data from a French nationwide cohort of 46 patients and review of the literature. Autoimmun Rev. 2017;16(4):377–84.
61. Chaigne B, et al. Corticosteroid-sparing benefit of intravenous immunoglobulin in systemic sclerosis-associated myopathy: a comparative study in 52 patients. Autoimmun Rev. 2020;19(1):102431.
62. Takehara K, Ihn H, Sato S. Intravenous immunoglobulin treatment in patients with diffuse cutaneous systemic sclerosis. Clin Exp Rheumatol. 2013;31(9):s151–6.
63. IVIG treatment in systemic sclerosis. ClinicalTrials.gov. NCT01785056 study. [Online]. https://clinicaltrials.gov/ct2/show/NCT01785056?term=NCT01785056&rank=1.
64. Nagaraja V, et al. Current and future outlook on disease modification and defining low disease activity in systemic sclerosis. Arthritis Rheumatol. 2020;72(7):1049–58.
65. Khanna D, et al. SYSTEMIC SCLEROSIS-ASSOCIATED INTERSTITIAL LUNG DISEASE: how to incorporate two Food and Drug Administration-approved therapies in clinical practice. Arthritis Rheumatol. 2021;
66. Roofeh D, et al. Tocilizumab prevents progression of early systemic sclerosis associated interstitial lung disease. Arthritis Rheumatol. 2021;73(7):1301–10.
67. Distler O, et al. Nintedanib for systemic sclerosis–associated interstitial lung disease. N Engl J Med. 2019:NEJMoa1903076.

Biologics in Idiopathic Inflammatory Myopathies

9

Rudra Prosad Goswami and Uma Kumar

9.1 Introduction

Idiopathic inflammatory myopathies (IIMs) comprise diverse autoimmune systemic diseases characterised by chronic skeletal, muscular inflammation [1]. Treatable subtype of IIM include (juvenile) dermatomyositis ((j)DM), antisynthetase syndrome (ASS), immune-mediated necrotizing myopathy (IMNM) and overlap/non-specific myositis [OM/NSM, formerly called polymyositis (PM)]. Treatment of Idiopathic inflammatory myositis (IIMs), is not only long and often arduous but is also stymied by a general lack of guidelines or therapeutic algorithms available and updated readily and regularly as for other rheumatologic diseases such as rheumatoid arthritis or systemic lupus erythematosus. Corticosteroids have traditionally been used as the first-line agent along with other agents like methotrexate, cyclosporine, azathioprine, mycophenolate mofetil and rituximab [2, 3]. Often, either in case of non-responsive patients or in recurrent flares, biologics are employed. In this chapter, we will summarise the evidence and practices of the biologics already in use and those in the pipeline in the treatment of IIMs (not including inclusion body myositis, IBM).

Despite various completed and ongoing trials, issues regarding patient composition, sample sizes, heterogeneity with regards to inclusion and exclusion criteria and most important, outcome measures have hampered uniform interpretation of myositis clinical trials and other observational studies. The strongest evidence till date is for intravenous immunoglobulin (IVIg), rituximab, and abatacept. However, evidence is emerging for other drugs like sifalimumab and other anti-interferon therapies, Janus kinase (JAK) inhibitors and corticotropin injection.

R. P. Goswami · U. Kumar (✉)
Department of Rheumatology, AIIMS, New Delhi, India

N. Jain, L. Duggal (eds.), *Handbook of Biologics for Rheumatological Disorders*, https://doi.org/10.1007/978-981-16-7200-2_9

9.2 Rituximab (Anti-CD 20)

Mechanism of Action and Evidence

- Rituximab, a monoclonal antibody targeting the CD-20 molecule on B lymphocytes, depletes peripheral blood B cell lineage up to plasmablasts and not only depletes B cells and reduces total and autoimmune antibody levels but also affect antigen-presenting function of B cells. Other major mechanisms of action of rituximab are altered B cell signal transduction through interaction at the lipid raft level; apoptosis of B lymphocytes; complement-dependent and antibody-dependent cell-mediated cytotoxicity (ADCC) [4]. It is well known that plasma cells play a major role in the pathogenesis of IIMs, especially DM. Autoantibodies, though not ubiquitously, are well-recognised features of the disease process. Increased intramuscular perivascular localisation of B cells are observed in many patients with DM, along with evidence for B cell-driven upregulation of interferon production and signalling, as well as antibody production and antigen presentation to T cells [5–7]. Evidence of use of rituximab in IIMs comes from the RIM trial [3]. This was a double blind randomised placebo controlled delayed start trial. Trial population included both adult PM/DM and jDM patients. Patients with refractory myositis were included. Definition of refractory myositis was intolerance or partial response to glucocorticoids and at least another second immunosuppressant like methotrexate, mycophenolate, azathioprine, cyclophosphamide, cyclosporine, tacrolimus, intravenous immunoglobulin [IVIG], etc. "Adequate" glucocorticoid dose was either 60-mg/day prednisolone equivalent (adults) or 1-mg/kg/day prednisolone equivalent (jDM) for ≥1-month. The duration criterion for the second immunosuppressant was 3 months. A muscle weakness criterion was bilateral Manual Muscle Testing 8 (MMT-8) ≤125 for adults along with two other International Myositis Assessment and Clinical Studies Group (IMACS) core set measures. For jDM, weakness criteria were similar, except if MMT-8 was exactly 125, then a third core set measure was needed for inclusion. The other cores set measures were: (1) Global assessment of disease activity by visual-analogue-scale (VAS) ≥2 mm (patients' or parents'); (2) physician's global assessment VAS ≥2 mm; (3) Health Assessment Questionnaire (HAQ) or Childhood HAQ (C-HAQ) ≥0.25; (4) elevated muscle enzyme ≥1.3 upper limit of normal; (5) Global extramuscular disease (investigator's composite of skeletal, constitutional, gastrointestinal, cutaneous, pulmonary, and cardiac scores of the Myositis Disease Activity Assessment Tool [MDAAT]) activity score ≥1.0 cm. The two treatment arms were: the early group (rituximab at weeks 0 and 1) and the late group (rituximab given at weeks 8 and 9). The primary outcome measure was time to achieve the preliminary IMACS definition of improvement (DOI).
- Overall 195 IIM patients (75 with PM, 72 with DM, and 48 with jDM) refractory to steroids and an average of 2 other immunosupressive drugs were included in the trial. The median time to achieve a DOI in the early treatment arm was 20 weeks (n = 93) and in the late treatment arm was 20.2 weeks (n = 102). This represents no significant difference, and the trial did not meet its primary end

point. But the most important statistic available from the RIM is that 161/195 (83%) of the entire study population achieved the DOI by 44 weeks. Interestingly the authors provided data for retreatment in some patients. Nine patients were retreated with rituximab out potential 17. The time to relapse was 16.5 weeks on average. Eight of the relapsed patients achieved repeat DOI after a mean of 19.9 weeks. This was the first and currently, the only randomised controlled trial (RCT) providing evidence of rituximab in the treatment of refractory IIMs and jDM. Several sub-studies were later published. The authors showed that patients with baseline higher interferon expression and positive Mi-2 autoantibody expression had a better clinical response [8]. In another analysis, and particularly in the absence of the interferon chemokine score, which is still a research tool, presence of anti-Jo-1 (hazard ratio (HR): 3.08), anti-Mi-2 (HR 2.5), jDM (HR 2.45) and lower damage score (HR 2.32) predicted a favourable outcome [9]. For cutaneous disease in DM, significant improvements were noted in both arms of rituximab regimens, but faster resolution was noted in the early treatment arm [9].

Dose children with a BSA ≤ 1.5 m^2: 575 mg/m^2 (0, 1 week); adults and children with a BSA > 1.5 m^2: 750 mg/m^2 (0, 1 week); max dose 1 g per infusion

Mode of Administration IV infusion

Frequency weeks 0, 1; repeat courses as per clinical guidance (generally not before 4–6 months)

Duration Evidence available for up to 1 year

Indication Refractory myositis

Can Be Used in JDM Yes

Adverse Effects Common: Infusion reaction; Infections (urinary tract, upper and lower respiratory tract, skin and soft tissue, herpes zoster); Less common: Hypogammaglobulinemia; Leucopenia; Fungal infections

9.3 Abatacept (CTLA-4 Agonist)

Mechanism of Action and Evidence

- Activated cytotoxic and helper T cells occupy a central role in the pathology and pathogenesis of IIMs. Abatacept acts by engaging co-receptor molecules expressed on effector T cells (CD80/86) and downregulating these and thereby suppressing T-cell activation, proliferation, and effector function [10]. Apart from this, abatacept also decreases the antigen-presenting capability of myocytes, inhibits macrophage migration and function, and decreases pro-inflammatory cytokines expression especially, interleukins (IL-) 6, and TNF-alpha [11].

- A phase 2b randomised, multicentre, delayed start trial has recently been published [12]. This trial included 20 patients with refractory IIM (9 patients with DM, the rest 11 with PM). The definition of refractory disease in this trial was the presence of active disease (Manual Muscle Test (MMT-8) <150) or low endurance (Functional Index for myositis (FI-2) <20% of upper limit), with elevated enzymes, recent biopsy evidence of active inflammation or MRI findings consistent with inflammation, or active extramuscular disease, while on ongoing treatment with glucocorticoids (≥0.5-mg/kg/day prednisolone equivalent for more than a month) and a second immunosuppressant (either methotrexate (≥15 mg/week) or azathioprine (≥100 mg/day) for more than 3 months). Patients were randomised to receive either immediate treatment or delayed start, i.e. after 3 months. The primary outcome measure was IMACS DOI at 6 months which was achieved by eight patients. The authors also observed a parallel increase in regulatory T cells in repeat muscle biopsy samples concomitant with clinical improvement. Certain parameters, like the global physician health, muscle enzyme and cardiovascular disease activity, fared better in the active early treatment arm. The drug was well tolerated.
- Similar results were reported from a sub-study of the ongoing ARTEMIS trial, with similar inclusion criteria and the authors reported that 7/12 patients had DOI at 6 months. The authors also suggested that CD4/CD8 ratio in blood sample may be a biomarker of treatment efficacy.

Dose <60 kg: 500 mg, 60–100 kg: 750 mg; >100 kg: 1000 mg

Mode of administration IV infusion

Frequency weeks 0, 2, 4, 8, 12, 16, 20, 24.

Duration Evidence available for up to 6 months

Indication Refractory myositis

Can Be Used in JDM Trial data not available, anecdotal evidence available

Adverse Effects Generally considered to be one of the safest biologics in terms of infections: pneumonia, skin and soft tissue infections and urinary tract infection and some reports on opportunistic infections like *Mycobacterium tuberculosis*, Aspergillosis, blastomycosis, and systemic candida infections are available from non-IIM studies; (0.01); Common: infusion reaction, headache; Uncommon: induction of autoimmune reactions: mostly mild to moderate, psoriasis being the most common; worsening of chronic obstructive pulmonary disease

9.4 Intravenous or Subcutaneous Immunoglobulin (IVIg/SCIg)

Mechanism of Action and Summary of Evidence

- Intravenous (and more recently subcutaneous) immunoglobulin preparations (IVIg/ScIg) work in various immunological diseases through multiple and often poorly defined mechanisms such as blocking cellular receptors, neutralisation of cytokines, complements, and autoantibodies (Fab dependent mechanisms) and blockage of activating Fcγ receptors and modulation of activation of activating versus inhibiting Fcγ receptors and selective upregulation of inhibiting Fcγ receptor FcγRIIB (Fc portion dependent mechanisms), etc. [13] There are multiple other mechanistic evidences which are closer at home when talking about idiopathic inflammatory myositis like decreasing deposition of complements and membrane attack complexes on capillaries as well as muscle fibres [14], downregulation of transforming growth factor (TGF-B) expression on muscle fibres [15], and downregulation of expression of adhesion molecules on myocytes and capillaries [16].
- The major study of any drug other than glucocorticoids shown to be effective in IIMs was on IVIg. This was shown in the pivotal trial by Dalakas et al. back in 1993 on 15 patients with refractory dermatomyositis (many of which would actually be classified as jDM nowadays) who were given IVIg (2-g/kg-bodyweight) or placebo monthly for 3 consecutive months in a randomised manner. Inclusion criteria were clinical active disease, active rash and positive biopsy. Patients needed to have at least 4–6 months of exposure to non-glucocorticoid immunosuppressive drugs like methotrexate, azathioprine, or cyclophosphamide and needed to have either poor response or poor tolerance to these agents to be eligible. Response was gauged clinically. The Medical Research Council (MRC) muscle strength score improved from 76.6 to 84.6 in the IVIg group (n = 8) and remained the same at 76.6 in the placebo group (n = 7). There was a cross—over portion of the trial after the initial 3 months, thereby increasing the number of patients in IVIg to 12, of whom 9 with severe disabilities experienced major improvements. The MRC scores improved from 74.5 to 84.7, an improvement hitherto almost unattainable in the field of IIM. Among the 11 patients treated with placebo, none had a major improvement, and 5 patients worsened with stable disease or mild improvement in the rest. This was the first trial that showed a marked response of refractory patients with DM to this drug. There were several later prospective cohorts and one RCT, some of which reproduced this result, and others provided data to the contrary. Several points need mentioned, like the continuous use of moderate to high dose steroids in the Dalakas trial, a trend which was not followed in later studies, patient population heterogeneity and most importantly, the point in which this drug is introduced and whether the "Goldilocks period" was lost or not in later studies [17–19]. One RCT later unsuccessfully used IVIg as first-line therapy in IIM [17].
- A 2012 systematic literature review of adult patients with PM/DM compiled data from 1985 to 2011 and concluded that given at a dose of 2 g/kg, divided into 2–5

individual daily doses, once monthly for 3–6 months, beneficial effects were notable in refractory, flare-up, rapidly progressive, or severe PM/DM and most therapeutic benefit are noted among patients with lung involvement and oesophageal involvement. Some steroid-sparing effect was also observed by the authors [2]. Despite this, the present authors warn the reader that the majority of the benefit of IVIg are seen in cases of DM, and there is a dearth of evidence in favour of its use in OM/NSM/PM are scanty [10]. One Cochrane review summarised evidence of various drugs in DM and found only one eligible study, discussed above on IVIg. The authors showed a non-significant relative risk of 4.44 of muscle power improvement with IVIg use [20].

- More recently, subcutaneous immunoglobulin preparation (ScIg) has been tested in several prospective studies [21, 22]. There are several advantages like home usage, lack of need for vascular access and subsequent reduction of infection risk, lesser hyperviscosity-related side effects like headache and visual disturbance and lower cost [10].

Dose 2 g/kg body weight

Mode of Administration IV infusion/SC infusion

Frequency Monthly

Duration Up to 6 months

Indication refractory myositis/Pharyngeal muscle weakness/Respiratory muscle weakness/Concomitant infection

Can Be Used in JDM Yes

Adverse Effects One of the safest if not the safest agent to use in terms of infectious side effects and often is used in patients with a concomitant active systemic infection where high doses of glucocorticoids or other biologics cannot be used; Common: infusion reactions like headache, fever, or asymptomatic laboratory changes like increased liver enzymes, dizziness, hypertension (generally mild, but may be severe, especially with older preparation which was rich with immunoglobulin A (IgA) given in patients with IgA deficiency, a problem which had largely been unnoticed with newer IgA poor preparations; these reactions, when occur could be resolved by reducing the infusion rate or with symptomatic therapy); Uncommon: aseptic meningitis; thromboembolic complications; hyperviscosity

9.5 Sifalimumab

Mechanism of Action and Evidence

- Sifalimumab is an anti-interferon alpha (IFN-α) monoclonal antibody. Increased interferon response and interferon gene signature, both systematic and localised to muscular tissue, has been described from yesteryears' studies back in 1980s to the most recent exponents [23, 24]. Interestingly, both jDM and DM have several mechanistic pathways common to lupus-like complement activation and vascular wall deposition of membrane attack complex, lymphocytic infiltration of target organ, plasmacytoid dendritic cell expression at the target site of inflammation and consequent type I interferon expression [25]. Recently, a fairly good number of studies on interferon blocking agents came in lupus, some failed like rontalizumab, but others succeeded like sifalimumab and anifrolumab. Recently a trial on sifalimumab came in the field of IIM [26].

- This was a pharmacodynamic study (phase Ib) in which neutralisation of a type I IFN gene signature (IFNGS) at blood and muscle level was assessed following drug exposure. At baseline, 72% of all patients had positive IFNGS. The IFNGS was suppressed by 53–66% on the various time points of measurements (4, 8, and 14 weeks) in the blood ($p = 0.019$) and by 47% (98th day) in muscle. Patients with 15% or greater improvement in manual muscle testing at day 98 from baseline showed greater neutralisation of the IFNGS. However, only 8 out of 24 patients experienced such clinical improvement. However, regarding the pharmacodynamic parameters, which were the primary outcome measure analysed in this study, this RCT reached its goals and is considered a success. In a subsequent sub-study, treated patients showed a significant reduction of several T-cell associated proteins, especially soluble interleukin-2 receptor chain alpha (IL-2RA) levels, which, apart from being of pathological importance, and the reader is drawn to its parallels with lupus, may also serve as a biomarker for response to therapy [27]. Unfortunately, further development of sifalimumab was blocked during a later trial on lupus due to an adverse event profile (NCT00979654). Recent report of a positive trial of anifrolumab in lupus has again rekindled hopes of targeting the interferon pathways [28], and trials on interferon pathways are ongoing, either in the developmental phase or recruitment phase (NCT02980198; NCT03181893).

Dose; Mode of administration; Frequency; Duration; Indication No extant drug available

Adverse Effects Primarily infections, especially herpes zoster infections, pharyngitis, and other viral infections (mostly available from trials on systemic lupus erythematosus rather than myositis trials)

9.6 Other Biologics

Several other biologics and targeted molecules have been tried PM/DM and are tabulated in Table 9.1 [29–36]. Of these, only tofacitinib and repository corticotropin injection have some potential and are being actively researched. TNF inhibitors may have some role, especially in jDM, however paradoxical worsening of myositis activity, especially dermatomyositis skin rash, is sometimes noticeable.

Table 9.1 Summary of evidence on various biologics in idiopathic inflammatory myopathies (IIMs)

Agent	Study design	Population	Summary of results	Current status
Infliximab	RCT	Adult polymyositis and dermatomyositis (n = 13)	• Nine patients completed the trial (three discontinued due to adverse effects and one due to a discovered malignancy) • Three of the completers improved by ≥20% in ≥3 core sets • Six remained unchanged or worsened • No patient improved in muscle strength by manual muscle test.	Not in contention in adult IIM
	Retrospective study	JDM (n = 39)	• Global disease activity increased at both 6 and 12 month time points • Muscle power also commensurately increased • 50% of patients had a reduction in the number and/or size of calcinosis lesions. • 25% switched from infliximab to adalimumab	Still a contender for JDM
Etanercept	RCT	Adult dermatomyositis (n = 16)	• Sixteen subjects were randomized, 11 to etanercept • Primary outcome was adverse effects • Five etanercept-treated and one placebo-treated subject developed the worsening rash. • All five subjects receiving placebo were treatment failures • Five were successfully weaned off prednisone	Generated some hope for a TNF inhibitor in DM
	Clinical Trial	JDM (n = 9)	• At the 12th week, seven patients had a mild decrease in disease activity, one remained stable, and one worsened • At the 24th week, one patient remained stable, two worsened, and three improved • There was no appreciable change in serum muscle enzymes or CMAS throughout the study.	Overall a negative study; found the TNF alpha 308 alleles to be associated with worsening DM skin rash

Table 9.1 (continued)

Agent	Study design	Population	Summary of results	Current status
Tocilizumab	RCT	Adult IIM (n = 40)	Ongoing	No results posted
Anakinra	Prospective study	Adult polymyositis, dermatomyositis and IBM (n = 15)	• Clinical response in 7/15 • Concomitant changes noted in repeat muscle biopsy	Still investigational
Tofacitinib	Prospective study	anti-MDA5 Ab+ DM-ILD (n = 5)	• Aggressive ILD with poor prognostic factor patients treated with triple therapy with high dose glucocorticoids, CSA and CYC were given additional TOF (10 mg/day). • Three survived, and two died. • The survival rate of patients who received TOF was significantly better than that of the historical controls.	Has definite potential both in cutaneous disease and lung disease
	Retrospective study	Multidrug-resistant cutaneous dermatomyositis (n = 3)	• Clinical response was observed after 4 weeks, and the mean treatment period was 9.6 months. • Clinical activity scores decreased in all three patients • No adverse events occurred • Tofacitinib was given as monotherapy in two patients, and one patient continued using hydroxychloroquine	

(continued)

Table 9.1 (continued)

Agent	Study design	Population	Summary of results	Current status
Repository Corticotropin Injection	Clinical trial	PM (n = 4)/DM (n = 6)	• 10/11 completed the study • 7/10 patients met primary end point at 8 weeks (IMACS definition of improvement) • Significant decrease in prednisolone dose from 18.5 mg/day to 2.3-mg/day • RCI was considered safe and tolerable. • No patient developed significant weight gain or an increase of haemoglobin A1c or cushingoid features.	Has definite potential, especially in cutaneous disease
	Clinical trial	DM patients with active cutaneous disease (n = 9)	• At 3 months, 7/9 patients had improved clinical cutaneous score and 8/9 improved global activity score • At 6 months, 7/7 patients had improved cutaneous score and global disease activity score	

Abbreviations used: *Ab* antibody, *CMAS* childhood myositis assessment scale, *CSA* cyclosporine, *CYC* cyclophosphamide, *DM* dermatomyositis, *IBM* inclusion body myositis, *IIM* idiopathic inflammatory myopathy, *ILD* interstitial lung disease, *IMACS* International Myositis Assessment and Clinical Studies, *JDM* juvenile dermatomyositis, *MDA* melanoma differentiation-associated protein, *PM* polymyositis, *RCI* repository corticotropin injection, *RCT* randomised controlled trial, *TNF* tumor necrosis factor, *TOF* tofacitinib

9.7 Conclusion

The niche of biologics in the treatment of adult PM/DM and jDM is restricted to mostly refractory patients who are either intolerant to conventional immunosuppressive drugs or are non-responsive or develop frequent flares, especially with glucocorticoid tapering. Exceptions to these exist in severe initial disease, especially with severe pharyngeal muscle weakness or respiratory muscle weakness where a definite role of IVIg is well known and practiced. In other cases, rituximab is till now the drug with the most promising evidence. The other especially promising drug is abatacept, but unfortunately, it is no more available in India. Tofacitinib and repository corticotropin injection are the two most "new kids in the block" which might prove to be game changers in the near future.

Conflict of interest None to declare

References

1. Lim J, Eftimov F, Verhamme C, Brusse E, Hoogendijk JE, Saris CGJ, et al. Intravenous immunoglobulins as first-line treatment in idiopathic inflammatory myopathies: a pilot study. Rheumatology (Oxford). 2021;60(4):1784–92.
2. Wang DX, Shu XM, Tian XL, Chen F, Zu N, Ma L, et al. Intravenous immunoglobulin therapy in adult patients with polymyositis/dermatomyositis: a systematic literature review. Clin Rheumatol. 2012;31(5):801–6.
3. Oddis CV, Reed AM, Aggarwal R, Rider LG, Ascherman DP, Levesque MC, et al. Rituximab in the treatment of refractory adult and juvenile dermatomyositis and adult polymyositis: a randomized, placebo-phase trial. Arthritis Rheum. 2013;65(2):314–24.
4. Smith MR. Rituximab (monoclonal anti-CD20 antibody): mechanisms of action and resistance. Oncogene. 2003;22(47):7359–68.
5. Chiu YE, Co DO. Juvenile dermatomyositis: immunopathogenesis, role of myositis-specific autoantibodies, and review of rituximab use. Pediatr Dermatol. 2011;28:357–67.
6. Kikuchi Y, Koarada S, Tada Y, Ushiyama O, Morito F, Suzuki N, et al. Difference in B cell activation between dermatomyositis and polymyositis: analysis of the expression of RP105 on peripheral blood B cells. Ann Rheum Dis. 2001;60(12):1137–40.
7. Oddis CV, Reed AM, Aggarwal R, Rider LG, Ascherman DP, Levesque MC, et al. Rituximab in the treatment of refractory adult and juvenile dermatomyositis and adult polymyositis: a randomized, placebo-phase trial. Arthritis Rheum. 2013;65(2):314–24.
8. Reed AM, Crowson CS, Hein M, de Padilla CL, Olazagasti JM, Aggarwal R, et al. Biologic predictors of clinical improvement in rituximab-treated refractory myositis. BMC Musculoskelet Disord. 2015;16:257.
9. Aggarwal R, Bandos A, Reed AM, Ascherman DP, Barohn RJ, Feldman BM, et al. Predictors of clinical improvement in rituximab-treated refractory adult and juvenile dermatomyositis and adult polymyositis. Arthritis Rheumatol. 2014;66(3):740–9.
10. Chandra T, Aggarwal R. Clinical trials and novel therapeutics in dermatomyositis. Expert Opin Emerg Drugs. 2020;25(3):213–28.
11. Cutolo M, Soldano S, Montagna P, Sulli A, Seriolo B, Villaggio B, et al. CTLA4-Ig interacts with cultured synovial macrophages from rheumatoid arthritis patients and downregulates cytokine production. Arthritis Res Ther. 2009;11(6):R176.
12. Tjärnlund A, Tang Q, Wick C, Dastmalchi M, Mann H, Tomasová Studýnková J, et al. Abatacept in the treatment of adult dermatomyositis and polymyositis: a randomised, phase IIb treatment delayed-start trial. Ann Rheum Dis. 2018;77(1):55–62.
13. Lünemann JD, Nimmerjahn F, Dalakas MC. Intravenous immunoglobulin in neurology–mode of action and clinical efficacy. Nat Rev Neurol. 2015;11(2):80–9.
14. Dalakas MC, Illa I, Dambrosia JM, Soueidan SA, Stein DP, Otero C, et al. A controlled trial of high-dose intravenous immune globulin infusions as treatment for dermatomyositis. N Engl J Med. 1993;329(27):1993–2000.
15. Amemiya K, Semino-Mora C, Granger RP, Dalakas MC. Downregulation of TGF-beta1 mRNA and protein in the muscles of patients with inflammatory myopathies after treatment with high-dose intravenous immunoglobulin. Clin Immunol. 2000;94(2):99–104.
16. Raju R, Dalakas MC. Gene expression profile in the muscles of patients with inflammatory myopathies: effect of therapy with IVIg and biological validation of clinically relevant genes. Brain. 2005;128(Pt 8):1887–96.
17. Cherin P, Piette JC, Wechsler B, Bletry O, Ziza JM, Laraki R, et al. Intravenous gamma globulin as first line therapy in polymyositis and dermatomyositis: an open study in 11 adult patients. J Rheumatol. 1994;21(6):1092–7.
18. Miyasaka N, Hara M, Koike T, Saito E, Yamada M, Tanaka Y, GB-0998 Study Group. Effects of intravenous immunoglobulin therapy in Japanese patients with polymyositis and dermatomyositis resistant to corticosteroids: a randomized double-blind placebo-controlled trial. Mod Rheumatol. 2012;22(3):382–93.

19. Anh-Tu Hoa S, Hudson M. Critical review of the role of intravenous immunoglobulins in idiopathic inflammatory myopathies. Semin Arthritis Rheum. 2017;46(4):488–508.
20. Gordon PA, Winer JB, Hoogendijk JE, Choy EH. Immunosuppressant and immunomodulatory treatment for dermatomyositis and polymyositis. Cochrane Database Syst Rev. 2012;2012(8):CD003643.
21. Danieli MG, Pettinari L, Moretti R, Logullo F, Gabrielli A. Subcutaneous immunoglobulin in polymyositis and dermatomyositis: a novel application. Autoimmun Rev. 2011;10(3):144–9.
22. Danieli MG, Gelardi C, Pedini V, Moretti R, Gabrielli A, Logullo F. Subcutaneous IgG in immune-mediate diseases: proposed mechanisms of action and literature review. Autoimmun Rev. 2014;13(12):1182–8.
23. Isenberg DA, Rowe D, Shearer M, Novick D, Beverley PC. Localization of interferons and interleukin 2 in polymyositis and muscular dystrophy. Clin Exp Immunol. 1986;63(2):450–8.
24. Baechler EC, Bilgic H, Reed AM. Type I interferon pathway in adult and juvenile dermatomyositis. Arthritis Res Ther. 2011;13(6):249.
25. Lundberg IE, Vencovsky J, Alexanderson H. Therapy of myositis: biological and physical. Curr Opin Rheumatol. 2014;26(6):704–11.
26. Higgs BW, Zhu W, Morehouse C, White WI, Brohawn P, Guo X, et al. A phase 1b clinical trial evaluating sifalimumab, an anti-IFN-alpha monoclonal antibody, shows target neutralisation of a type I IFN signature in blood of dermatomyositis and polymyositis patients. Ann Rheum Dis. 2014;73(1):256–62.
27. Guo X, Higgs BW, Rebelatto M, Zhu W, Greth W, Yao Y, et al. Suppression of soluble T cell-associated proteins by an anti-interferon-alpha monoclonal antibody in adult patients with dermatomyositis or polymyositis. Rheumatology (Oxford). 2014;53(4):686–95.
28. Morand EF, Furie R, Tanaka Y, Bruce IN, Askanase AD, Richez C, et al. Trial of anifrolumab in active systemic lupus erythematosus. N Engl J Med. 2020;382(3):211–21.
29. Dastmalchi M, Grundtman C, Alexanderson H, Mavragani CP, Einarsdottir H, Helmers SB, et al. A high incidence of disease flares in an open pilot study of infliximab in patients with refractory inflammatory myopathies. Ann Rheum Dis. 2008;67(12):1670–7.
30. Muscle Study Group. A randomized, pilot trial of etanercept in dermatomyositis. Ann Neurol. 2011;70(3):427–36.
31. Zong M, Dorph C, Dastmalchi M, Alexanderson H, Pieper J, Amoudruz P, et al. Anakinra treatment in patients with refractory inflammatory myopathies and possible predictive response biomarkers: a mechanistic study with 12 months follow-up. Ann Rheum Dis. 2014;73(5):913–20.
32. Rouster-Stevens KA, Ferguson L, Morgan G, Huang CC, Pachman LM. Pilot study of etanercept in patients with refractory juvenile dermatomyositis. Arthritis Care Res (Hoboken). 2014;66(5):783–7.
33. Kurasawa K, Arai S, Namiki Y, Tanaka A, Takamura Y, Owada T, et al. Tofacitinib for refractory interstitial lung diseases in anti-melanoma differentiation-associated 5 gene antibody-positive dermatomyositis. Rheumatology (Oxford). 2018;57(12):2114–9.
34. Kurtzman DJ, Wright NA, Lin J, Femia AN, Merola JF, Patel M, et al. Tofacitinib citrate for refractory cutaneous dermatomyositis: an alternative treatment. JAMA Dermatol. 2016;152(8):944–5.
35. Aggarwal R, Marder G, Koontz DC, Nandkumar P, Qi Z, Oddis CV. Efficacy and safety of adrenocorticotropic hormone gel in refractory dermatomyositis and polymyositis. Ann Rheum Dis. 2018;77(5):720–7.
36. Fernandez A. Interim results of an open-label study assessing efficacy and safety of adrenocorticotropic hormone gel for treatment of refractory cutaneous manifestations of dermatomyositis [abstract]. Arthritis Rheumatol. 2018;70(Suppl 10)

Biologics in ANCA-Associated Vasculitides

10

Saket Jha and Aman Sharma

> A 34 years old female presented with a history of hemoptysis, shortness of breath on exertion and fever. She had been on empirical anti-tubercular treatment for 3 months without relief in her symptoms. She also reported a history of multiple evaluations for epistaxis and nasal crusting. Examination showed a pulse rate of 110/min, respiratory rate of 26/min and blood pressure of 140/80 mmHg. She had pallor, and systemic examination revealed crepitations in bilateral lung fields. On laboratory evaluation, she had normocytic normochromic anemia (Hb—9 g/day) and thrombocytosis (Plt—540,000/L). Urine showed dysmorphic RBCs with proteinuria of 700 mg/24 h and creatinine of 0.9 mg/dL. Chest imaging showed nodules along with ground glass opacities in the middle and lower lung fields. Her Inflammatory markers were raised (ESR—60 mm/h and CRP—102 mg/dL). Immunological tests showed C-ANCA positive on immunofluorescence and high anti PR3 titers. She was diagnosed to have ANCA-associated vasculitis (granulomatous with polyangiitis).

The Chapel Hill Consensus Conference 2012 nomenclature system classifies anti-neutrophil cytoplasmic antibodies (ANCA) associated vasculitis (AAV) into Granulomatosis with polyangiitis (GPA), microscopic polyangiitis (MPA) and eosinophilic granulomatosis with polyangiitis (EGPA) [1]. The management of

S. Jha
Rheumatology Services, Department of Internal Medicine, Maharajgunj Medical Campus, Tribhuvan University Teaching Hospital, Kathmandu, Nepal

A. Sharma (✉)
Clinical Immunology and Rheumatology Services, Department of Internal Medicine, PGIMER, Chandigarh, India

N. Jain, L. Duggal (eds.), *Handbook of Biologics for Rheumatological Disorders*, https://doi.org/10.1007/978-981-16-7200-2_10

AAV has seen a turn in the last few decades with a change in status from a fatal disease to a manageable chronic disease [2].

10.1 Initial Management

- AAV is a multisystem disease; the initial onus of a clinician lies in finding out the disease burden and organ involvement.
- Depending on the organ involvement, the disease can be categorized into different subtypes. It was categorized by EUVAS, especially for the management of GPA/MPA (Table 10.1). This management classification has practical implications and helps in clinical decision-making.
- It is important to rule out mimics especially infections especially infective endocarditis.
- The management consists of two phases' (1) Remission Induction and (2) Remission Maintenance.
- Initial management in the induction phase consists of steroids either as pulse or oral depending upon the disease burden and disease subtypes.
- Steroid-sparing agents like cyclophosphamide, and biological drugs like rituximab are the mainstay of remission induction in most patients and these are given simultaneously along with steroids. Methotrexate and azathioprine is used as remission induction agents rarely in patients with very mild disease.
- The choice of steroid-sparing agent again depends upon the burden, severity, disease subtypes and choice of patients.

10.2 Remission Induction

10.2.1 The History

In the 1970s AAV was considered as a virtual death sentence with a mortality rate to the tune of 90% over 2 years [4]. The use of oral cyclophosphamide showered a ray of hope to this fatal disease bringing the down mortality significantly, however, this was at the cost of side effects like malignancies, cytopenias, infection, and

Table 10.1 EUVAS disease categorization for management of AAV [3]

EUVAS disease subtypes	Definitions
Limited	Upper and/or lower respiratory tract disease without other systemic involvement or constitutional symptoms
Early systemic	Without organ-threatening or life-threatening disease
Generalized	Renal or other life-threatening disease; serum creatinine <5.65 mg/dL
Severe	Renal or other vital organ failure; serum creatinine >5.65 mg/dL
Refractory	Progressive disease unresponsive to cyclophosphamide and glucocorticoids

hemorrhagic cystitis. To the rescue came pulse cyclophosphamide backed up by landmark CYCLOPS trial, which addressed the issues of side effects [5]. The use of other steroid-sparing agents like methotrexate and mycophenolate mofetil were restricted to remission induction in the only mild limited subtype of AAV [6, 7].

10.3 The Introduction of Biological Drug in AAV

- Biological drugs have been used on a compassionate basis since the 1980s. Biological drugs that have been used in the past and are being targeted for the future can be divided as:
  - Intravenous immunoglobulins (IVIG)
  - Cytokine blockade/therapy
    - TNF-α blocking agents
    - Interferon-γ
    - IL-5 (Mepolizumab)
  - Lymphocyte depletion
    - CD20 antibody (rituximab)
    - Anti B cell-activating factor
    - Anti-CD52 antibody
    - Antithymocyte globulin
- Amongst these, the most accepted and with the available evidence is rituximab.

10.4 Rituximab in AAV

Despite the use of cyclophosphamide, the relapse rate of AAV was still significant and was compounded by toxicity and fertility issues. There was a dire need for a new drug. Rituximab, a potent B cell depleting agent, had been in off-label use for severe AAV in various case reports, prospective, and retrospective clinical trials. RAVE and RITUXIVAS were two back-to-back trials published in 2010 which earned its FDA approval and established rituximab as a potent remission induction agent [8, 9]. Both RAVE and RITUXIVAS trials established non-inferiority of rituximab to cyclophosphamide. In addition, it was shown to be superior for relapsing disease. Apart from systemic involvement, rituximab has proved its worth against other agents for limited ear nose throat involvement [10]. Some of these manifestations though limited but could be life threatening, like sub-glottis stenosis.

Rituximab is the first anti-CD20 monoclonal antibody to be used in clinical practice. CD20 is expressed on the surface of naive B cells that have entered blood circulation after exiting bone marrow. The mechanism of action of rituximab for B cell depletion is postulated to be:

1. Complement mediated cytotoxicity
2. Induction of apoptosis
3. Antibody-dependent cell-mediated cytotoxicity

- Antibody-dependent cell-mediated cytotoxicity appears to be the most prominent mechanism for the action of rituximab.
- Rituximab is approved for remission induction in GPA and MPA. In EGPA though the evidence level is weak, however, it has been voted by 100% of experts as a favorable induction agent.
- Rituximab is preferred over cyclophosphamide in the following situation [11–16]:
  - When fertility preservation has to be done
  - Relapsing and PR3 positive disease
  - Limited life-threatening diseases like sub-glottis stenosis, midline destructive lesion
  - Inadequate response to cyclophosphamide
  - Refractory disease
- The caveat of rituximab is the granulomatous manifestation which appears to have an erratic response to treatment.
- Apart from the innovator biological molecules, several bio-similar and bio-mimic preparation of rituximab have been shown to be equally effective in AAV [17].
- The pre-infusion checklist of rituximab is shown in Table 10.2.
- The approved dosing regimen of rituximab is shown in Table 10.3.

Table 10.2 Showing pre-infusion investigation for rituximab

Pre-infusion checklist for rituximab
Complete blood count
Renal function test
Liver function test
Chest X-ray
Urine routine and microscopic examination
HBsAg, Anti HBc
Anti HCV
Rule out active infection
Serum Immunoglobulin G level (IgG)

Table 10.3 Showing approved dosing regimen of rituximab

Dosing regimen of rituximab
1. Rituximab IV 1 g on 0 and 15 days
2. Alternative regimen: Rituximab IV 375 mg/m^2 body surface area weekly for 4 weeks

10.5 Remission Maintenance

Relapses are the major concerns associated with AAV. Relapses were seen in one-half of the cases, and this rate could only be reduced to one-third with the use of steroid-sparing agents like methotrexate and azathioprine [18, 19]. Similar to induction, rituximab was also studied as a maintenance agent in various prospective and retrospective studies.

- The role of rituximab as the most prominent remission induction agent has been established by three landmark trials MAINRITSAN 1, 2, and 3.
- MAINRITSAN 1: It compared fixed-dose rituximab versus azathioprine and showed sustained remission with rituximab. At 28 months 5% relapse was seen in the rituximab arm as compared to 25% in the azathioprine arm [20].
- MAINRITSAN 2: No significant difference in the relapse rate was seen in fixed-dose rituximab (every 6 monthly) versus tailored dose rituximab (twofold rise in PR3 titers or clinical relapse) as studied in this trial [21].
- MAINRITSAN 3: It evaluated the efficacy of prolonged rituximab therapy in patients who achieved complete remission after the standard maintenance dosing. Lower rates of relapses were seen in patients who received extended biannual rituximab [22].
- The dosing and duration of rituximab during remission maintenance is shown in Table 10.4.

10.6 Other Biological Drugs in AAV

- Apart from rituximab, various other biological drugs have been investigated and tested in AAV
- The status of various other biological drugs is shown in Table 10.5.

Table 10.4 Dosing and duration regimen of rituximab

Dosing and duration
1. IV Rituximab 500 mg every 6 monthly
2. Duration: No definite data

Table 10.5 Biological agents in AAV

Drug and MOA	Disease	Remark
IgG antibodies against B cell activating factor (BAFF): Belimumab [23]	• GPA and MPA • Remission maintenance	• BREVAS Study: RCT to evaluate the efficacy and safety of belimumab in combination with azathioprine for the maintenance of remission in GPA and MPA • It did not reduce the risk of relapse • Not approved for use in AAV
Anti TNF: Infliximab [24]	• GPA • Remission induction • Refractory cases	• Four open-label studies have reported the use of infliximab in patients with AAV • With Infliximab use, remission was achieved in >80% (43 out of 53) of the patients • Not approved for use in AAV
Anti TNF: Etanercept [25]	• GPA • Remission maintenance	• WGET (Wegener's Granulomatosis Etanercept Trial) • It did not show an advantage of additional therapy with etanercept compared with standard therapy • Not approved for use in AAV
Interferon-α therapy [26]	• EGPA	• The data from patients showed that patients were able to reduce or drop steroid therapy or remain on low-dose steroids • Not approved for use in AAV
Anti-IL5 monoclonal antibody: Mepolizumab [27]	• EGPA	• Data from two open-label trials showed that the majority of EGPA patients treated with Mepolizumab achieved clinical remission and significant corticosteroid-sparing effect • Approved for use in EGPA
Anti-IgE monoclonal antibody: Omalizumab [28]	• EGPA	• Data from case reports shows clinical improvement and reduction in the peripheral eosinophil count • Not approved for use in AAV
Anti-CD52 monoclonal antibody: Alemtuzumab [29]	• AAV	• Data from small uncontrolled trials showed that around 85% of patients achieved clinical remission; however around 80% of them relapsed • Not approved for use in AAV

10.7 Conclusion

- The management of AAV remains a challenge despite advances in the diagnostics and therapeutics
- Various biological drugs have been studied in AAV, among them; only rituximab has established its use both in induction and remission maintenance of ANCA-associated vasculitis till date.
- Various other molecular targets needs/are being studied, which would answer several unanswered queries like; prevention of relapse, ideal duration and frequency of maintenance therapy and choice of drug for granulomatous versus vasculitic manifestations.

References

1. Jennette JC, Falk RJ, Bacon PA, Basu N, Cid MC, Ferrario F, et al. 2012 revised International Chapel Hill Consensus Conference Nomenclature of Vasculitides. Arthritis Rheum. 2013;65(1):1–11.
2. Sharma A, Naidu GS, Rathi M, Verma R, Modi M, Pinto B, et al. Clinical features and long term outcome of 105 patients of Granulomatosis with Polyangiitis: a single centre experience from north India. Int J Rheum Dis. 2018;21:278–84.
3. Mukhtyar C, Guillevin L, Cid MC, Dasgupta B, Groot K, Gross W, et al. EULAR recommendations for the management of primary small and medium vessel vasculitis. Ann Rheum Dis. 2009;68(3):310–7.
4. Novack SN, Pearson CM. Cyclophosphamide therapy in Wegener's granulomatosis. N Engl J Med. 1971;284(17):938–42.
5. de Groot K, Harper L, Jayne DRW, Flores Suarez LF, Gregorini G, Gross WL, et al. Pulse versus daily oral cyclophosphamide for induction of remission in antineutrophil cytoplasmic antibody-associated vasculitis: a randomized trial. Ann Intern Med. 2009;150(10):670–80.
6. Stone JH, Tun W, Hellman DB. Treatment of non-life threatening Wegener's granulomatosis with methotrexate and daily prednisone as the initial therapy of choice. J Rheumatol. 1999;26(5):1134–9.
7. Han F, Liu G, Zhang X, Li X, He Q, He X, et al. Effects of mycophenolate mofetil combined with corticosteroids for induction therapy of microscopic polyangiitis. Am J Nephrol. 2011;33(2):185–92.
8. Stone JH, Merkel PA, Spiera R, Seo P, Langford CA, Hoffman GS, et al. Rituximab versus cyclophosphamide for ANCA-associated vasculitis. N Engl J Med. 2010;363(3):221–32.
9. Jones RB, Cohen Tervaert JW, Hauser T, Luqmani R, Morgan MD, Peh CA, et al. Rituximab versus cyclophosphamide in ANCA-associated renal vasculitis. N Engl J Med. 2010;363(3):211–20.
10. Lally L, Lebovics RS, Huang W-T, Spiera RF. Effectiveness of rituximab for the otolaryngologic manifestations of granulomatosis with polyangiitis (Wegener's). Arthritis Care Res. 2014;66(9):1403–9.
11. Singh P, Dhooria A, Rathi M, Agarwal R, Sharma K, Dhir V, et al. Successful treatment outcomes in pregnant patients with ANCA-associated vasculitides: a systematic review of literature. Int J Rheum Dis. 2018;21(9):1734–40.
12. Sharma A, Kumar S, Wanchu A, Lal V, Singh R, Gupta V, et al. Successful treatment of hypertrophic pachymeningitis in refractory Wegener's granulomatosis with rituximab. Clin Rheumatol. 2010;29(1):107–10.
13. Lower EE, Baughman RP, Kaufman AH. Rituximab for refractory granulomatous eye disease. Clin Ophthalmol Auckl NZ. 2012;6:1613–8.
14. Holle JU, Dubrau C, Herlyn K, Heller M, Ambrosch P, Noelle B, et al. Rituximab for refractory granulomatosis with polyangiitis (Wegener's granulomatosis): comparison of efficacy in granulomatous versus vasculitic manifestations. Ann Rheum Dis. 2012;71(3):327–33.
15. Cartin-Ceba R, Golbin JM, Keogh KA, Peikert T, Sánchez-Menéndez M, Ytterberg SR, et al. Rituximab for remission induction and maintenance in refractory granulomatosis with polyangiitis (Wegener's): ten-year experience at a single center. Arthritis Rheum. 2012;64(11):3770–8.
16. Ayan G, Esatoglu SN, Hatemi G, Ugurlu S, Seyahi E, Melikoglu M, et al. Rituximab for anti-neutrophil cytoplasmic antibodies-associated vasculitis: experience of a single center and systematic review of non-randomized studies. Rheumatol Int. 2018;38(4):607–22.
17. Mittal S, Naidu GSRSNK, Jha S, Rathi M, Nada R, Minz RW, et al. Experience with similar biologic rituximab in 77 patients of granulomatosis with polyangiitis-a real-life experience. Clin Rheumatol. 2020;
18. Walsh M, Flossmann O, Berden A, Westman K, Höglund P, Stegeman C, et al. Risk factors for relapse of antineutrophil cytoplasmic antibody-associated vasculitis. Arthritis Rheum. 2012;64(2):542–8.

19. Pagnoux C, Mahr A, Hamidou MA, Boffa J-J, Ruivard M, Ducroix J-P, et al. Azathioprine or methotrexate maintenance for ANCA-associated vasculitis. N Engl J Med. 2008;359(26):2790–803.
20. Charles P, Guillevin L. S3. Rituximab for ANCA-associated vasculitides: the French experience. Presse Medicale Paris Fr 1983. 2013;42(4 Pt 2):534–6.
21. Charles P, Terrier B, Perrodeau É, Cohen P, Faguer S, Huart A, et al. Comparison of individually tailored versus fixed-schedule rituximab regimen to maintain ANCA-associated vasculitis remission: results of a multicentre, randomised controlled, phase III trial (MAINRITSAN2). Ann Rheum Dis. 2018;77(8):1143–9.
22. Charles P, Perrodeau É, Samson M, Bonnotte B, Néel A, Agard C, et al. Long-term rituximab use to maintain remission of antineutrophil cytoplasmic antibody-associated vasculitis: a randomized trial. Ann Intern Med. 2020;173(3):179–87.
23. Jayne D, Blockmans D, Luqmani R, Moiseev S, Ji B, Green Y, et al. Efficacy and safety of belimumab and azathioprine for maintenance of remission in antineutrophil cytoplasmic antibody-associated vasculitis: a randomized controlled study. Arthritis Rheumatol Hoboken NJ. 2019;71(6):952–63.
24. Mukhtyar C, Luqmani R. Current state of tumour necrosis factor α blockade in Wegener's granulomatosis. Ann Rheum Dis. 2005;64(Suppl 4):iv31–6.
25. Wegener's Granulomatosis Etanercept Trial (WGET) Research Group. Etanercept plus standard therapy for Wegener's granulomatosis. N Engl J Med. 2005;352(4):351–61.
26. Metzler C, Lamprecht P, Hellmich B, Reuter M, Arlt A, Gross W. Leucoencephalopathy after treatment of Churg-Strauss syndrome with interferon α. Ann Rheum Dis. 2005;64(8):1242–3.
27. Kim S, Marigowda G, Oren E, Israel E, Wechsler ME. Mepolizumab as a steroid-sparing treatment option in patients with Churg-Strauss syndrome. J Allergy Clin Immunol. 2010;125(6):1336–43.
28. Iglesias E, Camacho Lovillo M, Delgado Pecellín I, Lirola Cruz MJ, Falcón Neyra MD, Salazar Quero JC, et al. Successful management of Churg-Strauss syndrome using omalizumab as adjuvant immunomodulatory therapy: first documented pediatric case. Pediatr Pulmonol. 2014;49(3):E78–81.
29. Walsh M, Chaudhry A, Jayne D. Long-term follow-up of relapsing/refractory anti-neutrophil cytoplasm antibody associated vasculitis treated with the lymphocyte depleting antibody alemtuzumab (CAMPATH-1H). Ann Rheum Dis. 2008;67(9):1322–7.

Biologics in Behcet's syndrome

11

Rudrarpan Chatterjee, Sundeep Grover, and Vikas Agarwal

11.1 Introduction

Behcet's syndrome encompasses dysfunction in both the innate and the adaptive immune systems resulting in inflammation in a wide range of organ systems including the mucosal and epithelial barriers of the orogenital apparatus, blood vessels, eyes as well as relatively devastating effects in the brainstem and pulmonary vasculature. The mucocutaneous manifestations of oral and genital ulcers resemble autoinflammatory disorders and are associated with a high IL-1 beta signature. Similar observations have been made regarding the similarity of ulcers in the ileum in Behcet's and inflammatory bowel disease like Crohn's as well as enthesitis seen in the spondyloarthropathy spectrum of disorders. The inflammation of the blood vessels with manifestations such as superficial and deep venous thrombosis, pulmonary artery vasculitis, and resulting aneurysm and central nervous system inflammation bear similarities with adaptive immunity mediated by cytotoxic CD8 T cells. This flexible position in the continuum of innate and adaptive immunity provides us with both a challenge in terms of its widespread manifestations as well as an opportunity in the form of multiple plausible therapeutic targets in both arms of the immune system. With the advent of biologic therapies and small molecule inhibitors of the immunity, there is immense therapeutic potential for the targeted management of this elusive and often refractory disease.

R. Chatterjee · V. Agarwal (✉)
Department of Clinical Immunology and Rheumatology, Sanjay Gandhi Postgraduate Institute of Medical Sciences, Lucknow, India

S. Grover
Arthritis & Immunology Clinic, Meerut, India

N. Jain, L. Duggal (eds.), *Handbook of Biologics for Rheumatological Disorders*,
https://doi.org/10.1007/978-981-16-7200-2_11

11.2 Immune Dysfunction and Therapeutic Targets in Behcet's Syndrome

The pathogenesis of Behcet's syndrome starts with the innate immune cells that are primed as part of mucosal immunity. These cells include neutrophils which form the predominant inflammatory infiltrate in the aphthae, the NK cells which mediate inflammation and act as a bridge between the innate and adaptive immune systems. The cytokine milieu associated with these activated immune cells includes IL-6, IL-8, IFN-ɣ, and TNF as well as the inflammasome-mediated release of IL-1β. All these cytokines represent interesting possibilities for targeted biologic therapy but as a result of the redundancy in the pathways downstream of these cytokines, inhibition of anyone is often inadequate. The ɣδ-T cells were previously thought to be the only adaptive immune cells implicated in Behcet's due to their convenient location in the mucosal tissues as well as close parallels observed with the role these cells play in similar clinical manifestations of mucosal ulcers in inflammatory bowel disease and enthesitis in spondyloarthropathies. However, as our understanding of the pathogenesis of this disease has evolved with time, other adaptive immune cells such as the Th1 and Th17 polarized helper T cells and cytotoxic CD8 T cells have been found to play a role in subsets of the disease with severe manifestations such as vasculitis. This has been reflected in the classification of Behcet's syndrome as a variable vessel vasculitis in the Chapel Hill consensus definitions. The cytokine profile in Behcet's therefore also reflects these adaptive immune pathways with activation of the IL12–IL23–IL17 axis which is also a potential therapeutic target of biologics. Antigen presentation to these adaptive immune cells and the processing of antigens through the ERAP1 protein which is inadequately expressed in Behcet's is another interesting parallel to the spondyloarthropathies. This links to the major HLA association of Behcet's disease which is HLA-B51. Therefore, the treatment of Behcet's could potentially involve IL-1 inhibition with Anakinra or Canakinumab, TNF-α inhibition with infliximab, adalimumab, and a host of other available anti-TNF agents or even IL-17 inhibition with Secukinumab or inhibition of IL-23 with Ustekinumab upstream to it. The lack of development in targeted therapeutics to such a host of inviting targets stems from the fact that the syndrome itself is quite rare and even so has a wide variety of manifestations across geographic distributions and within phenotype variations in severity even among those in the same geographic cluster.

11.3 EULAR 2018 Update of Guidelines for Management of Behcet's Syndrome

In 2018, the need was felt to update the 2008 guidelines for the management of Behcet's syndrome with a major consideration being the emerging evidence for the role of biologics, especially anti-TNF therapies in these patients. The overarching principles advocated by EULAR do emphasize the need to individualize therapy

Table 11.1 Indications for biologics in the 2018 EULAR guidelines for management of Behcet's syndrome

Organ system involved	Indication for biologics (level of evidence)
Mucocutaneous	IFN-α, TNF-inhibitor for lesions refractory to colchicine, azathioprine, thalidomide, and short courses of systemic steroids (IB).
Eye	IFN-α, TNF-inhibitor for posterior segment uveitis refractory to Azathioprine and Cyclosporine (IIA). Upfront use in uveitis if recurrent severe and vision threatening (IIA).
Refractory venous thrombosis	TNF inhibitor for those refractory of azathioprine, cyclophosphamide, or cyclosporine (III).
Arterial	Pulmonary artery aneurysm refractory to cyclophosphamide and high dose glucocorticoids (III).
Gastrointestinal	Ileal ulcers refractory to Azathioprine or 5-aminosalicylic acid derivatives once IBD and tuberculosis have been ruled out (III).
Neurological	Acute parenchymal involvement with severe first attack or disease refractory to treatment with high dose glucocorticoids and cyclophosphamide (III).
Arthritis	IFN-α, TNF-inhibitor for chronic and recurrent arthritis.

Level of evidence: IA—meta-analysis of RCT, IB—at least one RCT, IIA—at least one controlled study sans randomization, IIB—at least one quasi-experimental study, III—descriptive studies such as case control studies, IV—expert consensus

based on patient characteristics and the poor prognosis associated with certain major organ involvements that warrant aggressive systemic therapy. The recommendations with respect to biologics are summarized in Table 11.1 [1].

11.4 Indications of Biologic Therapies in Behcet's Syndrome

- The thrust for the use of biologics in Behcet's is for disease refractory to conventional therapy. This stems from the fact that most mucocutaneous, as well as arthritic symptoms, respond well to colchicine alone which is safe, effective, and inexpensive as well as having a long track record for safety. Systemic immunosuppression is considered when the clinical manifestations are either recurrent or refractory to therapy with colchicine. A short course of glucocorticoids suffices to control acute flares of mucocutaneous disease. The use of anti-IL1 agents is an attractive option given their success in a host of other autoinflammatory illnesses. In this regard, Etanercept, a fusion protein of TNF receptor with the constant heavy chain of IgG1 has been found to reduce the mean number of oral ulcers as well as papulopustular skin lesions in a randomized controlled clinical trial [2]. Though randomized trials are lacking, the use of anakinra or canakinumab (both IL-1 antagonists) would also, therefore, be attractive therapeutic options in this setting and are approved for use in mucocutaneous manifestations of other autoinflammatory disorders.

- The role of biologics is better defined for disease that becomes refractory to conventional therapeutic options or when organ-threatening illness is present. Posterior uveitis is a potential such manifestation that may be asymptomatic and yet cause loss of vision and permanent disability to the patient. While azathioprine and cyclosporine are routinely advised for uveitis in Behcet's, it is prudent to rapidly escalate therapy to a TNF inhibitor such as infliximab (5 mg/kg every 2 months) or adalimumab (40 mg SC every 2 weeks). Interferon alpha (5 MU/day) is another option that has demonstrated efficacy in Behcet's related uveitis. Though data from randomized clinical trials is lacking, real-world evidence exists for earlier remission and decreased frequency of attacks with the early use of Infliximab for Behcet's related uveitis [3].
- Adalimumab, which has had success in the management of spondyloarthropathy-associated uveitis and is recommended as first-line drug for that indication is another attractive option for Behcet's associated uveitis. There are case series demonstrating the safety of adalimumab in this setting as well as evidence for visual preservation and complete resolution of ocular inflammation as well as a decrease in attack frequency [4]. Clinical trials of adalimumab in this setting of noninfectious uveitis including posterior uveitis have documented lesser treatment failures in those with uveitis and improvement in at least one patient-reported outcome in the form of visual acuity [5]. However, this was not a trial specifically for Behcet's and hence the treatment groups are far more heterogeneous and the data should be evaluated critically in this regard when it comes to Behcet's related uveitis.
- The other therapeutic targets in Behcet's syndrome include IL-17 and IL-23 as part of the Th17 immune pathway. Ustekinumab (90 mg SC at week 0, 4, and every 12 weeks thereafter), an inhibitor of the p40 subunit of the IL-23 molecule, has been evaluated in an open-label trial for mucocutaneous disease refractory to colchicine. The number of mucocutaneous ulcers was lower in those treated with ustekinumab along with decreased overall Behcet's syndrome activity scores. There were no safety signals associated with its use [6]. Secukinumab (150 mg or 300 mg SC every 4 weeks) has been studied in a multicenter retrospective study in patients with mucocutaneous and articular disease refractory to colchicine, disease-modifying anti-rheumatic drugs (DMARDs) and anti-TNF agents. This small study demonstrated the safety of Secukinumab as well as a complete or partial therapeutic response in two-thirds of the patients [7]. There was also a trend towards better response with the higher dose of Secukinumab with all patients on the higher dose achieving a complete response.
- For organ-threatening disease, considering the parallels of inflammatory bowel disease the use of anti-TNF agents is plausible in gastrointestinal involvement in the form of ileal ulcers. TNF inhibition with adalimumab (160 mg SC at week 0, 80 mg at week 2, and 40 mg SC every 2 weeks thereafter) has been shown to induce complete response in 20% of Japanese patients with intestinal Behcet's disease [8]. This data has to be evaluated keeping in mind the difference in disease severity across geographic regions as disease is known to be less severe in people of non-Turkish descent. The use of biologics in pulmonary artery involvement is not well studied mainly due to the rarity of the manifestation itself. In 13

patients with pulmonary artery involvement who were retrospectively reviewed, in those on TNF inhibition due to various indications that were all refractory to conventional immunosuppressives, 6 patients had a good response with continued TNF blockade, 4 could discontinue therapy completely due to response but 2 relapsed after withdrawal of TNF inhibition and azathioprine [9]. It is also important to note that one patient died of hemoptysis, two developed pulmonary artery involvement while using TNF inhibitor for another indication and one patient developed mesenteric vein thrombosis and new site of pulmonary artery involvement. More data is required to evaluate the safety and efficacy of TNF inhibition in this setting.

11.5 Conclusion

Biologic therapies are safe and effective in Behcet's syndrome with mucocutaneous and articular disease. The indications that have been studied at present include disease refractory to conventional therapy with colchicine and other DMARDs. For organ- or life-threatening illness, there is a lack of high-quality evidence for the use of biologics but important real-world data suggests they may have a role in disease refractory to conventional therapy.

References

1. Hatemi G, Christensen R, Bang D, Bodaghi B, Celik AF, Fortune F, et al. 2018 update of the EULAR recommendations for the management of Behçet's syndrome. Ann Rheum Dis. 2018;annrheumdis-2018-213225.
2. Melikoglu M, Fresko I, Mat C, Ozyazgan Y, Gogus F, Yurdakul S, et al. Short-term trial of etanercept in Behçet's disease: a double blind, placebo controlled study. J Rheumatol. 2005;32(1):98–105.
3. Guzelant G, Ucar D, Esatoglu SN, Hatemi G, Ozyazgan Y, Yurdakul S, et al. Infliximab for uveitis of Behçet's syndrome: a trend for earlier initiation. Clin Exp Rheumatol. 2017;35 Suppl 108(6):86–9.
4. Ho M, Chen LJ, Sin HPY, Iu LPL, Brelen M, Ho ACH, Lai TYY, Young AL. Experience of using adalimumab in treating sight-threatening paediatric or adolescent Behcet's disease-related uveitis. J Ophthalmic Inflamm Infect. 2019;9(1):14.
5. Jaffe GJ, Dick AD, Brézin AP, Nguyen QD, Thorne JE, Kestelyn P, et al. Adalimumab in patients with active noninfectious uveitis. N Engl J Med. 2016;375(10):932–43.
6. Mirouse A, Barete S, Desbois A-C, Comarmond C, Sène D, Domont F, et al. Long-term outcome of ustekinumab therapy for Behçet's disease. Arthritis Rheumatol (Hoboken, NJ). 2019;71(10):1727–32.
7. Fagni F, Bettiol A, Talarico R, Lopalco G, Silvestri E, Urban ML, et al. Long-term effectiveness and safety of secukinumab for treatment of refractory mucosal and articular Behçet's phenotype: a multicentre study. Ann Rheum Dis. 2020;79(8):1098–104.
8. Tanida S, Inoue N, Kobayashi K, Naganuma M, Hirai F, Iizuka B, et al. Adalimumab for the treatment of Japanese patients with intestinal Behçet's disease. Clin Gastroenterol Hepatol Off Clin Pract J Am Gastroenterol Assoc. 2015;13(5):940–948.e3.
9. Hamuryudan V, Seyahi E, Ugurlu S, Melikoglu M, Hatemi G, Ozguler Y, et al. Pulmonary artery involvement in Behçet's syndrome: effects of anti-Tnf treatment. Semin Arthritis Rheum. 2015;45(3):369–73.

12 Biologics in Takayasu's Arteritis

Avanish Jha and Debashish Danda

12.1 Introduction

Takayasu arteritis (TA) is an immune-mediated inflammatory disease of large arteries. Its pathological mechanisms are slowly unraveling and, in spite of paucity of biomarkers, some preliminary tools for assessing the disease like ITAS2010 and ITAS A (CRP) are being made available in day-to-day clinical practice. Hopefully, these ongoing advancements will make "treat to target" in TA a reality, sooner than later.

TA is a lifelong disease similar to most systemic autoimmune conditions. Spontaneous or off-treatment remission as well as rare monocyclic disease course, all put together, account for less than 20% of cases. Asymptomatic and slowly progressive nature of disease in TA can befool clinicians and falsely behave as silent or inactive disease. If left untreated because of apparent paucity of clinical features, TA only adds on cumulative damage due to ongoing, unsuspected, and untreated inflammatory process; and the unsuspecting clinicians are left in the dark and caught unaware with regretful, sudden surprises like irreversible major organ ischemia in the form of Myocardial infarction, stroke, renal failure, and several such devastating sequela including death.

While most people are treating TA using conventional immunomodulators and immunosuppressants, use of biological agents are coming into practice. Figure 12.1 depicts the biological basis of targeted treatment in TA. Considering their costs, we need a logical, rational, and economically tailored approach for prescribing biologics in TA.

A. Jha · D. Danda (✉)
Department of Clinical Immunology and Rheumatology, Christian Medical College, Vellore, India

N. Jain, L. Duggal (eds.), *Handbook of Biologics for Rheumatological Disorders*,
https://doi.org/10.1007/978-981-16-7200-2_12

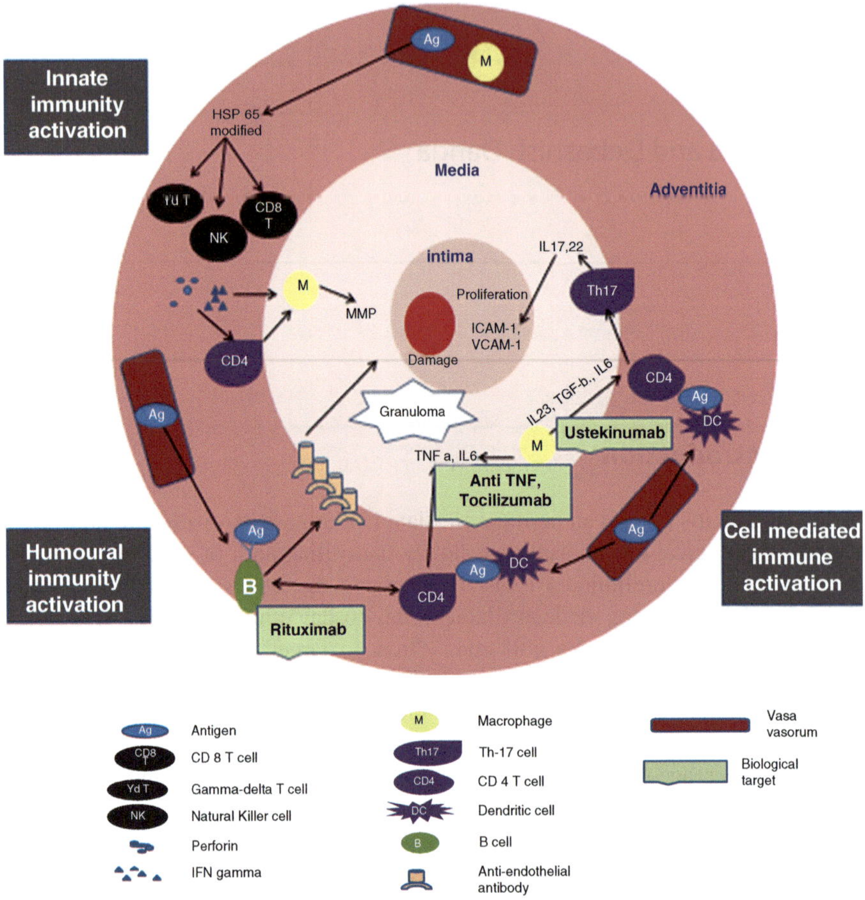

Fig. 12.1 Biological basis for targets of treatment in Takayasu arteritis

Here is a case-based scenario on the use of biological agents in a patient with TA from a resource-limited setup. This may offer learning steps for rheumatologists in this highly specialised area. We also have made a treatment algorithm for this purpose.

12.2 Case Scenario

A 19-year-old girl presented with a history of pain in her right arm, which occurs after a fixed amount of activity with her right upper limb. She also has unexplained weight loss and fatigue. Examination revealed absent right radial and brachial artery pulsations and a bruit over right subclavian artery.

12.3 Discussion

Takayasu arteritis is a large vessel granulomatous vasculitis involving predominantly aorta and its main branches at origin and sometimes pulmonary arteries. It can present with constitutional symptoms along with symptoms of ischemia in various systems; but presentations with pulse loss, hypertension, or claudication of limbs are among the commonest. Its varied manifestations include Reno-vascular hypertension, stroke, seizure, and cardiovascular symptoms like angina, myocardial infarction, and aortic incompetence. Acute phase reactants may be elevated, but these do not always increase in all patients with active disease.

12.4 STEP 1: Initial Assessment and Diagnosis

- Patient should be assessed by history taking and examination of all peripheral pulses and four limb blood pressure recordings to look for weakened, asymmetric or loss of pulse, blood pressure difference, and bruit over the major arteries.
- Laboratory investigations of raised acute phase reactants like CRP and ESR (may not be elevated in all cases).
- Imaging investigations include one of the following: conventional angiogram, Digital subtraction angiography, CT angiogram or MR angiogram, and most recently PET scan. The imaging might reveal stenosis, occlusion, or less commonly aneurysms. CT and MR angiography may also reveal wall thickening and enhancement with contrast. Contrast-enhanced ultrasound and color Doppler is an evolving modality in this area, although its use at the moment is restricted to expertise-dependent setups.
- Chest X-ray, electrocardiography (ECG), and echocardiogram are also done to assess cardiac and aortic root involvement.
- A confident diagnosis of Takayasu arteritis is based on a combination of Clinical, laboratory, and radiological investigations. Classification criteria have been proposed like 1990 ACR, Ishikawa, as well as Sharma's modification to Ishikawa criteria and these may be used for clinical guidance in diagnosis.
- After a patient fulfills classification and angiographic criteria (Hata's), disease activity scores like ITAS 2010 & ITAS-A (CRP), disease extent scores like DEI.TAK and damage scores like TADS must be documented and should be repeated in follow-up visits.

12.5 Step 2: Initiating Corticosteroids and Immunosuppression

- Patients are started on high dose steroids at 0.5 mg/kg body weight of prednisolone or equivalent dose of deflazacort, a derivative of prednisolone (authors prefer this due to its lesser metabolic side effects) and then steroids are gradually attempted to be tapered over 6 months to 5 mg/day or lesser.

- Glucocorticoids are good for remission induction but cause frequent relapse on tapering dosing in about 50% of cases.
- In view of the reason mentioned above, most Rheumatologists start a steroid sparing, conventional disease modifying agents (DMARD) or second-line immunosuppressant upfront along with steroids. These agents take several weeks to months to demonstrate efficacy. Therefore, upfront institution of second-line agents along with steroids right from the beginning help prevent relapse while tapering steroid. Mycophenolate mofetil (MMF) or Mycophenolate sodium (MMS), azathioprine, and Methotrexate are commonly used agents in routine practice; however, in some settings, cyclophosphamide, tacrolimus, leflunomide, and even JAK inhibitors like tofacitinib are also used based on anecdotal reports and biological basis.

12.6 Case Scenario

Our patient is diagnosed with Takayasu arteritis after assessment as per step 1 and started on 36 mg Deflazacort daily morning after breakfast and Methotrexate 15 mg/week and then built up to 25 mg subcutaneously over the next 2 months.

12.7 Step 3: Assessment of Disease Activity at Follow up

- Patients are followed up at 2 to 3 monthly intervals initially for response assessment and any features of relapse and damage after remission induction.
- In absence of any specific biomarker, combined clinical, laboratory, and radiological assessment tools are used.
- ITAS2010 and ITAS-A are validated tools for assessment of disease activity based on clinical features and acute phase reactants; these are easily doable unlike angiography that is unrealistic at frequent intervals in view of invasiveness and cost, unless interventions like stenting is indicated.
- Revascularization techniques like endovascular stenting are used for symptomatic significant stenosis or occlusion after control of active disease.

12.8 Case Scenario

Our patient does well on steroids initially but has worsening pain in the arm on dose reduction to less than 18 mg of Deflazacort at review visit. It is thus decided to increase the dose of the steroid to 36 mg and wait for 3 more months. However, she has a recurrence of symptoms at review at 6 months. She undergoes conventional angiogram and stenting of subclavian artery in view of worsening stenosis and symptoms. Methotrexate is changed to Mycophenolate mofetil and deflazacort is again increased to 60 mg and planned for slower taper.

Our patient comes back after 2 weeks with no pain in arm or any constitutional features, but complains of diarrhea, abdominal pain (that is, not like vasculitis or angina type), and has persistent nausea. Her examination shows no new findings. Her blood parameters show improving acute phase reactants and otherwise normal routine blood parameters. Her mycophenolate mofetil (MMF) is changed to an equivalent dose of the sodium salt of mycophenolic acid (MMS). She has improvement in diarrhea, abdominal pain, and nausea with the same.

12.9 Step 4: Step up to Biological Agents

- Patients with resistant disease or relapse on steroids and conventional DMARD or second-line immunosuppressant are considered for biological therapy.
  The following biological agents are being used in TA:

Tocilizumab

- Tocilizumab, an IL6 receptor blocker, has been utilized and proven effective as an add-on, steroid sparing, quick acting, and stopgap agent.
- One randomized controlled trial (TAKT study) using subcutaneous tocilizumab with small number of participants showed numerical benefit in attaining remission in relapsed disease, but failed to reach statistical significance probably due to small numbers recruited.
- In a cohort of 251 patients from India, monthly intravenous tocilizumab was used successfully in all 14 (5.6%) resistant, relapsed, or cases undergoing procedures to prevent restenosis as a stopgap and steroid sparing agent.
- TOCITAKA, a French open-labeled prospective study using tocilizumab in treatment naïve patients showed remission rates of 85%, but there was a relapse in 45% of them after discontinuation of tocilizumab.
- These data confirm the utility of Tocilizumab for short-term disease control; however, another maintenance agent like mycophenolate is needed to maintain remission.
- Table 12.1 summarizes some of the largest data on the use of biologics in TA.

Tumor necrosis factor (TNF) inhibitors

- There is no randomized controlled trial.
- Infliximab, a chimeric mouse and human monoclonal antibody against tumor necrosis factor has been used in observational studies involving resistant or relapsed cases.

Table 12.1 Selected published data on biologics in TA

Study	Disease status	Number of cases	Study type	Intervention	Primary outcome	Result	Comment
Tocilizumab studies							
TAKT study Nakaoka et al. (2017)	Relapse	36: 18 (I) vs 18 (C)	RCT	GC (at least 0.2 mg/kg/day) + TCZ 162 mg subcutaneously/week (started after ≥1 week from remission induction with steroid)	Time to relapse	HR, 0.41 95%CI 0.15–1.1	Small numbers, not met primary outcome; but tocilizumab may be useful
Ruchika Goel, Debashish Danda et al. (2012)	Resistant and difficult to treat	10 cases	Observational—Prospective	TCZ 8 mg/kg IV monthly for 6 doses + steroids 0.5–1 mg/kg in tapering dose (one patient was not on steroid and another on 2.5 mg prednisolone at baseline)	ITAS = 0, Normal APR, Radiological activity	Six (60%) had a clinical response with stable imaging and normal APR	Good reduction in steroid dose; good clinical response, but only 2 patients maintained stable disease state without upscaling of immunosuppressive treatment after TCZ was stopped; majority needed rescue therapy
TOCITAKA Arsene Mekinian et al. French Prospective cohort 2020	New, treatment naive	13 cases	Observational—Prospective	Steroids at the dose of 0.7 mg/kg/day and 7 infusions of 8 mg/kg/month of TCZ	Stopping of steroids at 7 months	Six (54%) patients met the primary end-point	Good reduction in steroid dose and activity but at 18 months 5 out of 11 had relapsed

H Liao et al. Chinese Cohort 2019	Details not available	27 TCZ and 22 Cyclophosphamide	Observational—two armed retrospective	Monthly TCZ 8 mg/kg Iv or Cyclophosphamide for 6 doses + steroids	Clinical response, APR and prednisolone dose reduction	Response significantly better in TCZ Group for all responses	Incidence of drug-related side effects in TCZ group was significantly lower (22 vs 54%)
Italian cohort Enrico Tombetti et al. (2013)	Refractory	7 cases	Observational—Retrospective	TCZ (8 mg/kg iv Monthly) + steroids	Response criteria and reduction of disease activity, as defined by acute-phase reactants and the US National Institutes of Health (NIH) criteria at 6 months	Four patients achieved clinical response. APR normalized in all	Response good in 4 patients, but vascular progression occurred overall in 4 patients
J. Loricera et al. (2016) Spanish group	7 out of 8 cases are Refractory	8 cases	Observational—Retrospective	TCZ (8 mg/kg iv) + steroids	Clinical symptom, CRP, ESR, and steroid dose reduction	7 were asymptomatic, APR normalized, reduction in steroid	1 patient developed SLE
Noémie Abisror et al. (2013)	Relapsed and resistant	5 cases and a total of 44 from literature were reviewed	Observational—Retrospective and literature review	TCZ (8 mg/kg) IV monthly + steroid	Clinical, biological, and radiological responses	All 5 had initial responses	2 out of 5 cases had relapse, one neutropenia; majority were doing well in the literature review

(continued)

Table 12.1 (continued)

Study	Disease status	Number of cases	Study type	Intervention	Primary outcome	Result	Comment
Catanoso et al. (2012)	Naïve and relapsed (2 GCA and 2 TAK)	2 cases of Takayasu arteritis	Observational—Retrospective	TCZ (8 mg/kg) IV monthly + steroid for 6 doses	Clinical, lab, and PET responses	All had improvement in all parameters	1 had mild liver enzyme elevation
Yoshikazu Nakaoka et al. (2013) Japanese case series	Steroid resistant	4 cases	Observational—Prospective	TCZ infusions (8 mg/kg) every 4 weeks a total of at least 24 times (range, 24–51) + steroid	Clinical remission, APR normalization, IL6 levels CT/MRI imaging	All had good clinical and APR response, 2 had imaging improvement in arterial lesion	Prednisolone could be reduced from 21.3 mg/day to 1.5 mg/day
TNF inhibitors studies							
Birgir Gudbrandsson et al. Norway cohort 2017	New and relapsing	78 patients from Southeast Norway TAK cohort and 19 cases from tertiary referral cohort	Observational—Retrospective cohort	32 TNF inhibitors (27 infliximab and 5 etanercept) and 40 on disease modifying agents (DMARDs)	NIH disease activity and prednisolone dose less than 10 mg at 6 months	Remission more in TNFi group, 44% sustained remission in TNF inhibitors vs 20% in DMARDs	10% in TNF inhibitors vs 40% in DMARDs had new lesions at 2 years
Arsene Mekinian et al. French Takayasu Network 2015	43 cases were resistant, relapsed or intolerant to DMARDs, 6 new cases	49 cases	Observational—Retrospective cohort	TNFi-80% [44 infliximab, 6 etanercept and 6 adalimumab] or tocilizumab [20%(n = 14)]	Clinical, laboratory, and imaging data and their treatments at least till 3 years	Relapse-free survival remained better after biological initiation compared with DMARDs period; hazard ratio 0.26 ($P = 0.01$)	TNF inhibitors and TCZ performed equally well 3-year relapse-free survival 91% and 85.7%, respectively

Hoffman et al. (2004)	Relapsing	15 cases	Interventional—Open labeled, prospective	7 received etanercept (later changed to infliximab in 3 patients), and 8 received infliximab	Complete remission and sustained remission No steroid use at 6 months	10 achieved complete and sustained response and 4 achieved partial response 6-month median prednisolone dose—0 mg/day	Two relapses during periods after anti-TNF therapy (etanercept) interrupted, remission was reestablished upon reinstitution
Jean Schmidt et al. (2012)	Refractory	20 cases	Observational—Retrospective	17 received infliximab, 2 received Adalimumab 1 etanercept Median duration of treatment 23 months (IQR 8.7–38.9 months)	Remission at 6 months with prednisolone dose less than 10 mg/day and sustained remission	Remission in 18 (90%) of 20 patients and sustained remission in 10 patients (50%)	6 out of 18 relapsed on discontinuation of TNFi
Molloy et al. (2008) US cohort	Refractory	25	Observational—Retrospective	21 with Infliximab and 9 with Etanercept, 5 patients switched from Etanercept to infliximab Treated up to 7 years	Achievement of partial or complete remission	Remission was achieved and prednisone was discontinued in 15 patients (60%) and successfully tapered below 10 mg/day in an additional 7 patients (28%)	Four patients suffered adverse events, including one with opportunistic infections and one with breast cancer

(continued)

Table 12.1 (continued)

Study	Disease status	Number of cases	Study type	Intervention	Primary outcome	Result	Comment
OTHERs							
Abatacept							
Carol A. Langford et al. (2017)	Newly diagnosed or relapsing		Randomized control trial	Abatacept 10 mg/kg IV on days 1, 15, 29, week 8, together with prednisone to all. Randomization to placebo vs abatacept from 12 weeks	Duration of remission (relapse-free survival).	At 12 months 22% of abatacept and 40% of placebo group were in remission	No significant benefit in use of abatacept ($p = 0.853$)

Abbreviations used: *I* intervention, *C* control, *RCT* randomized controlled trial, *GC* glucocorticoid, *TCZ* tocilizumab, *APR* acute phase reactants (CRP and ESR), *TNF* tumor necrosis factor, *DMARDs* disease modifying antirheumatic drugs

- A case series and review of observational data studied 84 cases of resistant Takayasu arteritis treated with TNF blockers.
- Infliximab (IFX) in 81% (68/84) and etanercept (ETA) in 19% (16/84) of patients were used.
- 31 (37%) had a complete remission and 45 (53.5%) were partial responders. There were 8 (9.5%) with no response.
- In a French Takayasu network cohort of patients on biological agents, TNF inhibitors achieved 3-year relapse-free survival similar to Tocilizumab (91% vs 85.7%).
- There is a paucity of data on Adalimumab and other newer TNF inhibitors.
- TNF blockers are generally considered as third line of treatment agents after:
  - Steroids+ conventional disease modifying agents/second-line immunosuppressants
  - Tocilizumab

  Also, the higher prevalence of latent TB in developing nations and the suspected association between TB and TA are concerns in using TNFi agents in such areas of the globe.

Case scenario

Patient presents back with increasing CRP and CT angiography show restenosis needing intervention. She also has been noted to have worsening cushingoid features and high blood glucose levels. Her blood MMF levels for 6 h Area under curve are performed and are found to be low.

She is initiated on monthly Tocilizumab 8 mg/kg IV and her MMS dose is increased to 2.16 g/day (equivalent of 3 g MMF) in two divided doses; it is also planned for more rapid and drastic taper of steroid to 9 mg deflazacort immediately after second dose of Tocilizumab and an endovascular intervention is done after 1 month.

12.10 Step 5: Experimental Therapy and Logistic Considerations

- Cyclophosphamide pulses [including oral pulses spacing over 3 days (i.e., day 1 to day 3 keeping the combined total dose of 3 days within 15 mg/kg body weight or 5 mg/kg body weight on each of the days from D1 to D3), initially once a month, and then it can be spaced to 3 monthly pulses after 4–6 pulses for 2 years as in lupus nephritis) and pulsed steroid therapy may be considered in this group of truly resistant disease, especially for economically constrained patients.
- Revascularization and antiplatelet agents with or without statins are used in this group of patients for symptomatic improvement as often advised by cardiologists.
- Ustekinumab, a humanized anti-p40 monoclonal antibody that targets both IL-12 and IL-23 pathways, thus disrupting the Th1 and Th17 immune responses may have a role.

- In a proof of concept study in three patients of Takayasu arteritis, all had improvement in acute phase reactants with Ustekinumab and benefit in pain and fatigue was noted with no severe side effects.
- IL-1 blockage has a theoretical role in Th17 cell activation and thus in pathogenesis, but has never been used in trials.
- Matrix metalloproteinase inhibitors, nitric oxide and Vascular endothelial growth factors may have a pathogenic role and their inhibitors may be used in future, but there is no clinical data on these agents till date.
- Patients with breakthrough flares and facing logistic difficulties of intravenous infusion, TCZ can be given subcutaneously at the dose of 162 mg, initially weekly or fortnightly and then tapered to monthly till disease activity is under control.

12.11 Case Scenario Completion

Our patient presented for review asymptomatic with equal pulses and blood pressure in limbs. Her ESR and CRP are within normal limits and are on stable dose of mycophenolate. Her Cushingoid features are improving and deflazacort dose is tapered to 6 mg/day at 6 months follow-up. Further tapering of steroid will be attempted very slowly, not faster than 1 mg/month under close monitoring of disease activity.

Patient is advised for a subcutaneous TCZ in case of a flare as a stopgap measure to avoid repeated hospitalization related logistic issues along with add on Tacrolimus (relatively expensive); however, if finance is an issue in the long run, she may be considered for any of the reserve agents like oral cyclophosphamide pulse, Leflunomide or generic Tofacitinib. Three to 6 monthly follow up, or earlier if there are symptoms of relapse, is mandatory throughout life. Treatment and follow up is lifelong with the lowest effective maintenance dose of immunosuppressant, as TA is rarely burnt out (contrary to belief); like most systemic autoimmune rheumatic diseases, TA is also burning all the time in absence of immunosuppression in vast majority of cases, even in absence of raised ESR/CRP. Figure 12.2 depicts the treatment algorithm that is followed by us.

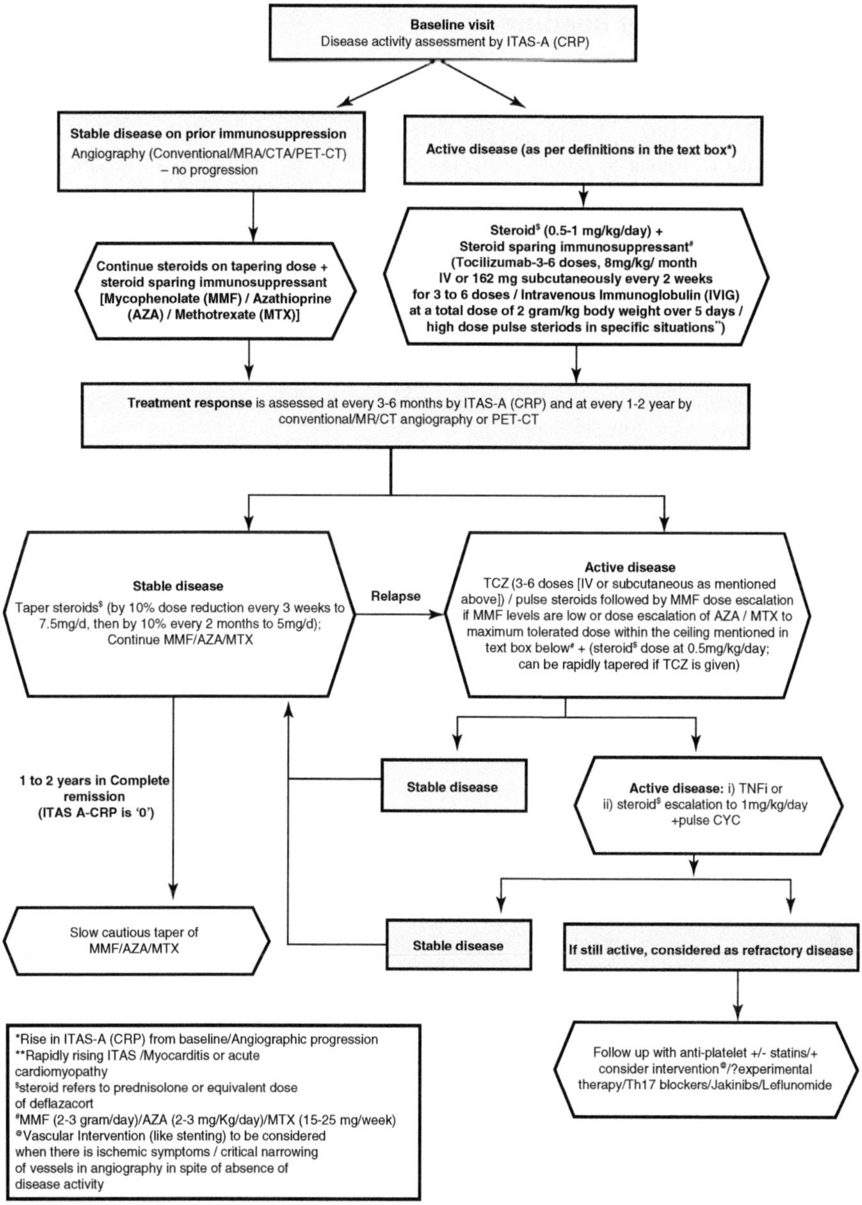

Fig. 12.2 Algorithm for treatment of Takayasu arteritis

Suggested Further Reading

Nakaoka Y, Isobe M, Takei S, et al. Efficacy and safety of tocilizumab in patients with refractory Takayasu arteritis: results from a randomised, double-blind, placebo-controlled, phase 3 trial in Japan (the TAKT study). Ann Rheum Dis. 2018;77:348–54.

Goel R, Danda D, Kumar S, Joseph G. Rapid control of disease activity by tocilizumab in 10 'difficult-to-treat' cases of Takayasu arteritis. Int J Rheum Dis. 2013;16:754–61.

Russo RAG, Katsicas MM. Takayasu arteritis. Front Pediatr. 2018;

Samsona M, Espígol-Frigoléc G, Terrades-García N, et al. Biological treatments in giant cell arteritis and Takayasu arteritis. Eur J Intern Med. 2018;

Misra R, Danda D, Rajappa SM, Ghosh A, et al. Indian Rheumatology Vasculitis (IRAVAS) group. Development and initial validation of the Indian Takayasu Clinical Activity Score (ITAS2010). Rheumatology (Oxford). 2013.

Sivakumar MR, Misra RN, Bacon PA, for the IRAVAS group, OP14. The Indian perspective of Takayasu arteritis and development of a disease extent index (dei.tak) to assess Takayasu arteritis. Rheumatology. 2005;44(Suppl_3).

Biologics in Interstitial Lung Diseases in Rheumatological Disorders

13

Ashish Sharma and Ashok Kumar

13.1 Introduction

- Interstitial lung disease (ILD) is a group of disorders, which affect the pulmonary interstitium by varying degrees of inflammation and fibrosis. Interstitium includes alveolar epithelium, connective tissue in perilymphatic and perivascular space, capillary basement membrane, and capillary endothelium. Although any part of the lung can be involved in systemic autoimmune rheumatic diseases (SARDs), including the pleura and the pulmonary vasculature, ILD remains the commonest form of lung involvement. Treatment of ILD is challenging and is further compounded by the potential pulmonary toxicity of various drugs used in the treatment of SARDs. Biologic drugs have gained popularity in the treatment of various SARDs because of their efficacy and safety. But their use in ILD remains restricted. We discuss in this chapter the current status of biologic disease modifying anti-rheumatic drugs (bDMARDs) in the treatment of ILD.
- Inflammation is the harbinger of ILD, which if not controlled timely, can lead to irreversible lung damage. Infiltration of inflammatory cells in the lung parenchyma leads to the release of pro-inflammatory cytokines. This also results in the transformation of resident pulmonary fibroblasts to myofibroblasts which leads to fibrosis.
- Inflammation predominates the initial stages (cellular stage) of ILD, which appears on chest computed tomography (CT) as non-specific interstitial pneumonia (NSIP). Advanced stage of ILD shows predominance of fibrosis (fibrotic stage), termed idiopathic pulmonary fibrosis or usual interstitial pneumonia (UIP) [the latter in cases of connective tissue disease-related ILD]. NSIP has a

A. Sharma · A. Kumar (✉)
Department of Rheumatology, Fortis Flt Lt Rajan Dhall Hospital, New Delhi, India
e-mail: ashok.kumar5@fortishealthcare.com

N. Jain, L. Duggal (eds.), *Handbook of Biologics for Rheumatological Disorders*,
https://doi.org/10.1007/978-981-16-7200-2_13

potential for significant improvement by immunosuppressive therapy. Once the patient reaches the fibrotic stage, medical treatment does not lead to significant improvement and lung transplantation remains the only treatment option.

- Various bDMARDs targeting different mediators of inflammation have been approved for use in the treatment of SARDs. bDMARDs have also been studied in patients with ILD but no formal guidelines exist. Most of the experience of bDMARDs for ILD has come from patients with ILD associated with systemic sclerosis (SSc) or rheumatoid arthritis (RA).

13.2 Tumor Necrosis Factor Inhibitors

- Tumor necrosis factor-α (TNF-α) is the master cytokine, which is implicated in the pathogenesis of many SARDs. TNF-α inhibitors are the most widely used bDMARDs in the treatment of various SARDs including RA, spondyloarthritis, and juvenile idiopathic arthritis. Five TNF-inhibitors (TNFi) have been approved for clinical use: infliximab (IFX), etanercept (ETN), adalimumab (ADA), golimumab (GOL), and certolizumab pegol (CZP). Because of the profibrotic potential of TNF, its inhibitors have been tried in the treatment of ILD [1].
- Stabilization of ILD has been observed after treatment with infliximab (IFX) in RA and SSc [2]. IFX has also been shown to be effective in sarcoidosis, with a more beneficial effect on extra-pulmonary manifestations [3]. Treatment with adalimumab (ADA) led to a marked improvement in drug-resistant ILD associated with dermatomyositis (DM) [4].
- On the other hand, Pervez-Alvarez et al. showed TNFi contributed to 96% of ILD developing in patients after initiation of a bDMARD [5]. Similar results were shown by the British Society for Rheumatology Biologics Register (BSRBR) where ILD was more frequently observed in patients receiving TNFi compared to those on conventional synthetic DMARDs (csDMARDs) [6]. Additionally, ILD was the cause of death more frequently in patients on TNFi as compared to the other group. Reports of acute exacerbations of ILD after TNFi therapy, severe enough to cause death have also been reported in the literature [7–9].
- ILD occurs early in the course after the initiation of ETN and IFX, as shown by Pervez-Alvarez et al. (mean 26 weeks) [5]. There are similar reports from Japan on IFX, ETN, and ADA [10–12].
- Mixed results are available in the literature regarding the use of TNFi in ILD. This is because TNF-α has both profibrotic and antifibrotic effects. TNF-α increases the expression of transforming growth factor-β (TGF-β), which is a potent profibrotic cytokine [1]. Animal studies have shown an increased incidence of development of lung fibrosis if TNF-α is depleted [13]. On the other hand, TNF-α has a significant role in repair of damaged lung tissue and controlling the inflammation [14, 15]. It leads to apoptosis of the cells giving rise to inflammation in the lungs and also promotes remodeling of the damaged alveoli and regeneration of the microvasculature. By blocking the latter effects of TNF-α, TNFi can theoretically lead to the development or progression of ILD due to persistent inflammation in the lungs.

- A study of more than 8000 patients with autoimmune diseases without ILD treated with TNFi or csDMARD did not show increased risk of development of ILD in those treated with TNFi as compared to csDMARD group [16].
- TNFi should be avoided in those with pre-existing ILD. Careful monitoring should be done in all patients who are started in TNFi, especially in the first 6 months after treatment initiation.

13.3 Anti-B-Cell Agents

- B-cells play an important role in the pathogenesis of various SARDs. B-cells contribute to inflammation by three mechanisms: production of antibodies, antigen presentation to T-cells and production of cytokines. Rituximab (RTX) is a humanized monoclonal antibody against CD-20, which has the widest use across many SARDs. It leads to a reduction in the number of B-cells by complement-mediated and antibody-dependent cell-mediated cytotoxicity. Because of potent anti-inflammatory effects, RTX has been tried in ILD.
- Fitzgerald et al. showed significant efficacy of RTX in CTD-associated ILD [17]. Treatment with RTX resulted in improvement in diffusion capacity of lungs for carbon monoxide (DLCO), forced vital capacity (FVC), and severity on CT scan over a median follow-up of 12.3 months. RTX has also been shown to maintain the stability of pre-existing ILD in patients with RA [18]. Similar results were shown in another study from the UK in more than 50% of patients with drug-resistant ILD associated with RA [19]. Stabilization of DLCO and FVC has also been in seen in patients with anti-synthetase syndrome, not responding to cyclophosphamide [20]. RTX is an attractive option for treatment of ILD, including drug-resistant cases.

13.4 Abatacept

Abatacept (ABT) is a fusion protein of cytotoxic T-lymphocyte-associated antigen 4 (CTLA-4) and Fc portion of IgG1. CTLA-4 is the ligand for CD-28 on T-cells, which prevents the binding of CD-80/CD-86 (on antigen-presenting cells) to CD-28, thereby inhibiting the co-stimulation of T-cells. Abatacept has found utility in various SARDs and has been used in patients with ILD.

Weinblatt et al. reported long-term safety of ABT in terms of development of ILD in patients with RA [21].

13.5 Other bDMARDs

Tocilizumab (TCZ) has been shown to be effective in ILD [22, 23]. Safety of TCZ in terms of ILD in patients with SSc was shown by Khanna et al. [24] On the other hand, deterioration of pre-existing ILD has been reported in patients with RA [25, 26]. High disease activity was observed to be a predictive factor for TCZ-induced acute exacerbation of pre-existing ILD in patients with RA [26]. Insufficient data are available for anakinra for its use in ILD. A trial of canakinumab in sarcoidosis is underway. Basiliximab is a chimeric monoclonal antibody against α-chain of IL-2 receptor on T-cells. Improvement in lung function and CT appearance has been shown in patients with anti-melanoma differentiation-associated protein 5 (anti-MDA 5) syndrome on treatment with basiliximab [27].

13.6 Idiopathic Pulmonary Fibrosis

Most of the drugs, including non-biologic and biologic DMARDs have shown negative results in the treatment of idiopathic pulmonary fibrosis (IPF). Rituximab has shown benefit in acute exacerbations of IPF [28]. ETN has failed to show any benefit compared to placebo after 48 weeks of treatment [29]. Tralokinumab is a monoclonal antibody against IL-13 which failed to show efficacy in IPF [30]. Lebrikizumab, another IL-13 antagonist, failed to show improvement in lung function [31]. Pamrevlumab, a monoclonal antibody against connective tissue growth factor (CTGF) is yet to enter phase III trials after showing encouraging results in phase II trials [32, 33]. SAR156597 is a bispecific antibody against IL-4 and IL-13 which failed in the treatment of IPF [34]. VAY736, a monoclonal antibody targeting B-lymphocyte stimulator (BLyS) is undergoing a phase II trial.

13.7 Conclusion

No formal guidelines exist regarding the use of bDMARDs in ILD. Most of the data on the use of bDMARDs in the treatment of ILD comes from case reports and case series. Although literature shows contradictory results in the efficacy and safety of bDMARDs, rituximab and abatacept seem to be effective with a favorable safety profile. TNF inhibitors have the potential to cause or exacerbate pre-existing ILD. Fatal cases of ILD have been reported with tocilizumab. No effective biologic therapy exists for IPF to date. Randomized controlled trials are needed to ascertain the true efficacy of bDMARDs in ILD and determine their exact role in managing ILD.

References

1. Sullivan DE, Ferris M, Nguyen H, Abboud E, Brody AR. TNF-alpha induces TGF-beta1 expression in lung fibroblasts at the transcriptional level via AP-1 activation. J Cell Mol Med. 2009;13:1866–76.
2. Antoniou KM, Mamoulaki M, Malagari K, et al. Infliximab therapy in pulmonary fibrosis associated with collagen vascular disease. Clin Exp Rheumatol. 2007;25:23–8.
3. Hostettler KE, Studler U, Tamm M, Brutsche MH. Long-term treatment with infliximab in patients with sarcoidosis. Respiration. 2012;83:218–2.

4. Park JK, Yoo HG, Ahn DS, Jeon HS, Yoo WH. Successful treatment for conventional treatment-resistant dermatomyositis-associated interstitial lung disease with adalimumab. Rheumatol Int. 2012;32:3587–90.
5. Perez-Alvarez R, Perez-de-Lis M, Diaz-Lagares C, et al. Interstitial lung disease induced or exacerbated by TNF-targeted therapies: analysis of 122 cases. Semin Arthritis. 2011;41:256–64.
6. Dixon WG, Hyrich KL, Watson KD, Lunt M. Influence of anti-TNF therapy on mortality in patients with rheumatoid arthritis-associated interstitial lung disease: results from the British Society for Rheumatology Biologics Register. Ann Rheum Dis. 2010;69:1086–91.
7. Ostor AJ, Chilvers ER, Somerville MF, et al. Pulmonary complications of infliximab therapy in patients with rheumatoid arthritis. J Rheumatol. 2006;33:622–8.
8. Horai Y, Miyamura T, Shimada K, et al. Eternacept for the treatment of patients with rheumatoid arthritis and concurrent interstitial lung disease. J Clin Pharm Ther. 2012;37:117–21.
9. Dias OM, Pereira DA, Baldi BG, et al. Adalimumab-induced acute interstitial lung disease in a patient with rheumatoid arthritis. J Bras Pneumol. 2014;40:77–81.
10. Takeuchi T, Tatsuki Y, Nogami Y, et al. Postmarketing surveillance of the safety profile of infliximab in 5000 Japanese patients with rheumatoid arthritis. Ann Rheum Dis. 2008;67:189–94.
11. Koike T, Harigai M, Inokuma S, et al. Postmarketing surveillance of safety and effectiveness of etanercept in Japanese patients with rheumatoid arthritis. Mod Rheumatol. 2011;21:343–51.
12. Koike T, Harigai M, Ishiguro N, et al. Safety and effectiveness of adalimumab in Japanese rheumatoid arthritis patients: postmarketing surveillance report of the first 3,000 patients. Mod Rheumatol. 2012;22:498–508.
13. Kuroki M, Noguchi Y, Shimono M, et al. Repression of bleomycin-induced pneumopathy by TNF. J Immunol. 2003;170:567–74.
14. Khasnis AA, Calabrese LH. Tumor necrosis factor inhibitors and lung disease: a paradox of efficacy and risk. Semin Arthritis Rheum. 2010;40:147–63.
15. Taki H, Kawagishi Y, Shinoda K, et al. Interstitial pneumonitis associated with infliximab therapy without methotrexate treatment. Rheumatol Int. 2009;30:275–6.
16. Herrinton LJ, Harrold LR, Liu L, et al. Association between anti-TNF-alpha therapy and interstitial lung disease. Pharmacoepidemiol Drug Saf. 2013;22:394–402.
17. Fitzgerald DB, Moloney F, Twomey M, et al. Efficacy and safety of rituximab in connective tissue disease related interstitial lung disease. Sarcoidosis Vasc Diffuse Lung Dis. 2015;32:215–21.
18. Kabia A, Md Yusof MY, Dass S, Vital E, Beirne P, Emery P. Efficacy and safety of rituximab in rheumatoid arthritis patients with concomitant interstitial lung disease. 10-year experience at single centre. Rheumatology. 2015;54:i86.
19. Sharp C, McCabe M, Dodds N, et al. Rituximab in autoimmune connective tissue disease-associated interstitial lung disease. Rheumatology. 2016;55:1318–24.
20. Keir GJ, Maher TM, Ming D, et al. Rituximab in severe, treatment refractory interstitial lung disease. Respirology. 2014;19:353–9.
21. Weinblatt ME, Moreland LW, Westhovens R, et al. Safety of abatacept administered intravenously in treatment of rheumatoid arthritis: integrated analyses of up to 8 years of treatment from the abatacept clinical trial program. J Rheumatol. 2013;40:787–97.
22. Keidel SM, Hoyles RK, Wilkinson NM. Efficacy of tocilizumab for interstitial lung disease in an undifferentiated autoinflammatory disorder partially responsive to anakinra. Rheumatology. 2014;53:573–4.
23. Mohr M, Jacobi AM. Interstitial lung disease in rheumatoid arthritis: response to IL-6R blockade. Scand J Rheumatol. 2011;40:400–1.
24. Khanna D, Denton CP, Lin CJF, et al. Safety and efficacy of subcutaneous tocilizumab in systemic sclerosis: results from the open-label period of a phase II randomised controlled trial (faSScinate). Ann Rheum Dis. 2018;77:212–20.
25. Kawashiri SY, Kawakami A, Sakamoto N, Ishimatsu Y, Eguchi K. A fatal case of acute exacerbation of interstitial lung disease in a patient with rheumatoid arthritis during treatment with tocilizumab. Rheumatol Int. 2012;32:4023–6.

26. Akiyama M, Kaneko Y, Yamaoka K, Kondo H, Takeuchi T. Association of disease activity with acute exacerbation of interstitial lung disease during tocilizumab treatment in patients with rheumatoid arthritis: a retrospective, case-control study. Rheumatol Int. 2016;36:881–9.
27. Zou J, Li T, Huang X, Chen S, Guo Q, Bao C. Basiliximab may improve the survival rate of rapidly progressive interstitial pneumonia in patients with clinically amyopathic dermatomyositis with anti-MDA5 antibody. Ann Rheum Dis. 2014;73:1591–3.
28. Donahoe M, Valentine VG, Chien N, et al. Autoantibody-targeted treatments for acute exacerbations of idiopathic pulmonary fibrosis. PLoS One. 2015;10:e0127771.
29. Raghu G, Brown KK, Costabel U, et al. Treatment of idiopathic pulmonary fibrosis with etanercept: an exploratory, placebo-controlled trial. Am J Respir Critic Care Med. 2008;178:948–55.
30. Parker JM, Glaspole IN, Lancaster LH, et al. A phase 2 randomized controlled study of tralokinumab in subjects with idiopathic pulmonary fibrosis. Am J Resp Crit Care Med. 2018;197:94–103.
31. Swigris JJ, Ogura T, Scholand MB, et al. The RIFF study (cohort A): a phase II, randomized, double-blind, placebo-controlled trial of Lebrikizumab as monotherapy in patients with idiopathic pulmonary fibrosis. Am J Resp Crit Care Med. 2018;197:A6167.
32. Raghu G, Scholand MB, de Andrade J, et al. FG-3019 anti-connective tissue growth factor monoclonal antibody: results of an open-label clinical trial in idiopathic pulmonary fibrosis. Eur Resp J. 2016;47:1481–91.
33. Raghu G, Scholand M, Andrade JDE, et al. Safety and efficacy of anti-CTGF monoclonal antibody FG-3019 for the treatment of idiopathic pulmonary fibrosis (IPF): results of Phase 2 clinical trial two years after initiation. Am J Resp Crit Care Med. 2014;189:A1426.
34. Raghu G, Richeldi L, Crestani B, et al. Safety and efficacy of SAR156597 in idiopathic pulmonary fibrosis (IPF): a phase 2, randomized, double-blind, placebo-controlled study. Am J Resp Crit Care Med. 2018;197:A2441.

14 Biologics in Osteoporosis

Ira Pande

14.1 Introduction

- Osteoporosis (OP) is a systemic skeletal disease characterised by low bone mass and microarchitectural deterioration of bone tissue. It is associated with increased risk of fracture due to bone fragility, in response to minimal or low-velocity force [1]. The sites commonly involved are vertebral, hip and distal radius, but can occur at any site within the skeletal system.
- Osteoporosis is a heterogeneous condition, involving interplay between endocrine, metabolic and mechanical factors. Osteoporosis can be classified into primary or secondary. Primary or idiopathic osteoporosis has been historically classified as postmenopausal. This accounts for 80% of women and 60% of men with osteoporosis. It results from a combination of factors including nutrition, peak bone mass, genetics, level of physical activity, age of menopause and oestrogen or testosterone levels. Secondary cause can be found in 20% of women and 40% of men [2, 3].
- Low trauma fractures associated with osteoporosis are important health issues because of their impact on morbidity, mortality and the significant socioeconomic burden [4, 5]. Delayed diagnosis and under treatment are common, particularly in patients who have already sustained a fragility fracture.

I. Pande (✉)
Rheumatology Department, Queens Medical Centre, Nottingham University Hospitals NHS Trust, Nottingham, UK
e-mail: ira.pande@nuh.nhs.uk

N. Jain, L. Duggal (eds.), *Handbook of Biologics for Rheumatological Disorders*,
https://doi.org/10.1007/978-981-16-7200-2_14

14.2 Therapeutic Options: Current and New

- The main goal of treatment is early identification of patients at risk of poor bone health and timely intervention using a combination of lifestyle advice and pharmacological treatment.
- The treatment of osteoporosis has evolved significantly, such that oestrogens are no longer the drug of choice; their use is now limited for a perimenopausal and postmenopausal women with co-existent menopausal symptoms. Similarly, use of drugs like strontium ranelate [6], calcitonin [7], etidronate is an exception, not the rule.
- The efficacy, as well as favourable safety profile, has made Bisphosphonates the mainstay of treatment [8]. But in real-world experience, issues have come up which affect their efficacy like lack of awareness among health care providers and poor adherence from patient side. In addition, there are limitations to what bisphosphonates, the most commonly used class of drugs, can achieve.
- Although bisphosphonates increase mineralisation of bone matrix and bone mineral density (BMD), they do this up to a certain point (average 3–6%). Most of the expected gain in BMD is seen in the first 3 years after starting the drug; following which there is stabilisation of BMD with no further increase [9].
- Post-marketing surveillance has shown adverse reactions with long-term use of these drugs including osteonecrosis of the jaw (ONJ) and atypical femoral fractures. Although these adverse events are not unique to bisphosphonate use, drug holiday, sequential therapy, combination therapy or emerging molecules mainly targeting the stimulation of bone formation have been proposed as ways to overcome these problems.
- In recent years, detailed knowledge of the molecular and cellular players has greatly improved our understanding of bone biology. These new findings have led to the development of drugs that act on the metabolic pathways of bone resorption and formation—such as the receptor activator of nuclear factor kappa beta (RANK) and its ligand (RANKL), osteoprotegerin (OPG), Cathepsin, Wnt, sclerostin, dickkopf-1, and beta-catenin proteins.
- Approaches are diverse and include enhancement of the synthesis or activity of a growth regulator or targeting a secreted growth factor antagonist. Development of drugs targeting intracellular proteins would require the product to cross the cell membrane making these molecules impractical targets for drug discovery.
- This handbook focuses on the use of biologics in the treatment of musculoskeletal disorders. In the field of osteoporosis, multiple novel drugs are in advanced stages of development in various clinical trials unlike the plethora of biologics already in use in inflammatory disorders like rheumatoid arthritis. This chapter will, therefore, cover traditional bone agents in current use and expand on newer agents with special emphasis on two biologics awaiting approval by regulatory bodies (abaloparatide and romosozumab).
- Patient education in the management of osteoporosis is very important to ensure compliance and adherence to change in lifestyle factors and use of bone agents as per product specifications.

- Fracture risk is not reduced with calcium intake only, but when combined with Vitamin D, there is a small reduction in hip and non-vertebral fractures, possibly extending to vertebral fractures.
- The commonest anti-resorptive drugs in use are bisphosphonates as they are efficacious in reducing vertebral and hip fracture [10, 11].
- Alendronic acid (70 mg) and risedronic acid (35 mg) are weekly oral tablets. For patients who are unable to tolerate oral bisphosphonates or in whom oral are contraindicated (patients with previous gastrointestinal bleed, oesophageal stricture, achalasia or ulcers), intravenous Zoledronic acid infusion (5 mg) is a good alternative. It is also a preferred option in patients in care or residential homes, the frail and elderly for whom travel to hospital is difficult as the infusion can be easily administered closer to home—in care homes, community setting or even patients' own home. The single infusion at intervals of 12 to 18 months has the added advantage of ensuring compliance with treatment over weekly or monthly preparations and one to consider in patients with multiple co-morbidities on polypharmacy. Unless a patient has significant renal impairment Cockgroft Gault GFR (CG GFR <35) intravenous zoledronate infusion is increasingly becoming a preferred first-line therapy in this group of patients.
- As data on the efficacy of ibandronate [12], another bisphosphonate available as monthly oral (150 mg) and 3 monthly intravenous preparation (3 mg), is limited to efficacy in reduction of vertebral fractures but not hip and non-vertebral fractures, this molecule is used in the exceptional circumstance where gain in spinal BMD with a view to prevent vertebral fracture is the primary end point and all other agents are either contraindicated or patient reports inability to tolerate or experiences side effects.
- Raloxifene, is a selective oestrogen receptor modulator (SERM). It is administered daily orally (60 mg). Raloxifene has a marketing authorisation in the UK for the treatment and prevention of osteoporosis in postmenopausal women [13]. Clinical trials have shown efficacy in vertebral fracture prevention only. Venous thromboembolism is a known adverse event with SERMs. Its use is therefore very limited. A good example where Raloxifene might be considered as an option to improve bone health in a woman in the sixth decade of life, at high risk of vertebral fracture with a family history of breast cancer.

14.3 Teriparatide

- The recombinant human parathyroid hormone [PTH] 1–34, teriparatide is available as a self-administered daily subcutaneous injection at a dose of 20 μg daily for 2 years. After completion of treatment, sequential therapy with another agent must follow. At present this is usually an antiresorptive agent.
- It is the first and most commonly used anabolic agent approved for the treatment of osteoporosis and causes a 65% reduction in the incidence of vertebral fractures and a 54% reduction in non-vertebral fractures [14].

- It is ideal for a subpopulation of patients with severe osteoporosis and or, multiple vertebral fractures. However, because of its high cost, its use is limited to patients at very high risk of fracture and hence in the UK not recommended for use as first-line therapy for osteoporosis.
- Biosimilar preparations have recently been introduced into the UK market but the persisting high cost compared to other bone agents has meant no change in guidelines for its use.
- Treatment is approximately for 24 months and it is co-prescribed with vitamin D (800–100 IU/day) and calcium (1000–1500 mg—if not adequate by diet).
- Its use is contraindicated in children, patients with active Paget's disease, hyperparathyroidism, pregnancy and lactation, severe renal impairment, metabolic bone disease other than osteoporosis, prior external beam or implant radiation or malignancies affecting the skeleton or hereditary disorders predisposing to osteosarcoma. Where indicated, it is best to use this drug as first-line agent followed by bisphosphonates (oral or IV) to maximise efficacy, gain in BMD and fracture risk reduction. Prior use of anti-resorptive tempers the response to teriparatide on BMD.
- Newer modes of administration of Teriparatide, such as oral, transdermal and intranasal are undergoing trials with a view to assess efficacy, tolerability and compliance compared to the subcutaneous route. Administration of both alendronate and teriparatide have not shown any benefits of the combination compared to either agent alone [15, 16]. However, simultaneous administration of intravenous zoledronate did not blunt the effect, and combination therapy resulted in a greater increase in hip BMD than teriparatide alone [17].
- Combination therapy with denosumab over a 2-year period also showed a substantial increase in BMD at all sites (spine, hip and femoral neck) that was greater than either agent alone [18, 19]. There is evidence to demonstrate that patients switching from teriparatide to denosumab continue to gain BMD, particularly at the hip [20]. Although combination therapy is currently not the norm, these observations need to be borne in mind and form the basis of useful discussions when considering sequential therapy in managing complex patients.

14.4 Abaloparatide

- It is an anabolic drug approved by the Food and Drug Administration (FDA) for clinical use in 2017 [21]. It is a 34-amino acid synthetic analogue of parathyroid hormone-related peptide (PTHrP). It shares 41% homology with human PTH 1–34 and 76% homology to human PTHrP (1–34). Its actions on bone are mediated through the same receptor of teriparatide, PTH type 1 receptor (PTH1R), which is expressed on the surface of osteoblasts and osteocytes. The PTH1R is a G-protein coupled receptor that acts with two different conformations: R0 and RG. This difference in the respective interaction with the PTHR1 leads to a more transient effect of PTHrP of abaloparatide over teriparatide [22, 23].

- This difference in mechanism of action could account for the favourable anabolic action of abaloparatide; with abaloparatide displaying more modest effects on bone resorption than teriparatide [23]. The drug has been studied in clinical trials compared to placebo and teriparatide in preventing fractures in patients with severe osteoporosis [24].
- In clinical trials treatment with abaloparatide at the licensed dose of 80 μg subcutaneous daily, had a greater effect on BMD at all sites (lumbar spine, femoral neck and total hip) compared to teriparatide but the reduction in major osteoporotic fractures was not significantly different.
- Exploratory analysis of major osteoporotic fractures revealed a favourable outcome for abaloparatide versus placebo (for vertebral fractures) and versus teriparatide and placebo (for non-vertebral fractures). Post hoc analysis of the trial underscored abalopartide's anti-fracture efficacy across a wide age range, baseline risk factors, independently of the presence or absence of previous fractures.
- Abalopartide is associated with adverse events like nausea, tachycardia and hypercalcaemia in approx. 3% of subjects. Like teriparatide, due to potential risk of osteosarcoma, the recommended cumulative use of abaloparatide is limited to 2 years during an individual's lifetime. However, the drug was not approved for use by the European Medicines Agency (EMA) as they had concerns about the medicine's effects on the heart, such as increases in heart rate and palpitations [24, 25]. The EMA could not identify a group of patients in whom the benefits would outweigh the risks. Abaloparatide, therefore, does not have marketing authorisation in the UK. I have no personal experience in using this drug. In countries where it is licensed for use, trials in men with osteoporosis and administration by other routes (dermal patch) are being evaluated.

14.5 Denosumab

- It is the first biologic licensed for both primary and secondary prevention of fragility fractures. It is a fully humanised monoclonal antibody against RANKL which blocks osteoclast maturation. It has proven efficacy in reducing risk of vertebral, non-vertebral and hip fractures [26].
- It is administered as a subcutaneous injection 6 monthly. It is an antiresorptive agent, similar to bisphosphonates, but due to its route of administration and 6 monthly dosing regimens, the adherence and persistence to treatment are higher than bisphosphonates. Unlike bisphosphonates its actions do not last in the bone matrix.
- Injection site cellulitis and hypocalcaemia are common side effects. It is a useful bone agent in patients where bisphosphonates are contraindicated due to poor renal function. As risk of hypocalcaemia with this drug is slightly high, it is recommended that serum calcium is checked prior to initiation of treatment, and 7–14 days after the drug is administered. Osteonecrosis of the jaw (ONJ) is also reported similar to other bone agents. Unlike bisphosphonates, BMD increases

year on year for the total duration of denosumab therapy making it the bone agent of choice in a subgroup of patients who have very low T scores at baseline.
- In contrast to bisphosphonates, on cessation of denosumab therapy, rebound rapid bone loss and increased risk of vertebral fracture have been reported. A single infusion of Zoledronic acid as sequential therapy to conserve the gain in BMD is often employed.

14.5.1 Newer Therapies

Drugs manipulating the canonical Wnt pathway are recent therapeutic advances for the treatment of osteoporosis. This pathway is a major regulator of osteoblast function [27, 28]. This key bone anabolic pathway is negatively regulated by sclerostin and dickkopf-1 (Dkk-1), which bind to LRP5/6 and kremen, respectively, inhibiting Wnt signalling. Wnts constitute a family of glycoproteins that play a fundamental role in the biology of many cells. Wnt/β-catenin signalling controls skeletal development and adult skeletal homeostasis. Wnt pathway is activated by the binding of a Wnt-protein ligand to a receptor complex composed of LRP-5/6 (low-density lipoprotein receptor-related protein) and a Frizzled protein (Fzd). Fzd recruits Axin and forms a complex which inhibits β-Catenin. Free β-catenin accumulates in the cytoplasm, translocates to the nucleus and regulates the transcription of target genes required for osteoblastogenesis thereby enhancing bone formation. Wnt signalling also has an inhibitory role in osteoclastogenesis and bone resorption by inducing OPG (osteoprotegerin), secreted by osteoblasts. In addition, Wnt suppresses adipogenesis.

14.6 Sclerostin

- Major Wnt inhibitor Sclerostin, is a glycoprotein secreted by osteocytes and encoded by the SOST gene [17q12–q21] [29]. Sclerostin binds to the LRP-5/6 receptors and prevents binding to the Fzd receptor leading to phosphorylation and degradation of β-catenin and disruption of the Wnt target gene expression [30]. In this way, the Wnt signalling pathway is inhibited, consequently inhibiting osteoblast proliferation, differentiation and function. Sclerostin also stimulates the production of RANKL from osteocytes thereby enhancing osteoclastogenesis.
- The Wnt/β-catenin canonical pathway is underscored by the identification of two inherited human diseases, van Buchem disease [31] and sclerosteosis [32], presenting with high bone mass, resistance to fractures and elevated levels of bone formation markers found to be due to impaired sclerostin expression and function, caused by inactivating mutations of SOST, the gene encoding sclerostin. Inactivating mutations of the LRP 5 causes osteoporosis-pseudoglioma syndrome characterised by fractures and severe bone loss.

- The pharmaceutical industry has recently developed three monoclonal antibodies against sclerostin: blosozumab (LY251546), setrusumab (BPS804) and romosozumab (AMG-785). In pre-clinical studies, sclerostin antibodies have been shown to increase bone mass at several skeletal sites and improve trabecular microarchitecture. There is an increase in bone formation followed by a decrease in bone resorption, thus uncoupling the two phases of bone metabolism.

14.7 Romosozumab

- It is a fully humanized monoclonal antibody that inhibits sclerostin and has recently been approved for use in women and men in a few countries [33]. It is a novel anabolic agent with dual effects thereby increasing bone formation and decreasing bone resorption. The drug development programme enrolled 14,000 patients in 19 clinical trials. It is administered subcutaneously at the monthly dose of 210 mg for 1 year. In trials, it has been studied using 12 months of the drug followed by 12 months of alendronate compared to 24 months of alendronate alone in postmenopausal women.
- Romosozumab use results in an increase in bone formation markers, reduction in bone resorption markers, increase in cortical thickness and BMD on high-resolution QCT scans of the spine.
- Treatment with Romosozumab, results in an early and rapid increase in bone formation markers (PINP) that peaks at 1–3 months, then return to baseline by month 6 and finally remains below baseline during the study duration. In parallel, there is a rapid decline CTX within the first month which remains suppressed during duration of study. Observed increases in BMD at both the spine and hip of 11.3% and 4.1%, respectively, were greater than those observed with teriparatide or alendronate.
- Phase 3 studies [34–36] have established the efficacy of Romosozumab in preventing new vertebral fractures (73%), clinical fractures (36%), while prevention of non-vertebral fractures was not significant. Neither study was powered to evaluate the effect on hip fracture risk. The gains in BMD at both the spine and the hip in 2 years exceeded the effects of 7 years of continuous denosumab therapy.
- In patients pre-treated with a bisphosphonate, sequential therapy with Romosozumab resulted in superior gains in BMD at lumbar spine, total hip and femoral neck compared to patients transitioning to teriparatide ((9.8% vs 5.4%, 2.6% vs −0.6%, and 3.2% vs −0.2%, respectively). This study (STRUCTURE—STudy evaluating effect of RomosozUmab Compared with Teriparatide in postmenopaUsal women with osteoporosis at high risk for fracture pReviously treated with bisphosphonate therapy) highlights differences in the effects observed in using an anabolic agent (Romosozumab versus Teriparatide) as sequential therapy after commonly used antiresorptive agent (bisphosphonates) [37].

- The main difference between romosozumab and teriparatide is dual anabolic and anti-resorptive action of romosozumab vis-a-vis exclusive anabolic effect of teriparatide.
- Most common adverse event observed was mild injection site reaction (5.2%) versus 2.9% placebo [34]. A rare occurrence of ONJ and few atypical femoral fractures have been reported with the drug. It is contraindicated in patients with a history of myocardial infarction or stroke as trials have shown around two times increase in the incidence of cardiovascular events in the romosozumab treated patients [36].
- Safety data in patients with severe renal impairment (estimated glomerular filtration rate [eGFR] 15–29 ml/min/1.73 m^2) or receiving dialysis is limited. As they are at greater risk of developing hypocalcaemia, caution needs to be taken if using the drug. Unlike, teriparatide and abalopartide, there is no concern about potential tumours. Romosozumab has been approved for use in Scotland and Northern Ireland; NICE has rejected the application for use in England. (personal communication Nov 2021).
- Additional sclerostin antibody drugs in development are Blosozumab [38] and BPS804. Other targets in drug development are antagonists to calcium-sensing receptor (CaSR) on parathyroid glands, antibodies against Dickkopf-1 (Dkk-1) and c-Src kinase inhibitors.
- Despite recent advances, development of new molecules and increased understanding of the drugs, there are various issues such as duration of treatment, duration of drug holiday, whether to use single agent or combination therapy, choice of sequential treatment that still have no evidence base and usage is guided by expert opinion.

14.8 Summary

Our better understanding of bone biology at the cellular level and signalling pathways has led to search and development of new agents, preferentially to obtain an anabolic response by targeting osteoblast differentiation and function. There is increasing evidence supporting the use of sequential therapy with an anabolic agent followed by an antiresorptive in patients at high risk of fragility fracture. Two agents, both anabolic (abaloparatide and romosozumab) have shown promising results in clinical trials with anti-fracture efficacy data. Although abaloparatide has not been approved by EMA and is currently not approved for marketing in the UK, FDA approval 3 years ago is likely to produce data on its use in the real world. Romosuzumab has been approved for use in men and women in a few countries including the European Commission, but its approval for use in England by NICE has been rejected. Other biological agents neutralising Dkk-1, sclerostin, c-Src kinase, cathepsin and caSR in various stages of clinical trials represent promising new therapeutic options.

References

1. NIH Consensus Development Panel on Osteoporosis Prevention, Diagnosis and Therapy. Osteoporosis prevention, diagnosis and therapy. J Am Med Ass. 2001;285:785–95.
2. Fitzpatrick LA. Secondary causes of osteoporosis. Mayo Clin Proc. 2002;77:453–68.
3. Adler RA. Laboratory testing for secondary osteoporosis evaluation. Clin Biochem. 2012;45:894–900.
4. Johnell O, Kanis JA. An estimate of the worldwide prevalence and disability associated with osteoporotic fractures. Osteoporosis Int. 2006;17:1726–33.
5. Nazrun AS, Tzar MN, Mokhtar SA, et al. A systematic review of the outcomes of osteoporotic fracture patients after hospital discharge: morbidity, subsequent fractures, and mortality. Ther Clin Risk Manag. 2014;10:937–48.
6. Bolland MJ, Grey A. Ten years too long: strontium ranelate, cardiac events, and the European Medicines Agency. BMJ. 2016;354:i5109.
7. Overman RA, Borse M, Gourlay ML. Salmon calcitonin use and associated cancer risk. Ann Pharmacother. 2013;47(12):1675–84.
8. Nogues X, Martinez-Laguna D. Review: update on osteoporosis treatment. Med Clin (Barc). 2028;150(12):479–86.
9. Black D, Schwartz A, Ensrud K, Cauley J, Levis S, Quandt S, et al. Effects of continuing or stopping alendronate after 5 years of treatment: the fracture intervention trial long-term extension (FLEX): a randomized trial. JAMA. 2006;296:2927–38.
10. Compston J, Bilezikian J. Bisphosphonate therapy for osteoporosis: the long and short of it. J Bone Miner Res. 2012;27:240–2.
11. Diab D, Watts N. Bisphosphonates in the treatment of osteoporosis. Endocrinol Metab Clin N Am. 2012;41:487–506.
12. Chesnut CH III, Skag A, Christiansen C, et al. Effects of oral ibandronate administered daily or intermittently on fracture risk in postmenopausal osteoporosis. J Bone Miner Res. 2004;19:1241–9.
13. Ettinger B, Black DM, Mitlak BH, Multiple Outcomes of Raloxifene Evaluation (MORE) Investigators, et al. Reduction of vertebral fracture risk in postmenopausal women with osteoporosis treated with raloxifene: results from a 3-year randomized clinical trial. JAMA. 1999;282(7):637–45.
14. Neer RM, Arnaud CD, Zanchetta JR, et al. Effect of parathyroid hormone (1–34) on fractures and bone mineral density in postmenopausal women with osteoporosis. N Engl J Med. 2001;344:1434–41.
15. Black DM, Greenspan SL, Ensrud KE, et al. The effects of parathyroid hormone and alendronate alone or in combination in postmenopausal osteoporosis. N Engl J Med. 2003;349(13):1207–15.
16. Finkelstein JS, Hayes A, Hunzelman JL, et al. The effects of parathyroid hormone, alendronate, or both in men with osteoporosis. N Engl J Med. 2003;349(13):1216–26.
17. Cosman F, Eriksen EF, Recknor C, et al. Effects of intravenous zoledronic acid plus subcutaneous teriparatide [rhPTH(1–34)] in postmenopausal osteoporosis. J Bone Miner Res. 2011;26(3):503–11.
18. Leder BZ, Tsai JN, Uihlein AV, et al. Two years of denosumab and teriparatide administration in postmenopausal women with osteoporosis (the DATA Extension Study): a randomized controlled trial. J Clin Endocrinol Metab. 2014;99(5):1694–700.
19. Tsai JN, Uihlein AV, Lee H, et al. Teriparatide and denosumab, alone or combined, in women with postmenopausal osteoporosis: the DATA study randomised trial. Lancet. 2013;382(9886):50–6.
20. Leder BZ, Tsai JN, Uihlein AV, et al. Denosumab and teriparatide transitions in postmenopausal osteoporosis (the DATA-switch study): extension of a randomised controlled trial. Lancet. 2015;386(9999):1147–55.

21. Chew CK, Clarke BL. Abaloparatide: recombinant human PTHrP (1–34) anabolic therapy for osteoporosis. Maturitas. 2017;97:53–60.
22. Hattersley G, Dean T, Corbin BA, et al. Binding selectivity of abaloparatide for PTH-type-1-receptor conformations and effects on downstream signaling. Endocrinology. 2016;157(1):141–9.
23. Canalis E. Management of endocrine disease: novel anabolic treatments for osteoporosis. Eur J Endocrinol. 2018;178(2):R33–44.
24. Miller PD, Hattersley G, Riis BJ, et al. Effect of abaloparatide vs placebo on new vertebral fractures in postmenopausal women with osteoporosis: a randomized clinical trial. JAMA. 2016;316(7):722–33.
25. Available from: https://www.ema.europa.eu/en/documents/smop-initial/questions-answers-refusal-marketing-authorisation-eladynos-abaloparatide_en.pdf. Accessed 14 Aug 2020.
26. Bone HG, Wagman RB, Brand ML, et al. 10 years of denosumab treatment in postmenopausal women with osteoporosis: results from the phase 3 randomised FREEDOM trial and open-label extension. Lancet Diabetes Endocrinol. 2017;5:513–23.
27. Gaur T, Lengner CJ, Hovhannisyan H, Bhat RA, Bodine PV, Komm BS, Javed A, van Wijnen AJ, Stein JL, Stein GS, et al. Canonical WNT signaling promotes osteogenesis by directly stimulating Runx2 gene expression. J Biol Chem. 2005;280:33132–40.
28. Boyden LM, Mao JH, Belsky J, Mitzner L, Farhi A, Mitnick MA, Wu D, Insogna K, Lifton RP. High bone density due to a mutation in LDL-receptor-related protein 5. N Engl J Med. 2002;346:1513–21.
29. Balemans W, Patel N, Ebeling M, Van Hul E, Wuyts W, Lacza C, Dioszegi M, Dikkers FG, Hildering P, Willems PJ, et al. Identification of a 52 kb deletion downstream of the SOST gene in patients with van Buchem disease. J Med Genet. 2002;39:91–7.
30. Li X, Zhang Y, Kang H, Liu W, Liu P, Zhang J, Harris SE, Wu D. Sclerostin binds to LRP5/6 and antagonizes canonical Wnt signaling. J Biol Chem. 2005;280:19883–7.
31. Staehling-Hampton K, Proll S, Paeper BW, Zhao L, Charmley P, Brown A, Gardner JC, Galas D, Schatzman RC, Beighton P, et al. A 52-kb deletion in the SOST-MEOX1 intergenic region on 17q12–q21 is associated with van Buchem disease in the Dutch population. Am J Med Genet. 2002;110:144–52.
32. Balemans W, Ebeling M, Patel N, Van Hul E, Olson P, Dioszegi M, Lacza C, Wuyts W, Van Den Ende J, Willems P, et al. Increased bone density in sclerosteosis is due to the deficiency of a novel secreted protein (SOST). Hum Mol Genet. 2001;10:537–43.
33. McClung M. Romosozumab for the treatment of osteoporosis. Review. Osteoporos Sarcopenia. 2018;4:11–5.
34. Cosman F, Crittenden DB, Ferrari S, et al. FRAME study: the foundation effect of building bone with 1 year of romosozumab leads to continued lower fracture risk after transition to denosumab. JBMR. 2018;33:1219–26.
35. Cosman F, Crittenden DB, Adachi JD, Binkley N, Czerwinski E, Ferrari S, et al. Romosozumab treatment in postmenopausal women with osteoporosis. N Engl J Med. 2016;375:1532–43.
36. Saag KG, Petersen J, Brandi ML, Karaplis AC, Lorentzon M, Thomas T, Maddox J, Fan M, Meisner PD, Grauer A. Romosozumab or alendronate for fracture prevention in women with osteoporosis. N Engl J Med. 2017;377:1417–27.
37. Langdahl BL, Libanati C, Crittenden DB, Bolognese MA, Brown JP, Daizadeh NS, Dokoupilova E, Engelke K, Finkelstein JS, Genant HK, et al. Romosozumab (sclerostin monoclonal antibody) versus teriparatide in postmenopausal women with osteoporosis transitioning from oral bisphosphonate therapy: a randomised, open-label, phase 3 trial. Lancet. 2017;390:1585–94.
38. Recker RR, Benson CT, Matsumoto T, et al. A randomized, double-blind phase 2 clinical trial of blosozumab, a sclerostin antibody, in postmenopausal women with low bone mineral density. J Bone Miner Res. 2015;30(2):216–24.

Biologics in Osteoarthritis

15

Siddharth Kumar Das

15.1 Introduction

Osteoarthritis is a non-glamourous disease for which generally neither rheumatologists nor orthopedicians, take any interest. The Rheumatologists love the disease to the extent that they can oblige their orthopedic colleagues and the Orthopedic surgeons love it for a chance to replace the joints. This is so because there is no pharmacological treatment available for Osteoarthritis. OA is a disease generally marked by a relentless course leading to disability and or joint replacement. Unfortunately, the disease is quite common and is possibly the fourth commonest cause of disability in India. It is also associated with increased mortality being associated with poor control of Diabetes and Heart disease. Osteoarthritis Research Society Internationale has labelled it as a "Serious disease" requiring urgent measures to tackle the disease.

Current Treatment options according to OARSI and the American College of Rheumatology mainly list non-pharmacological interventions. Pharmacological therapies are limited. The only pharmacological measures that are consistently effective in relieving symptoms are NSAIDS. Other pharmacological treatments are either considered of doubtful utility or outright rejected as useless. NSAIDS are believed to have high gastrointestinal, renal, and cardiac toxicity with wide publicity resulting in doctors not advising or patients not agreeing to start them. In such a setting, it is but natural to start thinking of biological therapies that may be useful in osteoarthritis patients. Biological therapies have been tried with a mixed bag of

S. K. Das (✉)
Department of Rheumatology, Era's Lucknow Medical College,
Lucknow, Uttar Pradesh, India

Formerly at Department of Rheumatology, KG Medical University,
Lucknow, Uttar Pradesh, India

N. Jain, L. Duggal (eds.), *Handbook of Biologics for Rheumatological Disorders*,
https://doi.org/10.1007/978-981-16-7200-2_15

results. There are two types of biological therapies, the first is cell-based therapies and other is monoclonals or other non-cell-based therapies. This chapter focuses on non-cell-based therapies.

It was previously believed that Osteoarthritis is a degenerative disease of the Cartilage. The two main proteins that make up the cartilage are Collagen and Aggrecan. Degeneration of these is mediated by Matrix Metalloproteinases—Aggrecanases and Collagenases. It is now widely believed that Osteoarthritis is a disease of the whole joint with well-defined biochemically mediated pathways. Secondly, it has been possible to identify many pathways that result in symptoms (pain), or pathways involved in joint inflammation and degeneration, or joint regeneration. The main cytokine involved in Osteoarthritis is Interleukin 1 beta (IL1β). IL1β is produced by conversion of Pro-IL1β by activated Caspase 1. Activated Caspase 1 is produced by activation of Inflammasome. How and why this inflammasome is activated is under investigation. IL1β leads to an inflammatory response and activates MMPs (Matrix Metalloproteinases) and Aggrecanases or ADMTS ("A Disintegrin and Metalloproteinase with Thrombospondin motifs"), prostanoids, nitric oxide, and free radicals, all believed to cause cartilage degeneration and inflammation in joint tissues. It also blocks the reparative process by inhibiting the synthesis of collagen-II and proteoglycans. Aggrecanases 1 (ADMTS-4) and 2 (ADMTS-5) are believed to proteolyze Aggrecan. ADMTS-5 is the main Aggrecanase to proteolyze Aggrecan. TNFα is another cytokine which is considered important for degeneration. Whereas the main substance thought to produce nociception is Nerve Growth factor.

Any treatment for Osteoarthritis including Biologicals would generally be acting predominantly on one or more of the three pathways:

1. Pain blocking.
2. Stopping degeneration.
3. Regeneration of tissues.

15.1.1 Biologics Targeting Pain Pathways

- Traditionally, it has been believed that since there can be no disease modification in Osteoarthritis hence only pain suppressants with least side effects are required. Paracetamol (acetaminophen) was initially advocated. It was seen that it does not help much. NSAIDs were then advocated but have been under a cloud because of side effect profile. Despite the adverse side effect profile, NSAIDs continue to be used maximally. Many advise opioid analgesics, but I am never in favor of them. The new kids on the block are new Monoclonals against Nerve Growth Factors.
- Nerve Growth factor (NGF) is elevated in patients with Osteoarthritis. Besides, there is an increase in Nociceptors and nociceptive nerve fibers in all tissues of the joints. This NGF may be responsible for the intractable pain in joint. To

Target NGF, Pfizer is actively pursuing Tanezumab for treatment of Osteoarthritis. Teva and Regeneron are developing Fasinumab. Initial clinical trials had to be stopped due to reports of Rapidly Progressive OA (RPOA) in some patients Hochberg. However, studies have continued using low-dose Tanezumab.

- The first study published on the efficacy of Tanezumab was published by Lane et al. [1]. There have been many Phase II and III studies, a Systemic review published in 2015 reviews many of these studies [2]. In a phase IIb/III study Daikin et al. [3] showed Fasinumab significantly improved pain and function in patients with hip and/or knee OA.
- In a lower dose phase 3 study in patients with unresponsive pain to standard therapy, 2.5 mg Subcutaneous Tanezumab at day 0 and Week 8 reduced pain, improved physical function and patient Global assessment [4]. Similar results were seen if 5 mg was given at 8 weeks. In another Phase III study Tanezumab 2.5 mg at Day 0 and 5 mg at every 8 weeks improved function and pain and Patients global assessment, however, 2.5 mg dose every 8 weeks did not improve patient global assessment. Both Tanezumab in doses of 2.5 to 10 mg and Fasinumab 3 to 9 mg resulted in RPOA, and Osteonecrosis in a dose-dependent manner [3, 5, 6]. Both therapies are yet to be approved by FDA for use.

15.1.2 Stopping Degeneration

IL1β and TNF α are the main Leukotrienes involved in the degenerative process. These leukotrienes besides producing inflammation also activate Matrix Metalloproteinases and Collagenases. These MMPs and Collagenases damage aggrecan and collagen. Degeneration and damage are believed to be due to inflammatory processes mediated by these inflammatory cytokines. Many Anti-IL1 monoclonals and anti-TNF monoclonals have been used. Monoclonals targeting MMPs are on the anvil.

15.2 IL-1 Countering Monoclonals

Anti-Interleukin-1 monoclonals are being tried since IL-1 is believed to be central to the pathogenesis of Osteoarthritis. In clinical settings, IL-1 blockers have been shown to reduce pain in OA.

15.2.1 Monoclonals Targeting IL1β Molecule

- **Canakinumab** is a recombinant monoclonal that binds to IL1β but not to IL1α nor to IL1 Receptor Antagonist (IL1ra). It prevents binding of IL1β to IL1 receptor. It is generally used in Cryopyrin-associated periodic syndromes. It has been recently tried for coronary artery disease in the CANTOS (Canakinumab Anti-Inflammatory Thrombosis Outcomes Study) Trial. The study looked for Cardiovascular events, in patients who already had a myocardial infarction, over 5 years. Osteoarthritis was not the aim of the trialists.

- In a post hoc analysis effect on Osteoarthritis was evaluated. Since Osteoarthritis was not the primary starting point the authors noted how many patients had a hip or knee replacement due to a diagnosis of Osteoarthritis as per their discharge records. This was the hardest evidence of diagnosis of Osteoarthritis in that study. They found that in the Canakinumab group there were fewer knee and hip joint replacements.
- Canakinumab was given in a dose of 50, 150, and 300 mg subcutaneously. The hazard ratios (HRs) for incident Joint replacements during median 3.5-year follow-up were 0.60 (95% CI, 0.38 to 0.95) for the 50-mg group, 0.53 (CI, 0.33 to 0.84) for the 150-mg group, and 0.60 (CI, 0.38 to 0.93) for the 300-mg group, suggestive of good activity in Osteoarthritis [7].
- Canakinumab was further tried as a single dose Intra-articular therapy in patients with Osteoarthritis of the knee. It was found that there was no difference in side effect profile nor efficacy from placebo (Clinical Trial number NCT01160822). A Phase 2 Clinical Trial of Intra-articular Canakinumab and another Novartis drug Intra-articular LNA034 (see below) is underway and has enrolled 133 patients.
- **Gevokizumab**, a monoclonal similar to canakinumab in mechanism of action has been tried in Hand OA, but results are not available so far (Clinicaltrialregistry.gov NCT02293564).

15.2.2 Drugs Acting on IL1 Receptor

- *AMG 108*, monoclonal antibody by Amgen, attaches to the IL-1 Receptor and blocks the activity of both IL-1β and IL-α. Given as Subcutaneous injection AMG 108 was well tolerated in human trials, but effect did not reach significance over 12 weeks compared to placebo. In another trial safety was again demonstrated but there was no significant relief. The development program for AMG 108 was terminated because of lack of efficacy [8].
- *Anakinra* also did not show significant improvement in symptoms in OA [9].
- *ABT-981 or Lutikizumab,* similar to AMG 108, blocks IL receptor for both IL1α and β. In a phase 1 trial, the monoclonal was found to be safe and well tolerated [10]. Fleishmann et al. [11] presented a Phase II trial of Lutikizumab in Knee Osteoarthritis wherein Pain relief was seen in WOMAC pain scores at 16 weeks with a 100-mg dose but not with 200 mg dose. There were no improvements in Synovitis on MRI at 26 and 52 weeks. Similarly, there was no significant improvement in Hand OA [12]. A Meta-analysis of various treatments in Osteoarthritis evaluating Lutikizumab also did not show any significant benefit of this monoclonal [13].

15.2.3 Anti TNF Therapies

TNF is supposed to play an important role in the damage and symptoms of Osteoarthritis. Anti TNF therapies have been tried in Osteoarthritis with mixed results.

- *Etanercept*, a recombinant TNF receptor fusion Protein, has been investigated. In knee osteoarthritis, Ohtori et al. [14] found improvement in knee pain. In the EHOA trial a double-blind placebo trial of etanercept in hand OA did not provide relief compared to placebo [15] but at 52 weeks there appeared to be some MRI evidence of fewer bone marrow lesions.
- *Infliximab*, a chimeric human–mouse monoclonal antibody directed against TNF showed some relief in symptoms and radiological pictures when directly injected in joints with inflammatory Hand OA [16]. No study in Knee osteoarthritis was found.
- *Adalimumab*, a fully human monoclonal directed against TNF was found to be effective in erosive hand OA [17]. But Adalimumab was not found effective in erosive hand OA in double-blind trial conducted by Chevalier et al. [18]. For knee OA, Grunke and Shulze-Koops [19] presented one patient who was given Adalimumab and had good responses. In an open-label study of subcutaneous 40 mg adalimumab fortnightly in 20 patients with knee OA 14 patients met the OARSI-OMERACT response criteria at 12 weeks [20]. Vasudeva et al. [21] 2019 reported good improvement in OA knee with10 mg Intra-articular Adalimumab in one patient. Wang [22] studied Intra-articular adalimumab in an open-label study comparing adalimumab and Hyaluronic acid and found it to be safe and effective as compared to hyaluronic acid.

15.2.4 Targeting Cartilage Breakdown

Cartilage breakdown occurs due to collagenases and Aggrecanases, hence they have been targets of treatment [23].

Collagenases Basically MMP-1, 13, and 14 are the important collagenases. Of these MMP-1 and MMP-14 are considered housekeeping collagenases. MMP-13 is the main enzyme that leads to joint damage. It has been found to be difficult to block MMP-13. General MMP blockers chelating Zinc have led to a "Musculoskeletal Syndrome" (MSS) due to excess formation of Collagen. Non-biological therapies, that block MMP 13 and do not lead to production of MSS, are currently in research phase. A monoclonal Ab 14D10 specific for active MMP-13 is still in infancy.

Aggrecanases Both non-biological therapies and biological therapies are being developed. Various biological therapies developed for Blocking ADAMTS-5 have so far not left the laboratory. Development of GSK 2394002 a humanized ADAMTS selective monoclonal was stopped because of unacceptable cardiovascular toxicity.

Another monoclonal CRB0017 targets the ancillary domain of ADAMTS and was found to be useful for delaying disease progression and some pain relief in mouse models. A nanobody (Single Domain antibody fragments) M6495 conjugated to half-life extension arm of S. albumin inhibited aggrecan turnover and has reached Phase I clinical trials. Two Phase 1 Human studies in normal healthy people and in patients with Osteoarthritis have been completed in 2019 (NCT03583346), however, no results have been posted yet.

15.2.5 Biologicals with Disease Modifying Properties in Osteoarthritis or Growth Factors

Growth factors are being studied with the aim to regenerate cartilage and other tissues. Current research may lead to the first disease modifying therapy for Osteoarthritis.

A. **Sprifermin**, a recombinant human fibroblast growth factor 18 (rhFGF18), binds to and activates Fibroblast growth factor receptor3. This promotes Chondrogenesis. Chondrogenesis, in turn, promotes matrix formation and cartilage repair [24]. Hochberg et al. [25] showed that Intra-articular Sprifermin is safe and well tolerated. Eckstein et al. [26], and Roemer et al. 2016 [27] by way of a post hoc analysis of the same data showed reduced cartilage loss, increased cartilage thickness, and improved BMLs. In a Phase II Drug trial (named Forward trial), Sprifermin, a dose of 100 ug is given Intra-articularly every 6 or 12 months, increased total knee joint cartilage after 2 years of treatment. It had a limited effect on pain [28]. In post hoc analysis Brett et al. [29], and Eckstein et al. [30] showed that not only did cartilage volume increase, the rate of deterioration of cartilage was slowed down to normal cartilage levels. A five-year follow-up study of the Forward trial showed that benefits of Sprifermin were maintained for at least 3.5 years in terms of increased cartilage and 50% improvement in pain [31].
B. **LNA043** is another compound being researched by Novartis. It is a modified human angiopoietin-like 3 (ANGPTL3) protein and is an inducer of Chondrogenesis. Phase 1 results on 30 patients given LNA043 Intra-articularly before Knee replacement therapy yielded overall good safety and tolerability [32]. The side effects were more related to total knee replacement surgery procedure than to LNA043. Biochemically there were chondro-anabolic changes though no clinical effects in this short study. A phase 2 trial with expected 138 participants has started this year (Clinical Trial number NCT04814368).

15.3 Summary

Though many biologicals are being investigated for Osteoarthritis none has come to clinical use. However, 2–3 biologicals are poised to come to the market in the next few years. The most promising ones are the pain-reducing Tanezumab. Despite reports of increased damage to articular tissues small doses of Tanezumab may be used in patients needing short duration relief from severe pain. The long-term use of Tanezumab is to be discouraged. The second is Sprifermin that has the potential for cartilage repair though has limited pain relieving properties. The third would be Canakinumab. It was given systemically in the large-scale "Cantos" trial. It was safe and a sub-analysis showed a reduction in joint replacement surgeries. It requires a phase 3 trial in patients with Osteoarthritis knee and or hip for critical evaluation. Current trials are focusing on Intra-articular use make making Phase 1 and 2 trials necessary for this new drug route. I have always believed that osteoarthritis is a systemic disease that involves all joints, though OA may be clinically evident in one joint only, hence it should be systemically treated. Another approach would be a combination of chondro-anabolic agent with a pain relief agent. Other biologicals are in phases of development, and we may be able to obtain one or more biologicals in near future.

References

1. Lane NE, Schnitzer TJ, Birbara CA, et al. Tanezumab for the treatment of pain from osteoarthritis of knee. N Engl J Med. 2010;363:1521–31.
2. Schnitzer TJ, Marks JA. A systemic review of the efficacy and general safety of antibodies to NGF in the treatment of OA of the knee. Osteoarthr Cartil. 2015;23(Suppl 1):58–17.
3. Dakin P, DiMartino SJ, Gao H, Maloney J, Kivitz AJ, et al. The efficacy, tolerability, and joint safety of fasinumab in osteoarthritis pain: a phase IIb/III double-blind, placebo-controlled, randomized clinical trial. Arthritis Rheumatol. 2019;71:1824–34.
4. Schnitzer TJ, Easton R, Pang S, et al. Effect of tanezumab on joint pain, physical function, and patient global assessment of osteoarthritis among patients with osteoarthritis of the hip or knee. JAMA. 2019;322:37–48.
5. Hochberg MC. Serious joint-related adverse events in randomized controlled trials of anti-nerve growth factor monoclonal antibodies. Osteoarthr Cartil. 2015;23(Suppl. 1):S18–21.
6. Lane NE, Corr M. Osteoarthritis in 2016: anti-NGF treatments for pain – two steps forward, one step back? Nat Rev Rheumatol. 2017;13:76–8.
7. Schieker M, Conaghan PG, Mindeholm L, et al. Effects of interleukin-1β inhibition on incident hip and knee replacement: exploratory analyses from a randomized, double-blind, placebo-controlled trial. Ann Intern Med. 2020;173:509–15.
8. Cohen SB, Proudman S, Kivitz AJ, et al. A randomized double-blind study of AMG108 in patients with osteoarthritis of the knee. Arthritis Res Ther. 2011;13:R125.
9. Chevalier X, Goupille P, Beaulieu AD, et al. Intraarticular injection of Anakinra in osteoarthritis of the knee: a multicenter, randomized, double-blind, placebo-controlled study. Arthritis Rheum (Arthritis Care Res). 2009;61:344–52.
10. Wang SX, Liu W, Jiang P, et al. Phase 1 studies Of anti-interleukin –1 dual- variable domain immunoglobulin in healthy subjects and patients with osteoarthritis. Osteoarthr Cartil. 2016;23:2.
11. Fleishmann RM, Bliddal H, Blanco FJ, et al. A phase II trial of Lutikizumab, an anti-interleukin-1α/β dual variable domain immunoglobulin, in knee osteoarthritis patients with synovitis. Arthritis Rheumatol. 2019;71:1056–69.
12. Kloppenburg M, Peterfy C, Haugen IK, et al. Phase IIa, placebo-controlled, randomised study of lutikizumab, ananti-interleukin-1α and anti-interleukin-1β dual variable domain immunoglobulin, in patients with erosive hand osteoarthritis. Ann Rheum Dis. 2019;78:413–20.
13. Cao Z, Li Y, Wang W, Jie S, et al. Is Lutikizumab, an anti-interleukin-1α/β dual variable domain immunoglobulin, efficacious for osteoarthritis? Results from a bayesian network meta-analysis. Biomed Res Int. 2020;2020. Article (II); 9013283:1–10.

14. Ohtori S, Orita S, Yamauchi K, et al. Efficacy of direct injection of etanercept into knee joints for pain in moderate and severe knee osteoarthritis. Yonsei Med J. 2015 Sep;56(5):1379–83.
15. Kloppenburg M, Ramonda R, Bobacz K, et al. Etanercept in patients with inflammatory hand osteoarthritis (EHOA): a multicentre, randomised, double-blind, placebo-controlled trial. Ann Rheum Dis. 2018;77:1757–64.
16. Güler-Yüksel M, Allaart CF. Watt I et al arthritis. Osteoarthr Cartil. 2010;18:1256–62.
17. Verbruggen G, Wittoek R, Cruyssen BV, Elewaut D. Tumour necrosis factor blockade for the treatment of erosive osteoarthritis of the interphalangeal finger joints: a double blind, randomised trial on structure modification. Ann Rheum Dis. 2012;71:891–8.
18. Chevalier X, Ravaud P, Maheu E. Adalimumab in patients with hand osteoarthritis refractory to analgesics and NSAIDs: a randomised, multicentre, double-blind, placebo-controlled trial. Ann Rheum Dis. 2015;74:1697–705.
19. Grunke M, Schulze-Koops H. Successful treatment of inflammatory knee osteoarthritis with tumour necrosis factor blockade. Ann Rheum Dis. 2006;65:555–6.
20. Maksymowych WP, Russell AS, Chiu P, Yan A, Jones N, Clare T, Lambert RG. Targeting tumour necrosis factor alleviates signs and symptoms of inflammatory osteoarthritis of the knee. Arthritis Res Ther. 2012;14(5):R206.
21. Yadav VA, Nanda SL, et al. Assessment of pain and structure after an intraarticular injection of adalimumab in osteoarthritis of the knee – a case report. Medicine. 2020;99:28.
22. Wang J. Efficacy and safety of adalimumab by intraarticular injection for moderate to severe knee osteoarthritis: an open label randomized controlled trial. J Int Med Res. 2018;46:326–34.
23. Malfait AM, Tortorella MD. The "elusive DMOAD": aggrecanase inhibition from laboratory to clinic. Clin Exp Rheumatol. 2019;37(Suppl 120 (5)):30–134.
24. Sennett ML, Meloni GR, Farran AJE, et al. Sprifermin treatment enhances cartilage integration in an in-vitro repair model. J Orthop Res. 2018;36:2648–56.
25. Hochberg MC, Lohmander LS, Hellot S, Dreher D, et al. Intraarticular sprifermin (recombinant human fibroblast growth factor 18) in knee osteoarthritis: a randomized, double-blind, placebo-controlled trial. Arthritis Rheumatol. 2014;66:1820–31.
26. Eckstein F, Wirth W, Guermazi A, et al. Brief report: intraarticular sprifermin not only increases cartilage thickness, but also reduces cartilage loss: location-independent post hoc analysis using magnetic resonance imaging. Arthritis Rheumatol. 2015;67:2916–22.
27. Roemer FW, Aydemir A, Lohmander S, et al. Structural effects of sprifermin in knee osteoarthritis: a post-hoc analysis on cartilage and non-cartilaginous tissue alterations in a randomized controlled trial. BMC Musculoskelet Disord. 2016;17:267.
28. Hochberg MC, Guermazi A, Guehring H, et al. Effect of intra-articular sprifermin vs placebo on Femorotibial joint cartilage thickness in patients with osteoarthritis. The FORWARD randomized clinical trial. JAMA. 2019;322:1360–70.
29. Brett A, Bowes MA, Conaghan PG, et al. Automated MRI assessment confirms cartilage thickness modification in patients with knee osteoarthritis: post-hoc analysis from a phase II sprifermin study. Osteoarthr Cartil. 2020;28(11):1432–6.
30. Eckstein F, Kraines JL, Aydemir A, et al. Intra-articular sprifermin reduces cartilage loss in addition to increasing cartilage gain independent of location in the femorotibial joint: post-hoc analysis of a randomised, placebo-controlled phase II clinical trial. Ann Rheum Dis. 2020;79:525–8.
31. Eckstein F, Hochberg MC, Guehring H, et al. Long-term structural and symptomatic effects of intra-articular sprifermin in patients with knee osteoarthritis: 5-year results from the FORWARD study. Ann Rheum Dis. 2021;80(8):1062–9. E-pub ahead of print. https://doi.org/10.1136/annrheumdis-2020-219181.
32. Scotti C, Gimbel J, Laurent D, et al. LNA043, a novel cartilage regenerative treatment for osteoarthritis: results from a first -in-human trial in patients with knee osteoarthritis. Osteoarthr Cartil. 2021;29:S10–S432.

Biologics in Juvenile Idiopathic Arthritis 16

Mehul P. Jariwala and Sujata Sawhney

16.1 Introduction

Juvenile idiopathic arthritis (JIA) is a heterogeneous disorder characterized by chronic arthritis of childhood with an unknown etiology starting before the age of 16 years and lasting for more than 6 weeks. Seven JIA subsets are proposed by the current International League of Associations for Rheumatology (ILAR) [1]. Though these groups were designed to be mutually exclusive, some degree of overlap does occur. The clinical presentation, course, prognosis, and response to treatment with disease modifying drugs differ between these groups. Insights into the biologic basis and pathogenesis of the disease subtype have led to the greatest improvements in care with improved efficacy and tolerability of treatments for JIA.

Multiple pro-inflammatory cytokines such as interleukin-1ß, interleukin-6, interleukin-17, and tumor necrosis factor-alpha (TNF) play a major role in the pathogenesis of inflammation in JIA [2]. Biologicals are defined as large, complex molecules (specific proteins) specifically targeting proinflammatory cytokines or cell surface antigens [3]. Some biologics inhibit cytokine function through nearly complete elimination or neutralization of the target cytokine while others interfere with cell-to-cell interaction and thereby inhibit T-cell activation or deplete the B cells. The inhibition of these cytokines or alteration in the mechanism of cell activity leads to an anti-inflammatory effect (Fig. 16.1) [4].

M. P. Jariwala (✉)
Division of Pediatric Rheumatology, University of Saskatchewan, Saskatoon, Saskatchewan, Canada
e-mail: mehul.jariwala@usask.ca

S. Sawhney
Pediatric Rheumatology Division, Institute of Child Health, Sir Ganga Ram Hospital, New Delhi, India

N. Jain, L. Duggal (eds.), *Handbook of Biologics for Rheumatological Disorders*,
https://doi.org/10.1007/978-981-16-7200-2_16

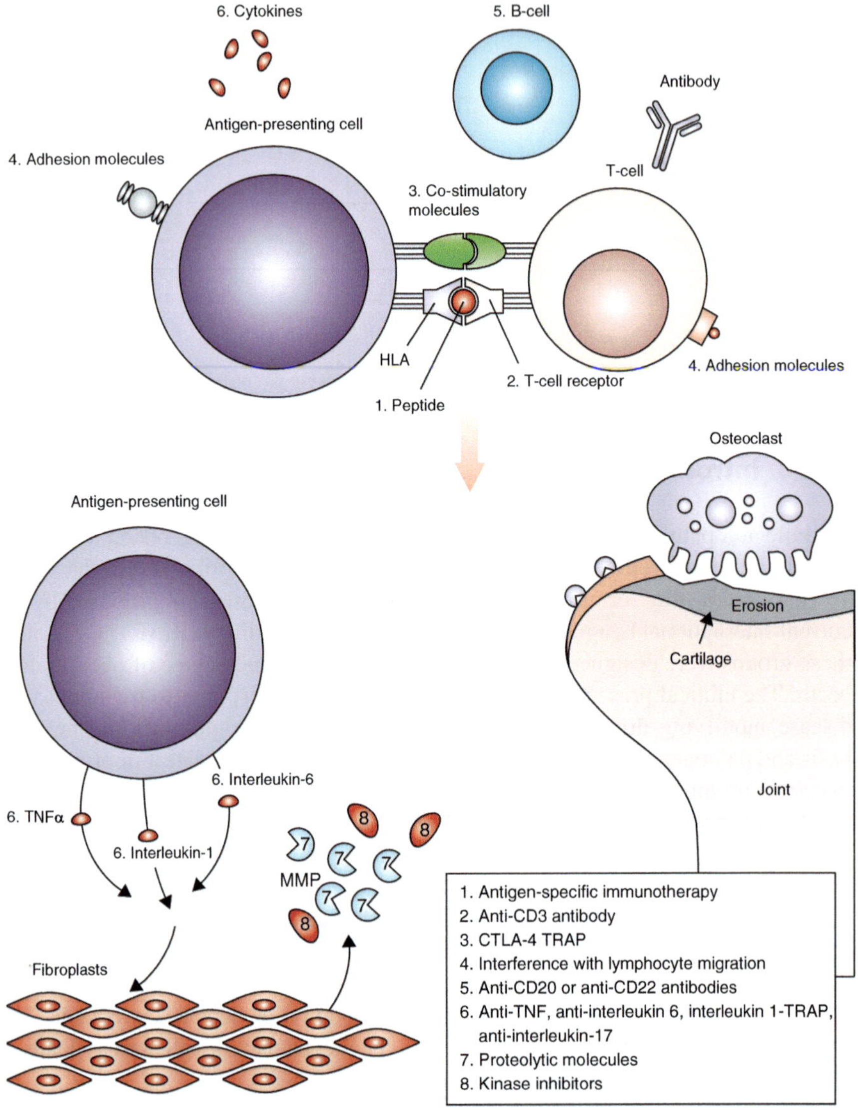

Fig. 16.1 Established and emerging biological treatment. Reprinted from Lancet, 377 (9783), Prakken, Berent, Albani, Salvatore, Martini, Alberto, Juvenile Idiopathic arthritis, 2138-49., Copyright (2011), with permission from Elsevier

16.2 Interference with Cytokines

Tumor necrosis factor-alpha (TNF-α): The cytokine TNF was first linked to rheumatoid arthritis, and elevated levels of TNF have been reported in JIA patients. TNF is a soluble 17 kD protein produced by T lymphocytes, monocytes, and macrophages. Post receptor binding, TNF is capable of synthesis of prostaglandins, prostacyclins, and other proinflammatory cytokines. Anti-TNF- α therapy (Etanercept, Adalimumab, and Infliximab) is usually used as the first biologic treatment in refractory oligoarticular or polyarticular JIA [5].

16.2.1 Soluble TNF Receptor Fusion Protein

16.2.1.1 Etanercept

- Etanercept (ETN) is fully human, a dimeric fusion protein of the human p75 TNF-α receptor and the Fc region of human IgG1. It binds to circulating soluble TNF-α, preventing its interaction with the cell surface receptor and the subsequent inflammatory response.
- It is the first TNF inhibitor approved for the treatment of JIA. It is administered subcutaneously once weekly in a dose of 0.8 mg/kg of body weight.
- ETN was first evaluated in a group of 69 children with polyarticular juvenile rheumatoid arthritis with over 70% responses (PedACR30 criteria) noted in the etanercept treatment group after 3 months of open-label treatment. No significant differences in the frequency of adverse events were identified between the two ETN and placebo groups.
- CLIPPER study: The efficacy and safety of ETN was reevaluated in phase 3b, open-label, multicenter study in patients with extended oligoarticular juvenile idiopathic arthritis, enthesitis-related arthritis (ERA), or psoriatic arthritis (PsA). ETN treatment for 12 weeks was effective [6] with higher proportions of patients achieving PedACR 50/70/90/100 responses and inactive disease status at week 12. The 2-year clinical benefit and safety of ETN demonstrated sustained efficacy at treating the clinical symptoms of all three JIA categories [7].
- TREAT trial: ETN was also evaluated for an early aggressive treatment of polyarticular JIA in a placebo-controlled study over 6 months in 85 children aged 2–16 years with a disease duration of fewer than 12 months. Aggressive treatment with methotrexate, ETN, and prednisolone were compared with methotrexate and placebo. This trial failed to reach its primary endpoint (clinical inactive disease at 6 months). The proportion of children in clinical remission on medication within 12 months of treatment was comparable in both the groups [8].

- Combined treatment with etanercept and MTX could improve the efficacy of the biologic drug [9].
- Adverse events (AE): Reported AE are generally mild and transient. Large national database studies [10] as well as long-term open-label studies [11, 12] have highlighted no increased risk of adverse events and infection with ETN. No apparent association is reported between the occurrence of malignancy and treatment with Etanercept [3, 13].

16.2.2 Monoclonal Anti-TNF Antibody

16.2.2.1 Adalimumab

Arthritis:

- Adalimumab (ADA) is a fully humanized monoclonal anti-TNF antibody approved for treatment in patients with polyarticular JIA and uveitis. It binds both soluble and membrane-bound TNF-α.
- It is administered as a subcutaneous injection given every other week. The dosing is weight based: 20 mg for children weighing <30 kg and 40 mg for children weighing >30 kg. ADA can be used weekly to treat juvenile idiopathic arthritis (JIA) and uveitis. The safety of weekly dosing was recently published [14, 15].
- Adalimumab demonstrated efficacy in treating polyarticular JIA with or without the concomitant use of methotrexate in 2008. In a randomized, double-blind, placebo-controlled withdrawal study in children with JIA, 74% percent of patients not receiving methotrexate (64 of 86) and 94% of those receiving methotrexate (80 of 85) had an ACRPed30 response at week 16. Eighty-eight percent, 80%, and 59% of patients on monotherapy and 95%, 92%, and 82% of patients on a combination with methotrexate showed a response according to PedACR 30, 50, and 70 criteria, respectively. In the "no methotrexate" arms of the study, the flare rate was 71% in the placebo group vs. 43% in the adalimumab group (P 1/4 0.031); in the "concomitant methotrexate" arms of the study the flare rates were 65% (adalimumab) vs. 37% (placebo) [16].
- Adalimumab also demonstrated efficacy in phase 3, multicenter, randomized double-blind study in patients aged ≥6 to <18 years with enthesitis-related arthritis (ERA). Significant reduction in the active joint count was noted at week 12 as compared to placebo and responses increased further with continued adalimumab therapy through week 52 [17].
- Though fully humanized, the development of anti-drug antibodies is known. A recent study identified a high incidence of anti-drug antibodies in a cohort of adalimumab-treated JIA patients observed over a mean period of 40 weeks, which also correlated with the number of relapses [18].
- In the German Biker registry, high percentages of patients in both ADA and ADA with MTX showed sufficient treatment response [19].
- SB5 is a biosimilar the reference anti-TNF monoclonal antibody adalimumab. It is approved for use in the indications for which reference ADA is approved. The

safety, tolerability, and efficacy profile is similar to that of reference ADA and its role in the management of JIA and non-infectious uveitis is well established [20].
- Adverse events: In a recent review evaluating the safety of ADA, commonly reported AE were upper respiratory tract infections, nasopharyngitis, and headache. No malignancies were reported and no new safety signals were identified in the treatment of pediatric patients with adalimumab [21].

Uveitis:
- SYCAMORE Trial: In a multicenter, double-blind, randomized, placebo-controlled trial, ADA was found to be safe and efficacious in the treatment of JIA-associated uveitis. In this trial children with active JIA-associated uveitis (on stable doses of methotrexate) were randomized in a 2:1 ratio to receive either ADA or placebo. Treatment failure of 16% was observed in the ADA group compared to 60% in the placebo group. Adverse events were reported more frequently in patients receiving adalimumab [15].
- In a retrospective interventional case series in participants enrolled from a single center in the SYCAMORE trial, the drug-induced remission of JIA-uveitis did not persist when ADA was withdrawn after 1-2 years of treatment. Children who continued on ADA tolerated the drug well with excellent visual acuity outcomes [22].
- ADJUVITE trial: It favored the use of using ADA in patients with early onset, chronic anterior uveitis associated with JIA, in case of inadequate response to topical therapy and MTX [23].
- A recent meta-analysis and systematic review provided evidence of ADA in reducing inflammatory activity, improving visual acuity with sparing corticosteroid use. ADA was associated with only minor adverse events [24].

16.2.2.2 Infliximab

Arthritis:
- Infliximab is a chimeric murine–human monoclonal anti-TNF antibody consisting of a mouse Fab fragment antibody and the constant region of human $IgG_{1.}$ It binds both soluble and membrane-bound TNF. It is not approved for the treatment of JIA.
- It is used as an intravenous infusion in a dose range of 3–6 mg/kg body weight and infusion intervals of 4 to 8 weeks. Higher dose of Infliximab >10 mg/kg has been found to be safe [25].
- Infliximab failed to show its efficacy in a multicenter, double-blind, placebo-controlled study in polyarticular JIA (primary endpoint by week 14) between patients who received infliximab (3 mg/kg) and placebo [26]. The lack of statistical significance in this trial was attributed to a smaller sample size, a higher rate of response in the placebo group and a smaller dose with a faster drug clearance in the pediatric age group. In a cross-over design patients initially treated with placebo later on received infliximab in a dose of 6 mg/kg body weight. A higher clinical response was achieved in this group with fewer infusion reactions. The long-term efficacy and safety of infliximab plus methotrexate were assessed in

the polyarticular course of juvenile rheumatoid arthritis in the open-label extension phase. Even though the high dropout rate was identified, infliximab was safe and effective (week 204) [27].

- ACUTE-JIA trial: A randomized open-label trial that compared methotrexate, methotrexate/sulfasalazine/hydroxychloroquine (COMBO), and infliximab (3–5 mg/kg) with methotrexate in disease modifying antirheumatic drug-naive patients. At week 54, ACRPed75 was achieved in 100% on infliximab, 65% on COMBO and 50% on methotrexate monotherapy. In this trial, patients on infliximab remained in a state of inactive disease for a longer duration than the other two treatment arms [28, 29].
- Concurrent use of MTX is advisable to prevent the development of human anti-chimeric antibodies. Higher infusion reactions and accelerated drug clearance are reported in patients with these anti-drug antibodies.
- Adverse events: The common AE reported were upper respiratory tract infections (viral/bacterial), pharyngitis, reactivation of latent tuberculosis, and headache. Infusion reactions have been reported in 32% of patients with a higher incidence in patients who have anti-drug antibodies [30].
- SB2 is a biosimilar of the reference anti-TNF-α antibody infliximab. Data regarding use in JIA is not available.

Uveitis:

- A high remission rate of 43% was reported in refractory JIA-uveitis from an Italian National Registry [31]. In patients with non-infectious uveitis (different etiology; 15/16 JIA associated uveitis) a higher remission of 82% was reported [32].
- In a retrospective study, higher than the recommended dose for infliximab have been suggested to achieve disease control in patients with uveitis [33].

16.2.3 Inhibition of Interleukin-1

Interleukin-1 (IL-1) is a pro-inflammatory cytokine produced by monocytes/macrophages, neutrophils, endothelial cells, and dendritic cells. IL-1ß seems to be a major mediator of the inflammatory response in systemic-onset JIA. Currently, three different biologic inhibitors of the IL-1ß pathway are available: anakinra, an interleukin-1 receptor antagonist; canakinumab, a human interleukin-1b antibody; and rilonacept, an interleukin-1 receptor fusion protein.

16.2.3.1 Anakinra

- Anakinra is a human recombinant form of interleukin-1 receptor antagonist identical to the physiological interleukin-1 receptor antagonist. It binds competitively to the interleukin-1 receptor. It has a short half-life of 4 to 6 hours and requires daily subcutaneous injection. It is administered at a dose of 1 to 2 mg/kg, but often higher doses are used in children with an incomplete response.
- Anakinra is recommended as a first-line therapy in children with systemic JIA with high disease burden and/or poor response to NSAIDs or glucocorticoids [29].

- ANAJIS trial: In this multicenter, randomized, double-blind, placebo-controlled trial, anakinra was shown to be efficacious in systemic JIA (sJIA) with normalization of blood gene expression profiles in clinical responders. Twenty-four patients were divided into two groups and treated with either anakinra or placebo for 1 month followed by patients in the placebo group started on anakinra. At month 1, 8/12 responders were receiving anakinra and 1 responder was receiving placebo ($p = 0.003$). Ten patients from the placebo group switched to anakinra and at month 2, nine were responders. Six patients discontinued treatment (between 1 and 12 months) due to an adverse event, lack of efficacy, or a disease flare [34].
- Anakinra was used as first-line therapy for sJIA (either as monotherapy or in conjunction with steroids and/or MTX) in a multicenter study with 46 patients. Excellent clinical efficacy was reported with the rapid resolution of systemic symptoms and refractory arthritis in almost 90% of patients. Within 1 month, fever and rash resolved in >95% of patients and C-reactive protein and ferritin normalized in >80% of patients. A complete response was noted in approximately 60% of patients without the need for therapy escalation [35].
- In a prospective cohort study, Anakinra was used as first-line therapy (before systemic steroid treatment was administered) in patients with sJIA with excellent responses in nearly all patients within 3 months. After 1 year, 85% of patients met the criteria for the clinically inactive disease. At two years, 12/14 (86%) of patients met the criteria for disease remission, 8 of which were not receiving the medication [36].
- Anakinra is safe and effective in controlling macrophage activation syndrome in children with systemic JIA [37, 38].
- Adverse events: Local injection site reactions are common composed of pain, redness, and erythema. Other adverse events include headaches, gastrointestinal complaints, upper respiratory infections, and infectious episodes [39]. Rare incidences of serious infection, nephrosis, sterile abscess, and transaminitis, have been reported. Anakinra use is associated with an increased incidence of infection, especially with concomitant use of corticosteroids and high-dose anakinra [40].

16.2.3.2 Rilonacept

- Rilonacept is a fully human dimeric fusion protein incorporating the extracellular domains of both the IL-1 receptor components. It acts as a soluble decoy receptor for IL-1, preventing the binding of IL-1ß to its cell-bound receptor. It has a half-life of approximately 1 week. Rilonacept is currently not approved for JIA.
- Rilonacept is administered as a subcutaneous injection given as a loading dose of 4.4 mg/kg (maximum 320 mg), followed by a weekly maintenance dose of 2.2 mg/kg (maximum 160 mg/week).
- Rilonacept has also demonstrated efficacy in systemic JIA. The efficacy of Rilonacept was evaluated in a 4-week, double-blind, placebo-controlled study with 23 systemic JIA patients first received rilonacept or placebo, followed by 23 months of open-label treatment. No significant difference was noted during

the double-blind phase, but fever and rash completely resolved in all patients by month 3 during the open-label treatment [41].

- Adverse events: Injection site reactions are common with other serious AE including arthritis flare, anemia, pulmonary fibrosis, and macrophage activation syndrome.

16.2.3.3 Canakinumab

- Canakinumab is a fully humanized IgG1 monoclonal antibody that binds to IL-1ß. It has a long half-life of 30 days and administered as a subcutaneous injection once monthly. It is administered at a dose of 4 mg/kg (maximum 300 mg/month).
- The efficacy of Canakinumab was evaluated in two phase III trials in children with systemic JIA with active systemic features. In the first trial, patients were randomized in a double-blind fashion, to a single subcutaneous dose of canakinumab (4 mg per kilogram) or placebo. In the first trial, on day 15, 84% of patients who received canakinumab achieved an ACRPed30 response versus 10% of patients who received a placebo. The second trial randomized 100 canakinumab responders to either continued treatment or placebo; 74% of patients who continued canakinumab had no flare versus 25% of patients who received placebo [42].
- Injection site reactions, infections, and abdominal pain were the most common adverse events observed in phase 3 clinical trials of canakinumab in systemic JIA [42].

16.3 Inhibition of Interleukin-6

IL-6 is an inflammatory cytokine that can then lead to intracellular signaling and result in cytokine production and release. It correlates with fever spikes, thrombocytosis, and joint involvement in patients with SJIA.

16.3.1 Tocilizumab

- Tocilizumab (TCZ) is a humanized antibody against the soluble and membrane-bound IL-6 receptor. TCZ is approved to be used in sJIA and refractory polyarticular JIA. It is an intravenous infusion. In systemic JIA it is given at a dose of 12 mg/kg (<30 kg) or 8 mg/kg (<30 kg) every 2 weeks. In children with polyarticular JIA, 8 mg/kg (>30 kg) and 10 mg/kg (<30 kg) is administered once every 4 weeks. TCZ is also available as a subcutaneous preparation.
- The safety and efficacy of TCZ were evaluated in a randomized, double-blind placebo control withdrawal design in 56 Japanese children with a diagnosis of sJIA. PedACR30 response was seen in 91% of patients during the initial 12 weeks open-label phase. Patients who had a PedACR30 and low CRP of less than 5 mg/L were randomized and received either placebo or to continue tocilizumab

treatment for 12 weeks. In this phase, patients receiving a placebo had significantly more flares. PedACR 30/50/70 of 98%, 94%, and 90%, respectively, was noted in patients who participate in an open-label extension study for an additional 48 weeks [43].

- TENDER trial: A similar trial design demonstrated the efficacy of Tocilizumab in a randomized double-blind phase at 12 weeks. In the open-label extension phase, 80% of patients who received tocilizumab achieved an ACR Pedi 70 with no fever [44].
- CHERISH study: In three parts, randomized, double-blind withdrawal trial, 188 patients received tocilizumab and then 163 of those patients were randomized to either continue tocilizumab or switch to placebo [38]. JIA flare occurred in 25.6% of patients who continued tocilizumab versus 48.1% of patients who received placebo [45].
- Tocilizumab is generally well tolerated in patients with sJIA and polyarticular JIA. The most frequently reported adverse events were upper respiratory tract infection and pharyngitis, nasopharyngitis, diarrhea, and headache. sJIA patients appeared to have an approximately 25% risk of a serious adverse event and an 11% risk of a serious infection per year of treatment. Neutropenia, thrombocytopenia, liver function abnormalities, anaphylactic reaction, and pulmonary hypertension were reported. In polyarticular JIA, similar but less serious adverse events were reported. No cases of malignancy or death have been reported [43, 44, 46].

16.4 Inhibition of T-cell Co-stimulation

16.4.1 Abatacept

- Abatacept is a fully human, soluble fusion protein composed of the Fc region of IgG_1 and the extracellular domain of CTLA-4. It competitively binds to CD80/86 on antigen-presenting cells and prevents the second signal required for T-cell activation. It is administered intravenously in a dosage of 10 mg/kg body weight at weeks 0, 2, 4, and then every 4 weeks. Abatacept is FDA approved for refractory polyarticular juvenile idiopathic arthritis with poor response to anti-TNF therapy.
- AWAKEN trail: Abatacept was used in a double-blind, randomized-controlled withdrawal trial in 190 patients with polyarticular JIA for 4 months. Those who responded were randomized in the second phase to receiving Abatacept or placebo for 6 months. In this phase, 20% of patients randomized to stay on abatacept experienced arthritis flares compared to 53% of patients switched over to placebo [47]. In the long-term extension phase, 90% achieved an ACRPed30 by day 589. Seventy-three percent of patients in phase 1, who did not achieve an ACRPed30 at the end of the 4-month, achieved ACRPed 30 by day 589 in open-label extension phase [48].
- Abatacept has been used in children with juvenile arthritis and uveitis refractory to topical and systemic corticosteroids, immunosuppressives, and at least one

anti-TNF therapy. It was shown not to have a sustained response in patients with severe and refractory uveitis [49]. Abatacept has been used in multiple case reports with good benefits.
- In terms of safety, the most frequent adverse events were nasopharyngitis, upper respiratory tract infection, and vomiting. A few cases of serious infections were noted. No cases of malignancy or tuberculosis were identified.

16.5 B-cell Depletion

- Rituximab is a chimeric anti-CD20 antibody that specifically binds and destroys CD20-positive B cells.
- ACR recommendations include the use of Rituximab for refractory polyarthritis despite receiving a TNF-α inhibitor and abatacept sequentially, especially in patients who are rheumatoid factor positive [50].
- Adverse events include infusion reactions, infections, leukopenia, neutropenia, prolonged hypogammaglobulinemia, and progressive multifocal leukoencephalopathy.

16.6 Treatment Guidelines for Juvenile Idiopathic Arthritis

Treatment recommendations in juvenile idiopathic arthritis were categorized per five treatment groups. These included oligoarticular JIA (4 or less joint involvement), polyarthritis (5 or more joints), active sacroiliac arthritis, and systemic juvenile arthritis [29, 50].

For Patients

1. Less than five affected joints, with an inability to reach inactive clinical disease after NSAIDs, intra-articular steroids, and methotrexate (depending on prognostic parameters after 3 or 6 months), a TNF inhibitor was recommended [50].
2. With five or more affected joints a TNF inhibitor is recommended with poor response to NSAIDS and synthetic DMARDS. If the patients continue to have a moderate or high clinical activity after 4 months of TNF inhibitor, either a switch to another TNF inhibitor or Abatacept is recommended [50]. These recommendations were made before the Tocilizumab trial was published.
3. For patients with active sacroiliac arthritis initiation of a TNF inhibitor was recommended for patients who have received an adequate trial of NSAIDs and have high disease activity and features of poor prognosis [50].
4. For patients with active systemic features and varying degrees of synovitis, anakinra was recommended as first-line therapy in accordance with glucocorticoid monotherapy or NSAIDs. If the patient had persistent active disease after one month of Anakinra, a switch to Tocilizumab, Canakinumab, or methotrexate was recommended. Those patients without active systemic features and varying

degrees of synovitis, Abatacept, Tocilizumab, Anakinra, or TNF-inhibitor was recommended after poor response to either methotrexate, NSAIDS, or intra-articular steroid injection [29].

16.7 Conclusion

There have been major advances during the last 10 years in the new therapeutic options available for children with JIA due to a better understanding of immune pathogenesis. The implementation of a treat to target (such as remission) with excellent effective and good response rates has been possible with newer more efficacious biologic therapy.

References

1. Petty RE, Southwood TR, Manners P, et al. International league of associations for rheumatology classification of juvenile idiopathic arthritis: second revision, edmonton, 2001. J Rheumatol. 2004;31(2):390–2.
2. Woo P. Cytokines and juvenile idiopathic arthritis. Curr Rheumatol Rep. 2002;4(6):452–7.
3. Horneff G. Update on biologicals for treatment of juvenile idiopathic arthritis. Expert Opin Biol Ther. 2013;13(3):361–76. https://doi.org/10.1517/14712598.2013.735657.
4. Prakken B, Albani S, Martini A. Juvenile idiopathic arthritis. Lancet. 2011;377(9783):2138–49. https://doi.org/10.1016/S0140-6736(11)60244-4.
5. Ringold S, Angeles-Han ST, Beukelman T, et al. 2019 american college of rheumatology/arthritis foundation guideline for the treatment of juvenile idiopathic arthritis: therapeutic approaches for non-systemic polyarthritis, sacroiliitis, and enthesitis. Arthritis Rheumatol. 2019;71(6):846–63. https://doi.org/10.1002/art.40884.
6. Horneff G, Burgos-Vargas R, Constantin T, et al. Efficacy and safety of open-label etanercept on extended oligoarticular juvenile idiopathic arthritis, enthesitis-related arthritis and psoriatic arthritis: Part 1 (week 12) of the clipper study. Ann Rheum Dis. 2014;73(6):1114–22. https://doi.org/10.1136/annrheumdis-2012-203046.
7. Constantin T, Foeldvari I, Vojinovic J, et al. Two-year efficacy and safety of etanercept in pediatric patients with extended oligoarthritis, enthesitis-related arthritis, or psoriatic arthritis. J Rheumatol. 2016;43(4):816–24. https://doi.org/10.3899/jrheum.150430.
8. Wallace CA, Giannini EH, Spalding SJ, et al. Trial of early aggressive therapy in polyarticular juvenile idiopathic arthritis. Arthritis Rheum. 2012;64(6):2012–21. https://doi.org/10.1002/art.34343.
9. Horneff G, De Bock F, Foeldvari I, et al. Safety and efficacy of combination of etanercept and methotrexate compared to treatment with etanercept only in patients with juvenile idiopathic arthritis (jia): preliminary data from the german jia registry. Ann Rheum Dis. 2009;68(4):519–25. https://doi.org/10.1136/ard.2007.087593.
10. Beukelman T, Xie F, Chen L, et al. Rates of hospitalized bacterial infection associated with juvenile idiopathic arthritis and its treatment. Arthritis Rheum. 2012;64(8):2773–80. https://doi.org/10.1002/art.34458.
11. Foeldvari I, Constantin T, Vojinovic J, et al. Etanercept treatment for extended oligoarticular juvenile idiopathic arthritis, enthesitis-related arthritis, or psoriatic arthritis: 6-year efficacy and safety data from an open-label trial. Arthritis Res Ther. 2019;21(1):125. https://doi.org/10.1186/s13075-019-1916-9.

12. Lovell DJ, Reiff A, Ilowite NT, et al. Safety and efficacy of up to eight years of continuous etanercept therapy in patients with juvenile rheumatoid arthritis. Arthritis Rheum. 2008;58(5):1496–504. https://doi.org/10.1002/art.23427.
13. Beukelman T, Haynes K, Curtis JR, et al. Rates of malignancy associated with juvenile idiopathic arthritis and its treatment. Arthritis Rheum. 2012;64(4):1263–71. https://doi.org/10.1002/art.34348.
14. Correll CK, Bullock DR, Cafferty RM, Vehe RK. Safety of weekly adalimumab in the treatment of juvenile idiopathic arthritis and pediatric chronic uveitis. Clin Rheumatol. 2018;37(2):549–53. https://doi.org/10.1007/s10067-017-3890-4.
15. Ramanan AV, Dick AD, Jones AP, et al. Adalimumab plus methotrexate for uveitis in juvenile idiopathic arthritis. N Engl J Med. 2017;376(17):1637–46. https://doi.org/10.1056/NEJMoa1614160.
16. Lovell DJ, Ruperto N, Goodman S, et al. Adalimumab with or without methotrexate in juvenile rheumatoid arthritis. N Engl J Med. 2008;359(8):810–20. https://doi.org/10.1056/NEJMoa0706290.
17. Burgos-Vargas R, Tse SM, Horneff G, et al. A randomized, double-blind, placebo-controlled multicenter study of adalimumab in pediatric patients with enthesitis-related arthritis. Arthritis Care Res (Hoboken). 2015;67(11):1503–12. https://doi.org/10.1002/acr.22657.
18. Marino A, Real-Fernandez F, Rovero P, et al. Anti-adalimumab antibodies in a cohort of patients with juvenile idiopathic arthritis: incidence and clinical correlations. Clin Rheumatol. 2018;37(5):1407–11. https://doi.org/10.1007/s10067-018-4057-7.
19. Klein A, Becker I, Minden K, Foeldvari I, Haas JP, Horneff G. Adalimumab versus adalimumab and methotrexate for the treatment of juvenile idiopathic arthritis: long-term data from the german biker registry. Scand J Rheumatol. 2019;48(2):95–104. https://doi.org/10.1080/03009742.2018.1488182.
20. Frampton JE. Sb5: An adalimumab biosimilar. Bio Drugs. 2018;32(5):507–10. https://doi.org/10.1007/s40259-018-0307-0.
21. Horneff G, Seyger MMB, Arikan D, et al. Safety of adalimumab in pediatric patients with polyarticular juvenile idiopathic arthritis, enthesitis-related arthritis, psoriasis, and crohn's disease. J Pediatr. 2018;201(166–175):e163. https://doi.org/10.1016/j.jpeds.2018.05.042.
22. Horton S, Jones AP, Guly CM, et al. Adalimumab in juvenile-idiopathic arthritis-associated uveitis (jia-u): 5-year follow-up of the Bristol participants of the sycamore trial. Am J Ophthalmol. 2019;207:170–4. https://doi.org/10.1016/j.ajo.2019.06.007.
23. Quartier P, Baptiste A, Despert V, et al. Adjuvite: a double-blind, randomised, placebo-controlled trial of adalimumab in early onset, chronic, juvenile idiopathic arthritis-associated anterior uveitis. Ann Rheum Dis. 2018;77(7):1003–11. https://doi.org/10.1136/annrheumdis-2017-212089.
24. Ming S, Xie K, He H, Li Y, Lei B. Efficacy and safety of adalimumab in the treatment of non-infectious uveitis: a meta-analysis and systematic review. Drug Des Devel Ther. 2018;12:2005–16. https://doi.org/10.2147/DDDT.S160431.
25. Tambralli A, Beukelman T, Weiser P, Atkinson TP, Cron RQ, Stoll ML. High doses of infliximab in the management of juvenile idiopathic arthritis. J Rheumatol. 2013;40(10):1749–55. https://doi.org/10.3899/jrheum.130133.
26. Ruperto N, Lovell DJ, Cuttica R, et al. A randomized, placebo-controlled trial of infliximab plus methotrexate for the treatment of polyarticular-course juvenile rheumatoid arthritis. Arthritis Rheum. 2007;56(9):3096–106. https://doi.org/10.1002/art.22838.
27. Ruperto N, Lovell DJ, Cuttica R, et al. Long-term efficacy and safety of infliximab plus methotrexate for the treatment of polyarticular-course juvenile rheumatoid arthritis: findings from an open-label treatment extension. Ann Rheum Dis. 2010;69(4):718–22. https://doi.org/10.1136/ard.2009.100354.
28. Tynjala P, Vahasalo P, Tarkiainen M, et al. Aggressive combination drug therapy in very early polyarticular juvenile idiopathic arthritis (acute-jia): a multicentre randomised open-label clinical trial. Ann Rheum Dis. 2011;70(9):1605–12. https://doi.org/10.1136/ard.2010.143347.

29. Ringold S, Weiss PF, Beukelman T, et al. 2013 update of the 2011 american college of rheumatology recommendations for the treatment of juvenile idiopathic arthritis: recommendations for the medical therapy of children with systemic juvenile idiopathic arthritis and tuberculosis screening among children receiving biologic medications. Arthritis Rheum. 2013;65(10):2499–512. https://doi.org/10.1002/art.38092.
30. Cecchin V, Zannin ME, Ferrari D, et al. Longterm safety and efficacy of adalimumab and infliximab for uveitis associated with juvenile idiopathic arthritis. J Rheumatol. 2018;45(8):1167–72. https://doi.org/10.3899/jrheum.171006.
31. Zannin ME, Birolo C, Gerloni VM, et al. Safety and efficacy of infliximab and adalimumab for refractory uveitis in juvenile idiopathic arthritis: 1-year followup data from the italian registry. J Rheumatol. 2013;40(1):74–9. https://doi.org/10.3899/jrheum.120583.
32. Kruh JN, Yang P, Suelves AM, Foster CS. Infliximab for the treatment of refractory noninfectious uveitis: a study of 88 patients with long-term follow-up. Ophthalmology. 2014;121(1):358–64. https://doi.org/10.1016/j.ophtha.2013.07.019.
33. Sukumaran S, Marzan K, Shaham B, Reiff A. High dose infliximab in the treatment of refractory uveitis: does dose matter? ISRN Rheumatol. 2012;2012:765380. https://doi.org/10.5402/2012/765380.
34. Quartier P, Allantaz F, Cimaz R, et al. A multicentre, randomised, double-blind, placebo-controlled trial with the interleukin-1 receptor antagonist anakinra in patients with systemic-onset juvenile idiopathic arthritis (anajis trial). Ann Rheum Dis. 2011;70(5):747–54. https://doi.org/10.1136/ard.2010.134254.
35. Nigrovic PA, Mannion M, Prince FH, et al. Anakinra as first-line disease-modifying therapy in systemic juvenile idiopathic arthritis: report of forty-six patients from an international multicenter series. Arthritis Rheum. 2011;63(2):545–55. https://doi.org/10.1002/art.30128.
36. Vastert SJ, de Jager W, Noordman BJ, et al. Effectiveness of first-line treatment with recombinant interleukin-1 receptor antagonist in steroid-naive patients with new-onset systemic juvenile idiopathic arthritis: results of a prospective cohort study. Arthritis Rheumatol. 2014;66(4):1034–43. https://doi.org/10.1002/art.38296.
37. Bruck N, Suttorp M, Kabus M, Heubner G, Gahr M, Pessler F. Rapid and sustained remission of systemic juvenile idiopathic arthritis-associated macrophage activation syndrome through treatment with anakinra and corticosteroids. J Clin Rheumatol. 2011;17(1):23–7. https://doi.org/10.1097/RHU.0b013e318205092d.
38. Sonmez HE, Demir S, Bilginer Y, Ozen S. Anakinra treatment in macrophage activation syndrome: a single center experience and systemic review of literature. Clin Rheumatol. 2018;37(12):3329–35. https://doi.org/10.1007/s10067-018-4095-1.
39. Ilowite N, Porras O, Reiff A, et al. Anakinra in the treatment of polyarticular-course juvenile rheumatoid arthritis: safety and preliminary efficacy results of a randomized multicenter study. Clin Rheumatol. 2009;28(2):129–37. https://doi.org/10.1007/s10067-008-0995-9.
40. Fleischmann RM, Tesser J, Schiff MH, et al. Safety of extended treatment with anakinra in patients with rheumatoid arthritis. Ann Rheum Dis. 2006;65(8):1006–12. https://doi.org/10.1136/ard.2005.048371.
41. Lovell DJ, Giannini EH, Reiff AO, et al. Long-term safety and efficacy of rilonacept in patients with systemic juvenile idiopathic arthritis. Arthritis Rheum. 2013;65(9):2486–96. https://doi.org/10.1002/art.38042.
42. Ruperto N, Brunner HI, Quartier P, et al. Two randomized trials of canakinumab in systemic juvenile idiopathic arthritis. N Engl J Med. 2012;367(25):2396–406. https://doi.org/10.1056/NEJMoa1205099.
43. Yokota S, Imagawa T, Mori M, et al. Efficacy and safety of tocilizumab in patients with systemic-onset juvenile idiopathic arthritis: a randomised, double-blind, placebo-controlled, withdrawal phase iii trial. Lancet. 2008;371(9617):998–1006. https://doi.org/10.1016/S0140-6736(08)60454-7.
44. De Benedetti F, Brunner HI, Ruperto N, et al. Randomized trial of tocilizumab in systemic juvenile idiopathic arthritis. N Engl J Med. 2012;367(25):2385–95. https://doi.org/10.1056/NEJMoa1112802.

45. Brunner HI, Ruperto N, Zuber Z, et al. Efficacy and safety of tocilizumab in patients with polyarticular-course juvenile idiopathic arthritis: results from a phase 3, randomised, double-blind withdrawal trial. Ann Rheum Dis. 2015;74(6):1110–7. https://doi.org/10.1136/annrheumdis-2014-205351.
46. Yokota S, Imagawa T, Mori M, et al. Longterm safety and effectiveness of the anti-interleukin 6 receptor monoclonal antibody tocilizumab in patients with systemic juvenile idiopathic arthritis in Japan. J Rheumatol. 2014;41(4):759–67. https://doi.org/10.3899/jrheum.130690.
47. Ruperto N, Lovell DJ, Quartier P, et al. Abatacept in children with juvenile idiopathic arthritis: a randomised, double-blind, placebo-controlled withdrawal trial. Lancet. 2008;372(9636):383–91. https://doi.org/10.1016/S0140-6736(08)60998-8.
48. Ruperto N, Lovell DJ, Quartier P, et al. Long-term safety and efficacy of abatacept in children with juvenile idiopathic arthritis. Arthritis Rheum. 2010;62(6):1792–802. https://doi.org/10.1002/art.27431.
49. Tappeiner C, Miserocchi E, Bodaghi B, et al. Abatacept in the treatment of severe, long-standing, and refractory uveitis associated with juvenile idiopathic arthritis. J Rheumatol. 2015;42(4):706–11. https://doi.org/10.3899/jrheum.140410.
50. Beukelman T, Patkar NM, Saag KG, et al. 2011 american college of rheumatology recommendations for the treatment of juvenile idiopathic arthritis: initiation and safety monitoring of therapeutic agents for the treatment of arthritis and systemic features. Arthritis Care Res (Hoboken). 2011;63(4):465–82. https://doi.org/10.1002/acr.20460.

Biologics in Pediatric Connective Tissue Disorders

17

Sarit Sekhar Pattanaik and Amita Aggarwal

17.1 Introduction

Early diagnosis and treatment of pediatric connective tissue diseases (CTD) like SLE, juvenile dermatomyositis (JDM), and vasculitis have considerably reduced mortality in these rare diseases. However, this has led to significant treatment-related adverse events that impact quality of life. Corticosteroids continue to be the first-line therapy for most of CTDs but they result in short stature, delayed puberty, avascular necrosis, osteoporosis, and increased infection risk. Thus, steroid sparing therapies are the need of the hour.

Better understanding of disease pathogenesis has led to identification of specific pathways for targeting therapy. Biologics are potent addition in the armamentarium of rheumatologists over the past decade. Evidence for the use of biologics in the pediatric population is mostly from case reports, case series, or registry data. Low prevalence of diseases and ethical constraints precludes randomized control trials in children with life-threatening diseases.

Biologics have a potential role in treatment of refractory pediatric CTDs and their use in management is likely to increase in the near future. Herein, we review the use of biologics in pediatric SLEJDM and vasculitis.

S. S. Pattanaik · A. Aggarwal (✉)
Department of Clinical Immunology & Rheumatology,
Sanjay Gandhi Postgraduate Institute of Medical Sciences, Lucknow, India
e-mail: amita@sgpgi.ac.in

N. Jain, L. Duggal (eds.), *Handbook of Biologics for Rheumatological Disorders*,
https://doi.org/10.1007/978-981-16-7200-2_17

17.2 Biologics in SLE

- SLE is an multisystemic autoimmune disease in which both innate and adaptive immune systems play an important role in its pathogenesis. Juvenile SLE has a more severe phenotype with higher prevalence of nephritis compared to adults with SLE [1].
- The major role of B cells in production of autoantibodies and demonstration of association between pathogenic B cells and disease activity has made B cell depletion therapy an attractive option in SLE [2]. Though there are many biologics that target B cells, but antibodies to CD20 (Rituximab [RTX]) and B lymphocyte stimulator (Blys) have been used for management of SLE.
- Although results from phase III clinical trials of RTX in adults, both LUNAR and EXPLORER failed to meet their primary end points the enthusiasm to treat refractory disease with RTX has not faded away. With encouraging results of RITUXILUP study showing the efficacy of "steroid free" combination of RTX and Mycophenolate regimen in management of active nephritis there is a renewed interest in RTX in management of SLE [3].
- Rituximab is used in pediatric population in refractory cytopenias, lupus nephritis, and neuropsychiatric lupus. Rituximab at a dose of 750 mg/m^2 two weeks apart shows good response with complete remission in 75–90% cases along with steroid sparing effect [4, 5].
- In a retrospective data of 44 pediatric active lupus nephritis patients from India RTX led to decrease in flares resulting in a significantly higher 36-month flare-free survival compared with MMF and CYC (100% vs. 83% and 53%, respectively; $p = 0.006$), increased rate of complete remission and steroid sparing effect (0.3 mg/kg/day in RTX arm compared to 0.7–0.9 mg/kg/day in MMF and CYC arm at the end of 3 years) as compared to mycophenolate and cyclophosphamide. The RTX group demonstrated better long-term treatment outcomes despite the presence of poorer baseline disease characteristics [6].
- Belimumab is a BLyS-specific inhibitor that blocks the binding of soluble BLyS, to its receptors on B cells. Patients with SLE, both adults and children have increased levels of BLyS in their sera and this is believed to drive pathogenic B cells and promote inflammation.
- In 2011, FDA approved Belimumab for treatment of adults with non-organ threatening SLE. Although studies have shown a potential role of Belimumab in decreasing rates of renal flare but its role in organ-threatening disease remains to be still defined. Data from recently concluded Phase II PLUTO trial [7], looking at the efficacy of Belimumab in pediatric population ($N = 93$) the results have been encouraging with a significant proportion of patients attaining SLEDAI responder index (SRI-4) compared to standard of care. They also had less flare rate and almost double the time to severe flare (160 days versus 82 days). In addition, there were no new safety signals.
- In April 2019 based on trial data, Belimumab was approved by FDA as first drug for pediatric lupus. Cost of therapy, availability, prolonged duration of treatment, and potential increased prevalence of psychiatric symptoms and malignancy on

long-term use have to be considered before prescribing Belimumab in pediatric population.

- CALIBRATE (NCT02260934), a phase II study designed to administer Belimumab after 2 doses of RTX and cyclophosphamide in refractory or relapsed lupus nephritis found Belimumab to be safe but did not show any therapeutic benefit [8]. The trials of other B cell depleting therapy like Tabalumab, Epratuzumab, and Blisibimod have not shown any benefit in adult SLE and thus have not been studied in the pediatric population [9].

17.3 Biologics in JDM

- JDM is a systemic autoimmune disease characterized by vasculopathy affecting the skin and muscles. It can also involve the lungs, heart, gastrointestinal system, joints, and other organs. B cells play a critical role in the initiation and propagation of the immune response and are implicated in the pathogenesis of myositis. In addition to functioning as the precursor of autoantibody-producing plasma cells, B cells present antigen to T cells and secrete proinflammatory cytokines.
- Corticosteroids are the mainstay of therapy in JDM, however, to reduce toxicity of steroids it is recommended to start IS agent like methotrexate upfront. This has considerably reduced mortality and morbidity but there remains a subgroup of patients who have suboptimal responses.
- The RTX in myositis (RIM) study had 200 patients with refractory myositis, which also included 46 patients with JDM [10]. Although the study did not meet its primary endpoint but 83% of refractory adult and juvenile myositis patients met the definition of improvement, suggesting that RTX has a potential role in JDM. While analyzing predictors of response to RTX in RIM trial, autoantibodies (anti-synthetase, anti Mi2), JDM category of myositis, and lower disease damage were associated with better response [11]. Other than RTX, a study from North America (CARRA registry) shows some benefit with anti-TNF agents, abatacept and tocilizumab in patients with JDM, but RTX is still the preferred biologic in refractory cases [12]. Ongoing trial of Abatacept (AID) will further define its role in therapy of JDM (NCT02594735).

17.4 Biologics in Pediatric Vasculitis

Primary systemic vasculitis although rare in childhood has the potential to cause significant morbidity and mortality [13]. Kawasaki disease and IgA vasculitis are the most common vasculitis in children. Corticosteroids, cyclophosphamide, and IVIG have been the mainstay of therapy in this subgroup. Better understanding of pathogenesis of disease, encouraging results from the use of biologics in adults, toxicity concerns with long-term steroids, cyclophosphamide, and prohibitive cost of IVIG has led to exploring the use of biologics in pediatric vasculitis.

17.4.1 Takayasu Arteritis

- Although rare, it is an important cause of renovascular hypertension in pediatric age group. The lack of validated outcome measures makes clinical trials more difficult in TA.
- Case series of anti-TNF agents in pediatric TA which included 4 patients treated with IFX showed some benefit in refractory cases albeit with side effects [14]. Similarly, double-blind trial of Tocilizumab which included 6 pediatric patients did not show any difference between treatment groups though it had a steroid sparing effect as median glucocorticoid dose reduced from 0.223 mg/kg/day at the time of relapse before study to 0.105 mg/kg/day after 96 weeks [15].

17.4.2 Kawasaki Disease

- The rationale for use of anti-TNF agents stems from studies showing elevated TNFα and TNFα soluble receptors I and II concentrations in the acute phase of KD, and the levels are highest in children who subsequently develop coronary artery aneurysms.
- With reports from case studies showing successful treatment of recrudescent fever in Kawasaki disease with anti-TNF agents, a double-blind randomized trial enrolling 196 children with KD was designed combining upfront use of Infliximab, single dose of 5 mg/kg with standard of care compared to IVIg [16]. There was no difference in development of treatment resistance between either groups. Although the group on infliximab showed a marked reduction in ESR and Z score of left anterior descending coronary artery at 2 weeks, there was no difference at the end of 5 weeks. However, a pilot study looking at IFX as compared to IVIG second dose in 24 patients with treatment-resistant disease found similar outcomes in both groups with no new safety signals [17].
- In another Japanese trial of IVIG-resistant KD, fever defervescence rate within 2 days was better for infliximab as compared to second dose of IVIG (76.7% vs 37%; $p < 0.05$). In addition, time to defervescence was shorted for IFX [17]. The fact that a single dose of Infliximab is equivalent to IVIG in resistant cases makes it a potential therapeutic target in resource-poor countries like India where cost of IVIG is very high. Further studies are underway with Etanercept (NCT00841789) and Anti IL-1 (NCT02179853) based therapy in Kawasaki disease.

17.4.3 DADA2 Deficiency and PAN

- DADA2 deficiency is a recently described autoinflammatory syndrome characterized by intermittent fevers, early-onset lacunar strokes, and other neurovascular manifestations, livedoid rash, hepatosplenomegaly, and systemic PAN-like vasculopathy.

- The suggestion of skewing of macrophage toward M1 phenotype leading to increased TNF production as the mechanism of inflammation in DADA2 deficiency has led to use of anti-TNF agents in its management with success [18]. Based on efficacy of TNF blockade in DADA2 deficiency there has been a postulated role in sporadic PAN, however, there are no trials to support such hypothesis.

17.4.4 ANCA Vasculitis (AAV)

- With the results of RITUXIVAS and RAVE study establishing the role of Rituximab as an inducing agent in AAV, PEPRS study (Pediatric Polyangiitis Rituximab Study) an open-label study which enrolled 25 children was designed [19].
- Newly diagnosed or relapsing granulomatosis with polyangiitis (19 patients) or microscopic polyangiitis (6 patients) were included. Patients received weekly intravenous RTX 375 mg/m^2 for 4 weeks and glucocorticoids 1 mg/kg/day (max 60 mg/day) tapered to 0.2 mg/kg/day (max 10 mg/kg/day) by 6 months in addition to 3 pulse doses of methylprednisolone.
- In the first six months of the study, RTX was safe and well tolerated, with 52% of patients achieving remission. Although encouraging the long-term results will define the use of RTX in pediatric AAV. There is no data for use of other biologics like anti-TNF agents, abatacept, or tocilizumab in children with AAV.

17.4.5 IgA Vasculitis

- IgA vasculitis in children usually has a benign course and can be easily managed with corticosteroids. However, in children with significant renal disease there is a need to add other immunosuppressive drugs. In patients with refractory nephritis, biologics are being tried. In a systematic review where RTX was used for refractory nephritis almost 95% had some clinical improvement and nearly 75% had remission. Further the dose of other drugs reduced [20].

17.5 Conclusions

- The indication and choice of biologics in pediatric vasculitis are summarized in Table 17.1.
- With the current paradigm shift in treating rheumatic disease from saving lives to having complete remission and good quality of life, need for targeted therapy is being felt. A better understanding of the disease pathogenesis and importance of immune cells and cytokines have led to the development of biologic therapy. The potential of blocking an important pathway has not always translated to results in trials again highlighting the multiple redundant pathways operative in autoimmune diseases.

Table 17.1 Biologics in vasculitis

Type	Biologic agent	Remarks
AAV	RTX Anti-TNF	Relapsing and refractory disease No data
KD	IFX Etanercept and Anakinra TCZ	KD refractory to standard therapy Trials ongoing May worsen coronary artery aneurysms
TA	Anti-TNF	Selected cases, increased infection risk
DADA2 sporadic PAN	Anti-TNF	First-line therapy No reports in sporadic PAN
HSP	RTX	Adult IgA vasculitis with refractory nephritis anti-TNFα can induce HSP in some patients

AAV-ANCA associated vasculitis; KD-Kawasaki Disease; TA-Takayasu arteritis; DADA2-Deficiency of ADA2; PAN-Polyarteritis Nodosa; HSP-Henoch Scholein Purpura; RTX-Rituximab; TNF-Tumor necrosis factor; IFX-Infliximab; TCZ-Tocilizumab

- The use of biologics in pediatric connective tissue disease is limited to treatment of refractory cases unlike in adults where they can be used as first-line therapy. However, RTX in myositis, lupus nephritis, AAV, and IFX in KD show promise.
- Belimumab despite being approved is not used much for pediatric lupus. With the ongoing clinical trials in pediatric population and promising new molecules in the pipeline, the day is not far when biologics will play an important role in management of pediatric connective tissue diseases.

References

1. Tucker LB, Uribe AG, Fernández M, Vilá LM, McGwin G, Apte M, et al. Adolescent onset of lupus results in more aggressive disease and worse outcomes: results of a nested matched case-control study within LUMINA, a multiethnic US cohort (LUMINA LVII). Lupus. 2008;17:314–22.
2. El-Hallak M, Binstadt BA, Leichtner AM, Bennett CM, Neufeld EJ, Fuhlbrigge RC, et al. Clinical effects and safety of rituximab for treatment of refractory pediatric autoimmune diseases. J Pediatr. 2007;150:376–82.
3. Condon MB, Ashby D, Pepper RJ, et al. Prospective observational single-Centre cohort study to evaluate the effectiveness of treating lupus nephritis with rituximab and mycophenolate mofetil but no oral steroids. Ann Rheum Dis. 2013;72:1280–6.
4. Tambralli A, Beukelman T, Cron RQ, Stoll ML. Safety and efficacy of rituximab in childhood-onset systemic lupus erythematosus and other rheumatic diseases. J Rheumatol. 2015;42:541–6.
5. Olfat M, Silverman ED, Levy DM. Rituximab therapy has a rapid and durable response for refractory cytopenia in childhood-onset systemic lupus erythematosus. Lupus. 2015;24:966–72.
6. Basu B, Roy B, Babu BG. Efficacy and safety of rituximab in comparison with common induction therapies in pediatric active lupus nephritis. Pediatr Nephrol. 2017;32:1013–21.

7. Brunner HI, Abud-Mendoza C, Viola DO, Calvo Penades I, Levy D, Anton J. For Paediatric Rheumatology International Trials Organisation (PRINTO) and the Pediatric Rheumatology Collaborative Study Group (PRCSG). Safety and efficacy of intravenous belimumab in children with systemic lupus erythematosus: results from a randomised, placebo-controlled trial. Ann Rheum Dis. 2020;79:1340–8.
8. Atisha-Fregoso Y, Malkiel S, Harris KM, Byron M, Ding L, Kanaparthi S, et al. Phase II randomized trial of rituximab plus cyclophosphamide followed by Belimumab for the treatment of lupus nephritis. Arthritis Rheumatol. 2021;73:121–31.
9. Yuen JH, Nguyen SC, Askanase AD. Targeted B cell therapies in adult and pediatric systemic lupus erythematosus. Lupus. 2016;25:1086–96.
10. Oddis CV, Reed AM, RIM study group. Rituximab in the treatment of refractory adult and juvenile dermatomyositis and adult polymyositis: a randomized, placebo-phase trial. Arthritis Rheum. 2013;65:314–24.
11. Aggarwal R, BandosA RAM, et al. Predictors of clinical improvement in rituximab treated refractory juvenile and adult dermatomyositis and adult polymyositis. Arthritis Rheumatol. 2014;66:740–9.
12. Spencer CH, Rouster-Stevens K, Gewanter H, Syverson G, Modica R, Schmidt K, et al. Pediatric rheumatologist collaborators. Biologic therapies for refractory juvenile dermatomyositis: five years of experience of the childhood arthritis and rheumatology research Alliance in North America. Pediatr Rheumatol Online J. 2017 Jun 13;15:50. https://doi.org/10.1186/s12969-017-0174-0.
13. Akamine K, Punaro M. Biologics for childhood systemic vasculitis. Pediatr Nephrol. 2019;34:2295–309.
14. Filocamo G, Buoncompagni A, Viola S, Loy A, Malattia C, Ravelli A, Martini A. Treatment of Takayasu's arteritis with tumor necrosis factor antagonists. J Pediatr. 2008;153:432–4.
15. Nakaoka Y, Isobe M, Tanaka Y, Ishii T, Ooka S, Niiro H, et al. Long-term efficacy and safety of tocilizumab in refractory Takayasu arteritis: final results of the randomized controlled phase 3 TAKT study. Rheumatology (Oxford). 2020;59:2427–34.
16. Tremoulet AH, Jain S, Jaggi P, Jimenez-Fernandez S, Pancheri JM, Sun X, et al. Infliximab for intensification of primary therapy for Kawasaki disease: a phase 3 randomised, double-blind, placebo-controlled trial. Lancet. 2014;383:1731–8.
17. Mori M, Hara T, Kikuchi M, Shimizu H, Miyamoto T, Iwashima S, et al. Fuse S. Infliximab versus intravenous immunoglobulin for refractory Kawasaki disease: a phase 3, randomized, open-label, active-controlled, parallel-group, multicenter trial. Sci Rep. 2018 Jan 31;8(1):1994.
18. MeytsI AI. Deficiency of adenosine deaminase 2 (DADA2): updates on the phenotype, genetics, pathogenesis, and treatment. J Clin Immunol. 2018;38:569–78.
19. Brogan P, Cleary G, Kasapcopur O, Rangaraj S, Yeung R, Brunetta P, Cooper J, Pordeli P. Lehane PB OP0332 Paediatric open label clinical study of rituximab for the treatment of granulomatosis with polyangiitis (GPA) and microscopic polyangiitis (MPA). Ann Rheum Dis. 2018;77:212–6.
20. Hernández-Rodríguez J, Carbonell C, Mirón-Canelo JA, Diez-Ruiz S, Marcos M, Chamorro AJ. Rituximab treatment for IgA vasculitis: a systematic review. Autoimmun Rev. 2020 Apr;19(4):102490. https://doi.org/10.1016/j.autrev.2020.102490.

18 JAK Inhibitors in Rheumatic Disease

P. D. Rath, S. S. Nelson, and A. K. Khan

18.1 Introduction

Jak inhibitors are small molecules with a low molecular weight. They were developed for the treatment of autoimmune inflammatory diseases like Rheumatoid Arthritis (RA). They target and inhibit components of the intracellular inflammatory signalling cascade. Among the Jak inhibitors, the most successful are the Janus kinase (JAK) enzymes inhibitors. They consist of four members, which are JAK1, JAK2, JAK3 and TYK2.

In clinical practice, patients of RA are treated with conventional synthetic DMARDs (csDMARDs) and bridging therapy with glucocorticoids, followed by parenterally administered biologic DMARDs (bDMARDs) in patients with poor prognosis and refractory disease. However, only 30–50% of patients treated with this combination achieve remission within few months. Moreover, bDMARDs can potentially induce immunogenicity by developing anti-drug antibodies, with a loss of its efficacy. Another disadvantage with bDMARDs is that they require subcutaneous or intravenous use as they are digestible following oral administration.

P. D. Rath (✉)
Max Super Speciality Hospital, New Delhi, India

S. S. Nelson
Department of Medicine, Division of Rheumatology, NSCB Medical College, Jabalpur, MP, India

A. K. Khan
Center for Rheumatic Diseases and Pain Management, Shifa Medical Center, Jammu and Kashmir, India

N. Jain, L. Duggal (eds.), *Handbook of Biologics for Rheumatological Disorders*,
https://doi.org/10.1007/978-981-16-7200-2_18

18.2 The JAK/STAT Pathway

- JAKs, which are cytoplasmic non-receptor tyrosine kinases, have the ability to phosphorylate tyrosine residues both alone (autophosphorylation) and on neighbouring molecules (transphosphorylation), including STATs.
- The STATs, area family of transcription factors, with seven members and act downstream of JAKs [1].
- The JAK/STAT pathway regulates the action of many types of molecules such as ILs, IFNs, colony-stimulating factors, growth factors and hormones (also called hormone-like cytokines), which then operate through type I and type II receptors.
- Type I receptors are used by many ILs, colony-stimulating factors and hormones, whereas IFNs and IL-10related cytokines (IL-10, IL-19, IL-20, IL-22, IL-22 and IL-26) use type II receptors. These receptors are made up of various subunits, each of them associated with a JAK molecule.

As the effector protein binds to its receptor, which oligomerizes, it activates the corresponding JAK, which is then autophosphorylated and transfers a phosphate to the tyrosine residue in the receptor's subunit, creating a docking site for the STAT molecule.

The JAK phosphorylates the STAT molecule, which are dimerized and translocated from the cytosol to the nucleus, thereby regulating gene expression (Table 18.1).

- The subunits of a receptor can be associated with only one specific JAK or more than one JAK, and many different cytokines may carry out their actions through the same JAK. Therefore, inhibiting a JAK molecule may inhibit more than a

Table 18.1 JAK heterodimers and homodimers important for the signalling of particular cytokines

Cytokines		IL-2 IL4, IL7, IL-9, IL-15, IL-21	EPO, TPO, GH	1 L-3, IL5, GM-CSF	IL-13, IL-6,	IL12, L-23’	Type 1 IFN (a/f’)	Type 2 IFN (y)
JAK heterodimers And homodimers[a]		JAK1 JAK3	JAK2 JAK3	JAK2 JAK2	JAK1 TYK2 JAK2	JAK2 TYK2	JAK1 TYK2	JAK1 JAK2
Inhibitiont1	JAK1	+	–	–	+	–	+	+
	JAK2	–	+	+	+	+	–	+
	JAK3	+	–	–	–	–	–	–
	JAK4	–	–	–	+	+	+	–

EPO erythropoietin, *GH* growth hormone, *GM-CSF* granulocyte-macrophage, colony-stimulating factor, *TPO* thrombopoietin

[a]Different cytokines signal through different JAk combinations. A particular JAk must be inhibited to stop the signalling started by these cytokines. This provides opportunities to design specific JAk inhibitors that reduce signalling from particular cytokines

single pathway, explaining both the beneficial and the adverse effects are seen with JAK inhibitors [2].

During the past few years, many JAKinibs have been subcategorised as first-generation and newer JAKinibs.

- The first-generation JAKinibs, also called pan-JAK inhibitors, do not show high specificity, having activity against three or even all four of the JAK family members.

The newer JAKinibs, are selective against specific JAKs with fewer side effects. Currently, three JAKinibs have been approved for the treatment of RA and PsA.

18.3 Evaluation of Efficacy of JAKinibs in RA Clinical Trials

Tofacitinib was the first jakinib developed for the treatment of autoimmune disease. In adult RA patients, multiple randomised-controlled trials (RCTs) demonstrated the efficacy of tofacitinib in both early and established disease, as monotherapy, in combination with csDMARDs, including MTX, and in both treatment-naive and treatment-refractory patients (Table 18.2).

- In the phase III tofacitinib trials in RA, patients achieved statistically significant and clinical improvements in disease activity as evaluated by the categorical criteria of the American College of Rheumatology response criteria (ACR20, 50 and 70) and other measures as well as improvements in functional status assessed by the Health Assessment Disability Index (HAQ-DI) and 36-Item Short Form Survey (SF-36). Tofacitinib has been shown to be disease modifying and prevents the progression of structural damage to joints as assessed both by conventional radiography and MRI.
- It also results in a rapid improvement in a range of patient-reported outcomes (PROs).
- Tofacitinib in RA was superior to MTX in Phase III clinical trials, efficacious in MTX- and csDMARD-refractory, active RA, non-inferior in combination with MTX to the anti-TNF agent adalimumab plus MTX. It was also efficacious in patients with active RA who did not respond to multiple bDMARDs with different mechanisms of action.
- In 2012, the Federal Drug Administration (FDA) approved tofacitinib in a dose regime of 5 mg twice daily for the treatment of RA in patients who were intolerant or unresponsive to MTX [3].
- In 2017 the European Medicines Agency approved **Baricitinib** for the treatment of adult RA patients as 2 mg and 4 mg doses once daily with moderate to severe active disease. These patients had either responded inadequately or had an intolerance to one or more csDMARDs (Table 18.3).
- Baricitinib is a selective inhibitor of the JAK family that does not affect other enzyme kinases. It inhibits JAK1 and JAK2 and to a much lesser extent TYK2,

Table 18.2 Tofacitinib: phase III clinical trials for moderate to severe RA

	ORAL Start (25) MTX-naive (*n* = 958)	ORAL Solo (11) csDMARD-IR (*n* = 611)	ORAL Sync (12) csDMARD-IR (*n* = 797)	ORAL Scan (14) MTX-IR (*n* = 797)	ORAL Standard (15) MTX-IR (*n* = 717)	ORAL Standard (27) MTX-IR (*n* = 1148)	ORAL Step (10) TNF-IR (*n* = 339)
Duration, months background treatment Arms	24 None (1) 5 mg bd (2) 10 mg bd (3) MTX	6 None (1) 5 mg bd (2) 10 mg bd (3) placebo Advancing at 3 months to 5 mg bd or 10 mg bd	12 csDMARDs (1) 5 mg bd (2) 10 mg bd (3) placebo Advancing at 6 months to 5 mg bd or 10 mg bd	24 MTX (1) 5 mg bd (2) 10 mg bd (3) placebo Advancing at 6 months to 5 mg bd or 10 mg bd	12 MTX (1) 5 mg bd (2) 10 mg bd (3) placebo Advancing at 6 months to 5 mg bd or 10 mg bd (4) ADA	12 None (1) 5 mg bd (2) 5 mg bd-MTX (3) ADA + MTX	6 MTX (1) 5 mg bd (2) 10 mg bd (3) placebo Advancing at 6 months to 5 mg bd or 10 mg bd
Feature	X-ray with monotherapy	Monotherapy	Background DMARDs	X-ray	Active control (adalimumab)	Active control (adalimumab non-inferiority)	TNFi failure
Coprimary end points	AmTSS ACR70	ACR20 HAQ-DI DAS28(ESR) < 2.6	ACR20 HAQ-DI DAS28–4 (ESR) < 2.6	ACR20 mTSS HAQ-DI DAS28(ESR) < 2.6	(1) ACR20 (2) HAO-dl (3) DAS28(ESR) (4) DAS28(ESR) <2.6	ACR50 ACR20 SDAI	ACR20 HAQ-DI DAS28(ESR)

The table summarises the wide range of RA patient types studied in tofacitinib phase III confirmatory studies. *ADA* adalimumab, *csDMARD* conventional synthetic, DMARD, *HAQ-DI* Health Assessment Disability Index, *IR* inadequate response, *mTSS* modified Total Sharp Score, *SDAI* Simplified Disease Activity Index, *TNF* TNF inhibitor

Table 18.3 Baricitinib: phase III clinical trials for moderate to severe RA

	RA BEGIN [4] MTX-naive ($n = 588$)	RA-BEAM [5] MTX-IR ($n = 1307$)	RABUILD [6] csDMARD-IR ($n = 684$)	RA-BEACON [7] bDMARD-IR ($n = 527$)	RABEYOND [34] OLE study ($n = 3073$)
Type of therapy	Monotherapy + combination therapy	Combination therapy	Combination therapy	Combination therapy	Monotherapy-patients Who completed previous BARI RA study
Background active comparator Arms	None/MTX MTX (1) 4 mg qd + MTX (2) 4 mg qd monotherapy (3) MTX	MTX ADA+ MTX (1) PBO (2) 4 mg qd (3) ADA	csDMARD (1) 2 mg qd (2) 4 mg qd (3) PBO	csDMARD (1) 2 mg qd (2) 4 mg qd (3) PBO	csDMARD (1) 2 mg qd (2) 4 mg qd
Duration, weeks Primary end point Key secondary End point	24 ACR20 (week 24) Week 24 DAS28-CRP HAQ-DI mTSS SDAI remission	52 ACR20 (week 12) Week 12: DAS28-CRP HAQ-DI mTSS (week 24) SDAI remission Morning joint stiffness	24 ACR20 (week 12) Week 12: DAS28-CRP HAQ-DI SDAI remission Morning joint stiffness	24 ACR20 (week 12) Week 12: DAS28-CRP HAQ-DI SDAI remission	52, with optional Extension to 104 weeks Safety & efficacy Currently recruiting Estimated completion December 2020

The table summarises the broad range of RA patient types studied in baricitinib phase III confirmatory studies, *ADA* adalimumab, *csDMARD* conventional synthetic. DMARD, *HAQ-DI* Health Assessment Disability Index, *IR* inadequate response, *mTSS* modified Total Sharp Score, *SDAI* Simplified Disease Activity Index, *TNF* TNF inhibitor

with the result that JAK3 is preserved with a 100-fold selectivity for JAK1 and JAK2.

- In phase II and III RCTs, Baricitinib was seen to be efficacious and those patients who successfully completed the phase III RCTs like RA-BEGIN, RABUILD, RA-BEAM and RA-BEACON have enrolled for the long term extension studies RABEYOND and RA-BALANCE in countries like Argentina, Brazil and China.
- Upadacitinib is a selective JAK-1 inhibitor that has been approved by the FDA in 2019 for RA.
- In the SELECT-EARLY and SELECT-MONOTHERAPY RCTs, upadacitinib 15 mg and 30 mg showed a significantly higher clinical response than methotrexate in theACR50 response (52.1%, 56.4% and 28.3%, p 0.001) and DAS28-CRP < 2.6(35.6%, 40.8%, and 13.7%) at week 12 [8, 9].

SELECT-COMPARE compared upadacitinib + methotrexate with adalimumab + methotrexate in patients with RA with a previously inadequate response to methotrexate.

After 12 weeks, upadacitinib + methotrexate was superior to adalimumab + methotrexate with ACR 20 (70.5% vs. 63%, $p < 0.05$), ACR50 (45.2% vs. 29.1%, $p < 0.01$) and DAS28-CRP < 3.2 (45.0% vs. 28.7%).

Patients receiving upadacitinib (86%) or adalimumab (88%), had no radio graphic progression compared to placebo (74%). (<0.001) [10].

18.4 JAKinibs in PsA

- The JAK/STAT pathway is associated with the IL-23/−17 axis, which in turn plays a key role in the underlying pathogenesis of PsA and spondyloarthropathies. However, the mode of action of JAKinibs in psoriatic arthritis is not fully understood. Although IL-17 per se does not seem to employ the JAK/STAT pathway, IL-23 (which is an upstream driver of IL-17A release) exerts its function through the JAK2-TYK2/STAT3-STAT4 system [11]. Additionally, IL-22 (also a key player in the pathogenesis of SpAs and an important mediator of the IL-23/−17 axis) uses the JAK/STAT pathway.

18.4.1 Tofacitinib

- The efficacy of oral tofacitinib 5 mg twice daily in patients with PsA having previously received DMARD therapy was evaluated in two randomised, multinational, double-blind, placebo-controlled phase III trials: the 12-month OPAL Broaden ($n = 422$) [12] and 6-month OPAL Beyond ($n = 394$) trials [13].
- It was used in combination with methotrexate in patients who had an inadequate response or who have been intolerant to a prior DMARD therapy. It was shown to improve the clinical symptoms of PsA and PsA-related disability in TNFi-naïve patients and in patients with an inadequate response to prior TNFi therapy. It was also efficacious across multiple PsA domains with an acceptable tolerability profile.

18.4.2 Upadacitinib

- In a 24-week randomised, placebo-controlled, double-blind, phase 3 trial, 642 patients were randomised to once per day upadacitinib 15 mg or 30 mg, placebo followed by upadacitinib 15 mg or placebo followed by upadacitinib 30 mg at week 24 [14]. The primary endpoint was the proportion of patients achieving ACR 20 response at week 12 along with the achievement of minimal disease activity (MDA) assessed at week 24.

- At week 12, significantly more patients receiving upadacitinib 15 mg and 30 mg vs. placebo achieved ACR20 (56.9% and 63.8% vs. 24.1%; $p < 0.001$ for both comparisons). At week 24, MDA was achieved by more upadacitinib 15 mg-treated (25.1%) and 30 mg-treated patients (28.9%) vs. placebo (2.8%; $p < 0.001$ for both comparisons). The incidence of treatment-emergent adverse events was similar with placebo and upadacitinib 15 mg and higher with upadacitinib 30 mg at week 24, and the incidence of serious infections were 0.5%, 0.5% and 2.8% with placebo, upadacitinib 15 mg and upadacitinib 30 mg, respectively.
- The selective TYK2 inhibitor BMS-986165 has shown the highest efficacy towards psoriasis of any JAK inhibitor to date, with a PASI75 response of 75% after 12 weeks of treatment in a phase 2 trial [15].

18.5 Giant Cell Arteritis

- A phase 2 study, testing the safety and efficacy of baricitinib in relapsing GCA, is ongoing backing the theory that JAK inhibitors could be potentially efficacious in patients with GCA. In a chimeric model, treatment with tofacitinib reduced proliferation rates of lesional T cells, microangiogenesis, intimal outgrowth and the production of IFN-g, IL-17, IL-21 and CD4 + CD103+ T memory cells.

18.6 Safety of JAKinibs

- Most of the safety data was obtained from the clinical trials of tofacitinib in RA and appears to be acceptable and similar to those of the biological drugs.

18.6.1 Infections

- For Tofacitinib, the incidence rate for severe infections has been estimated to be 2.7 per 100 patient-years [16] and 2.9/100 patient-years for baricitinib [17]. An increased incidence of reactivation of herpes zoster was associated with both tofacitinib and baricitinib, which may be due to inhibition of IFN and IL-15, the important anti-viral cytokines that signal through JAK1, JAK2 and JAK3.

18.6.2 Malignancies

- Despite the increased exposure to tofacitinib, the incidence of malignancies (with the exception of non-melanoma skin cancer) remained stable over time and was in the same range as RA treatment with biologics [16].

18.6.3 Gastrointestinal Perforation

- Inhibition of IL-6, which signals via JAK1, JAK2 and TYK2 may be associated with gastrointestinal perforation. For tofacitinib, the IR of gastrointestinal perforation was 0.11/100 patient-years, and 0.05/100 patient-years for baricitinib. However, this was lower than that of 0.27/100 patient-years with tocilizumab.

18.6.4 Deep Vein Thrombosis and Pulmonary Embolus

The IR of DVT and PE related to tofacitinib have not been reported. However, five cases of deep vein thrombosis and pulmonary embolus (DVT/PE) were seen with baricitinib in RCTs (IR 1.2/100 patient-years), but none in the placebo-treated group [18], with the overall IR of DVT/PE being 0.5/100 patient-years.

18.6.5 Laboratory Abnormalities

- JAK2 inhibition can reduced erythropoiesis as haemopoietic cytokines, including erythropoietin signal via JAK2. This is seen by Hb changes associated with baricitinib [19], in which a statistically significant greater reduction ($P = 0.02$) in Hb occurred in patients treated with baricitinib (0.17 ± 0.02) when compared with placebo-treated patients (0.12 ± 0.02). Anaemia occurred in 29% of baricitinib-treated vs. 26% of placebo-treatment patients. However, a mild increase in Hb was observed with tofacitinib, which has a less inhibitory effect on JAK2: 0.47 g/dl and 0.28 g/dl with 5 and 10 mg, respectively. The mild increase in Hb with tofacitinib 10 mg is dose-dependent inhibition of JAK2, i.e. at a low dose (5 mg) tofacitinib is selective for JAK1 and JAK3 but at 10 mg, this selectivity is diminished and JAK2 is inhibited.
- Tofacitinib and baricitinib should not be used in patients who are anaemic (Hb < 8 g/dl), and treatment should be withdrawn when haemoglobin drops below 8 g/dl.
- A decrease in the neutrophil count with occasional neutropenia and lymphopenia has been observed with all JAKi.
- An increase in both high-density lipoprotein and low-density lipoprotein cholesterol occurred after treatment with both tofacitinib and baricitinib, without a change in high-density lipoprotein/low-density lipoprotein ratio.
- IR of major adverse cardiovascular events was 0.58/100 patient-years for tofacitinib [20] and 0.5/100 patient-years for baricitinib [18]. The cholesterol ester fractional catabolic rate was higher in RA patients, indicating increased cholesterol catabolism. Treatment with tofacitinib reduced inflammation and restored cholesterol catabolism.
- Liver transaminases elevation (>3 times upper limit of normal) occurred in 2% of patients receiving tofacitinib [6] and 1.4% of patients being treated with bar-

icitinib [4]. The increase was transient and asymptomatic and has to be monitored but temporarily stopped when liver transaminases increase significantly.
- A small increase in serum creatinine by 2–4 mmol/l was observed in RCTs when compared with placebo for tofacitinib [7] and baricitinib [5]. This stabilised after 3 months and did not have any significant renal side effects.
- Arise in creatine phosphokinase levels(more than five times the upper limit of normal) was seen in 1% of patients who received tofacitinib or baricitinib. In most of the patients, the increase in creatine phosphokinase was temporary, asymptomatic and did not require treatment discontinuation.

18.7 Newer JAKinibs (Table 18.4)

18.7.1 Filgotinib

Filgotinib (GLPG0634)—a selective JAK1 inhibitor—is an investigational drug for RA.

- In the DARWIN 1 study, filgotinib 100 or 200 mg per day in patients who received a stable dose of methotrexate showed significantly more ACR20 responses at week 12 than placebo [21]. These improvements were sustained up to week 24.
- The results of the DARWIN 2 trial suggest that filgotinib monotherapy could improve the signs and symptoms of RA compared to placebo, with 12-week ACR20 responses of 67%, 66%, 73% and 29% in the filgotinib 50, 100 or 200 mg per day, and placebo groups, respectively [22].

18.7.2 Peficitinib

- The JAK1/3 inhibitor peficitinib (ASP015K), another study drug, was shown to improve RA outcomes in two phase IIb placebo-controlled studies.
- These studies showed that in Japanese patients with moderate to severe RA, peficitinib monotherapy at daily doses of 25, 50, 100 and 150 mg resulted in a dose-dependent improvement in ACR20 response scores compared to placebo [23].

Another study also found that peficitinib treatment resulted in dose-dependent improvements in ACR20 responses relative to placebo among patients with moderate to severe RA.

Table 18.4 JAK inhibitors that are currently in clinical development

Drug/Compound	Current stage of development
Filgotinib	Phase III
Peficitinib	Phase III
Decernotinib	Phase II (currently on hold)

18.7.3 Decernotinib

Another JAK3 inhibitor decernotinib was shown to be superior to placebo in a phase IIa trial in patients who had been failed treatment with at least one DMARD, and a following dose-escalating phase IIb study found that decernotinib significantly improved ACR20 response rates at weeks 12 and 24 compared with placebo [24]. The clinical development of decernotinib is at present discontinued.

18.8 Conclusion

JAK inhibitors are novel, orally administered, effective and rapidly acting agents for the treatment of RA. After the advent of biologics, the introduction of the first non-selective JAK inhibitors constitutes a major breakthrough, overcoming the limitations of antagonising a single target through a broader magnitude of response.

The oral route of administration of JAK inhibitors has the potential to minimise drug discontinuation. Further head-to-head comparative studies may show their superiority to biologics.

The manufacturing cost of JAKi is substantially less than biologics. This has made access to more effective treatment for RA.

References

1. O'Shea JJ, Kontzias A, Yamaoka K, et al. Janus kinase inhibitors in autoimmune diseases. Ann Rheum Dis. 2013;72(Suppl 2):ii111–5.
2. Banerjee S, Biehl A, Gadina M, Hasni S, Schwartz DM. JAK-STAT signaling as a target for inflammatory and autoimmune diseases: current and future prospects. Drugs. 2017;77:521–46.
3. Traynor K. FDA approves tofacitinib for rheumatoid arthritis. Am J Health Syst Pharm. 2012;69:2120.
4. Baricitinib. Summary of product characteristics. London: European Medicine Agency; 2017.
5. Keystone EC, Taylor PC, Drescher E, et al. Safety and efficacy of baricitinib at 24 weeks in patients with rheumatoid arthritis who have had an inadequate response to methotrexate. Ann Rheum Dis. 2015;74:333–40.
6. Fleischmann R, Wollenhaupt J, Takiya L, et al. Safety and maintenance of response for tofacitinib monotherapy and combination therapy in rheumatoid arthritis: an analysis of pooled data from open-label long-term extension studies. RMD Open. 2017;3:e000491.
7. Isaacs JD, Zuckerman A, Krishnaswami S, et al. Changes in serum creatinine in patients with active rheumatoid arthritis treated with tofacitinib: results from clinical trials. Arthritis Res Ther. 2014;16:R158.
8. Van Vollenhoven R, Takeuchi T, Pangan AL, et al. A phase 3, randomized, controlled trial comparing upadacitinib monotherapy to MTX monotherapy in MTX-naïve patients with active rheumatoid arthritis. Arthritis Rheumatol. 2018;70(Suppl 10):990–2.
9. Smolen JS, Cohen S, Emery P, et al. Upadacitinib as monotherapy: a phase 3 randomized controlled double-blind study in patients with active rheumatoid arthritis and inadequate response to methotrexate. Arthritis Rheumatol. 2018;70(Suppl 10):886–91.
10. Fleischmann R, Pangan AL, Mysler E, et al. A phase 3, randomized, double-blind study comparing upadacitinib to placebo and to adalimumab, in patients with active rheumatoid arthritis with inadequate response to methotrexate. Arthritis Rheumatol. 2018;70(Suppl 10):1788–800.

11. Raychaudhuri SK, Abria C, Raychaudhuri SP. Regulatory role of the JAK STAT kinase signalling system on the IL-23/IL-17 cytokine axis in psoriatic arthritis. Ann Rheum Dis. 2017;76:e36.
12. Mease P, Hall S, FitzGerald O, et al. Tofacitinib or adalimumab versus placebo for psoriatic arthritis. N Engl J Med. 2017;377(16):1537–50.
13. Gladman D, Rigby W, Azevedo VF, et al. Tofacitinib for psoriatic arthritis in patients with an inadequate response to TNF inhibitors. N Engl J Med. 2017;377(16):1525–36.
14. Mease PJ, Lertratanakul A, Anderson JK, et al. Upadacitinib for psoriatic arthritis refractory to biologics: SELECT-PsA 2. Ann Rheum Dis. 2021;80:312–20.
15. Papp K, Gordon K, Thaçi D, et al. Phase 2 trial of selective tyrosine kinase 2 inhibition in psoriasis. N Engl J Med. 2018;379:1313–21.
16. Curtis JR, Lee EB, Kaplan IV, et al. Tofacitinib, an oral Janus kinase inhibitor: analysis of malignancies across the rheumatoid arthritis clinical development programme. Ann Rheum Dis. 2016;75:831–41.
17. Genovese MC, Smolen JS, Takeuchi T et al. Safety profile of baricitinib for the treatment of rheumatoid arthritis up to 5.5 years: an updated integrated safety analysis. Presented at the ACR/ARHP Annual Meeting, San Diego, CA, USA, 38 November 2017; Abstr. 511.
18. Weinblatt M, Taylor PC, Burmester G et al. Cardiovascular safety during treatment with baricitinib in patients with rheumatoid arthritis. Presented at the ACR/ARHP Annual Meeting, San Diego, CA, USA, 38 November 2017; Abstr. 499.
19. Smolen JS, Genovese MC, Takeuchi T. Safety profile of baricitinib in patients with active rheumatoid arthritis: an integrated analysis. Presented at European League Against Rheumatism (EULAR), London, UK, 811 June 2016; Poster THU0166.
20. Charles-Schoeman C, Wicker P, Gonzalez-Gay MA, et al. Cardiovascular safety findings in patients with rheumatoid arthritis treated with tofacitinib, an oral Janus kinase inhibitor. Semin Arthritis Rheum. 2016;46:261–71.
21. Westhovens R, Taylor PC, et al. Filgotinib (GLPG0634/GS-6034), an oral JAK1 selective inhibitor, is effective in combination with methotrexate (MTX) in patients with active rheumatoid arthritis and insufficient response to MTX: results from a randomised, dose-finding study (DARWIN 1). Ann Rheum Dis. 2017;76:998–1008.
22. Kavanaugh A, Kremer J, Ponce L, et al. Filgotinib (GLPG0634/GS-6034), an oral selective JAK1 inhibitor, is effective as monotherapy in patients with active rheumatoid arthritis: results from a randomised, dose-finding study (DARWIN 2). Ann Rheum Dis. 2017;76:1009–19.
23. Takeuchi T, Tanaka Y, Iwasaki M, et al. Efficacy and safety of the oral Janus kinase inhibitor peficitinib (ASP015K) monotherapy in patients with moderate to severe rheumatoid arthritis in Japan: a 12-week, randomised, double-blind, placebo-controlled phase IIb study. Ann Rheum Dis. 2016;75:1057–64.
24. Genovese MC, van Vollenhoven RF, Pacheco-Tena C, Zhang Y, Kinnman N. VX-509 (Decernotinib), an Oral selective Janus kinase 3 inhibitor, in combination with methotrexate in patients with rheumatoid arthritis. Arthritis Rheumatol. 2016;68(1):46–55.

Biologics in Rheumatic Diseases in the Presence of Infection

19

Padmanabha Shenoy and Kaveri K. Nalianda

19.1 Introduction

The treatment of autoimmune rheumatic diseases has been revolutionized by the introduction of biologic therapy. These target key components of the immune system and suppress the pathological cascade of inflammation. Cytokines like TNF-α and IL-6 play a vital role in integrated host defenses. Hence treatment with biologicals leads to a degree of immunosuppression, thereby increasing patient's susceptibility to infection.

TNFI (TNF α inhibitors) have been in use clinically for the longest period of time. Hence studies evaluating the association between TNF inhibitors and infection are the most numerous. Data regarding other biologicals is comparatively less.

Infectious complications related to treatment with biological agents include bacterial infections like *Streptococcus pneumoniae*, *Mycobacterium tuberculosis*, diph theria monocytogenes, and the potential reactivation of viral infections like herpes, Varicella zoster, and hepatitis B and C [1].

Rheumatology guidelines from various international societies universally advocate the need to screen patients with rheumatic diseases for TB and other infections prior to commencing treatment with biological DMARDs [2].

P. Shenoy (✉) · K. K. Nalianda
Centre for Arthritis and Rheumatism Excellence (CARE), Kochi, India

N. Jain, L. Duggal (eds.), *Handbook of Biologics for Rheumatological Disorders*,
https://doi.org/10.1007/978-981-16-7200-2_19

19.2 Latent TB Infection

- The burden of tuberculosis varies greatly around the world. The regions of South-East Asia (35%), Western Pacific Region (21%), and Africa (30%) account for the highest risk of infection. The WHO in 2015 estimated 9.6% million cases of TB globally. 2.2 million cases were from India [2].
- Only 5–10% of people infected by mycobacterium tuberculosis develop active disease. Replication of Mycobacterium tuberculosis (Mtb) is inhibited by the host immune response [3].
- TNF plays a significant role in this immune response and, along with Interferon-gamma stimulates macrophagic phagocytosis of bacteria and enhances mycobacterium killing. It recruits inflammatory cytokines, stimulates the production of chemokines, and contains the mycobacteria within the granulomas. This achieves a latent state of the disease [1].
- Most patients infected with Mtb carry latent tuberculosis infection (LTBI) and are asymptomatic and non-infectious [3]. The prevalence of LTBI in India in various populations is in the range of 9% to 80%. The lifetime risk of a latent infection developing into active TB is 5–10% [2].
- LTBI is defined as a positive tuberculin skin test or a positive Interferon-Gamma Release Assay in the absence of evidence of active tuberculosis (clinical symptoms and signs for TB of cough, fever, and microbiological isolation of mycobacteria, and normal chest radiograph).
- During treatment with biologicals such as anti-TNF, the risk of developing active tuberculosis in patients with LTBI is high. Hence screening and investigations to detect LTBI are recommended [3].
- Among the anti-TNF antibodies, the risk of TB has been found to be higher with infliximab and adalimumab [1]. The incidence of TB with certolizumab pegol and golimumab is less conclusive, but they have been cases of active TB reported in patients with rheumatic diseases treated with certolizumab and golimumab.

19.2.1 Non-anti-TNF Biologics

- Due to its targeted action on B-lymphocytes the data of rituximab risk of TB reactivation is very reassuring [4]. Only two cases of pulmonary tuberculosis were reported among 3595 rheumatoid arthritis patients who had received rituximab over follow-up of 11 years [5].
- A low TB risk has been recorded in patients treated with abatacept, tocilizumab, secukinumab, ustekinumab, and anakinra [4].

19.2.2 Screening for Latent TB

The two tests used to screen and diagnose LTBI are the in vivo tuberculin skin test (TST) and the ex vivo Interferon-Gamma Release Assays (IGRA) [2]. Both the tests detect an adaptive immune response of T-lymphocytes to mycobacterial antigens but are unable to identify if the disease is latent or active [1].

(a) *TST Or Purified Protein Derivative (PPD) Test:*
   - The TST, also known as the Mantoux test, is based on T-cell mediated delayed hypersensitivity reaction to *M. tuberculosis*. It involves intradermal injection into the inner surface of the forearm of either PPD or tuberculin and assessment at 48–72 h for skin induration measured with a ruler [2].
   - The WHO study has concluded that either 5 TU or 10 TU doses can be suitable for use in Mantoux testing [6]. In India, 1 TU PPD-RT23 (equivalent to 5 TU PPDs) in 0.1 mL is the standard commercial preparation routinely used [2].

(b) *Interferon-Gamma Release Assays (IGRA)*:
   - IGRA is measured by ELISA. The Interferon-gamma is released by T-lymphocytes of a patient with tuberculosis when re-exposed to TB-specific antigens.
   - The three assays are QuantiFERON-TB Gold assay (QFT-G), QuantiFERON-TB Gold in-tube assay (QFT-GIT) and T-SPOT TB assay. The antigenic targets in these assays are ESAT-6, CFP10, and TB7.7. The T-SPOT TB test is an ELISPOT assay that estimates the number of interferon gamma-producing cells.
   - ACR guidelines advise that if either the TST or IGRA is positive, then a chest x-ray should be done. If the chest X-ray is negative, the patient should receive treatment for latent tuberculosis infection. If the chest X-ray is positive, then a sputum test for AFB should be done. If the sputum test is positive for AFB, then treatment for active TB to be commenced. If the sputum is negative for AFB, then the patient should be treated for latent tuberculosis.
   - IGRA testing is more sensitive than TST but can give indeterminate results and, taking into consideration the risk of TB activation with biologics use and the high cost of therapy, using both the tests to optimize the sensitivity for detecting LTBI would be logical.
   - WHO guidelines mandate that the patients testing positive on either TST or IGRA should have a chest radiograph done to look for active disease. If the chest radiograph is abnormal, then depending on the clinical picture, treatment for either active TB or latent TB infection is commenced. If there is a high risk of TB exposure, then a negative screening test and a normal chest radiograph notwithstanding, CECT scan of the chest may be done to be certain before starting biologicals [2].
   - Malaviya et al. have recommended a screening strategy for LTBI in India whereby patients are first screened clinically with the 4S (four symptoms) complex of fever, cough, night sweats and weight loss. If positive, then confirm active TB infection, treat with standard ATT and start biologics after TB is fully treated. If clinical screening is negative, then assess for LTBI with a 10TU Mantoux and QuantiFERON-TB Gold (QTBG) and a chest radio-

graph. If Mantoux is less than 10 mm and QTBG is negative, and chest radiograph is normal, then LTBI is ruled out, and biologics can be commenced. If either Mantoux is >/= 10 mm or QTBG is positive, or chest radiograph is positive, then chemoprophylaxis for LTBI should be given before commencing biologics [7].

- Biologics can be commenced after the completion of one month of treatment for latent tuberculosis and should be resumed after the completion of treatment of active tuberculosis [8].

19.2.3 Treatment

19.2.3.1 One of the Following Treatment Regimens can be Chosen for LTBI

(a) Isoniazid—in adults 5 mg/kg (maximum dose 300 mg) for six or nine months (advised by both CDC and WHO). In children (2–11 years), nine months of therapy is preferred.
(b) Rifampicin—10 mg/kg in adults (maximum dose 600 mg) for four months. 5 mg/kg for children.
(c) INH plus Rifampicin—300 mg INH and 600 mg Rifampicin daily for 3–4 months.

Recently, the guidelines for the treatment of Latent Tuberculosis infection have been updated by the National Tuberculosis Controllers Association and CDC in 2020 for people with LTBI who live in the USA.

The preferred regimens are:

(i) Isoniazid (15 mg/kg rounded up to the nearest 50 or 100 mg: 900 mg maximum) plus Rifapentine (25.1–32 Kg: 600 mg, 32.1–49.9 Kg: 750 mg, >/= 50 Kg: 900 mg Max): given once weekly for three months.
(ii) Rifampin (10 mg/kg adults, Children: 15–20 mg/kg): given daily for 4 months.
(iii) Isoniazid (5 mg/kg; Max 300 mg in adults; 10–20 mg/kg in children) and Rifampin (10 mg/kg in adults; 15–20 mg /kg in children): given daily for 3 months [9].

- In patients with LTBI, biological agents can be commenced or continued after one month of LTBI treatment with anti-TB medication. In patients with rheumatic diseases and diagnosed also to have active tuberculosis, biologics should be given after the completion of treatment for active tuberculosis [4].
- If active TB disease occurs while the patient is on treatment with biologics, especially TNF I, biologics should be stopped immediately, and anti-TB treatment commenced (two months of induction with Isoniazid, Rifampicin, Pyrazinamide Ethambutol) followed by four months' maintenance with Isoniazid and Rifampicin.
- General expert opinion is to postpone restarting biologics especially anti- TNF, until after the full course of TB therapy is completed.

- There are no guidelines or recommendations for the treatment of flare of underlying rheumatic disease in patients who are on ATT for active TB. Therefore, adjusting treatment according to disease activity scores has been suggested.
- In patients with RA, who have high disease activity, low-risk biologics such rituximab, abatacept, tocilizumab, or anakinra can be started after completion of first two months of ATT. In those who fail to respond to the low-risk biologics, etanercept can be initiated as it has the lowest risk of TB reactivation among the anti-TNF agents.
- In severe psoriatic arthritis, ustekinumab can be started after two months of ATT and in those who do not respond to ustekinumab, etanercept. Analysis of pooled data from 21 RCTs of Secukinumab (fully human anti-IL-17A) in PsO (14 phase 3 trials and 1 phase 4 trial), PsA (3 phase 3 trials) and AS (3 phase 3 trials) along with post-marketing surveillance data did not reveal any cases of TB reactivation [10]. The risk of mycobacterial infection or TB reactivation based on clinical, animal and in vitro studies is low with Secukinumab therapy in contrast to anti-TNF [11].
- In ankylosing spondylitis with a high ASDAS score, anti-TNF, preferably etanercept can be restarted after the first two months of TB induction therapy [3].

19.3 HBV and HCV Infection

- Chronic HBV and HCV infections affect nearly 500 million people globally, making them a global health problem. Worldwide, they also are the most common causes of cirrhosis and liver cancer. Most patients with chronic HBV or HCV infections are asymptomatic and therefore are undiagnosed.
- Biologic therapies, if administered to patients infected with HBV or HCV, can lead to reactivation, resulting in asymptomatic hepatic flares to hepatocellular failure and death [12]. Up to 20–50% of HBV carriers have HBV reactivation while undergoing immunosuppressive treatment. While reactivation of HCV is rarer, if severe hepatitis occurs, then mortality rates are similar to those with HBV.
- Rituximab, TNF α inhibitors, Abatacept with or without combination therapy (including corticosteroids) are some of the biologics associated with the risk of HBV and HCV reactivation [13].
- Therefore, it is imperative that the patients with rheumatic diseases, before the initiation of biologic therapy, should be screened for HBC and HCV infections.

19.4 Hepatitis B

19.4.1 Natural Course

A complex interplay between host, virus, and environmental factors determines the progression from acute to chronic HBV infection. This, in adults, is less than 5% [13].

All patients with chronic HBV infection do not have chronic hepatitis B. The natural history of chronic HBV infections is divided into five phases, not necessarily sequential. These 5 phases are determined by taking into account the presence of HBe-antigen, levels of HBV DNA, alanine aminotransferase (ALT) levels, and the absence or presence of liver inflammation.

Phase 1—HBe-antigen-positive, chronic HBV infection. The old nomenclature was the immune tolerant phase [14]. There is active virus replication in the liver, and hence it is characterized by the presence of elevated serum levels of HBV DNA (>20,000 IU/mL), presence of serum HBe-antigen and normal levels ALT. There is minimal host immune response hence minimal or no liver necroinflammation or fibrosis.

Phase 2—HBe-antigen-positive, chronic hepatitis B. The old nomenclature was the immune active phase. In this phase, clearance of the virus is attempted by a vigorous host response against hepatocytes infected with HBV. This causes transaminitis and immune-mediated hepatocyte injury. The characteristics of this phase are serum HBe-antigen positivity, high levels of serum HBV DNA (>20,000 IU/mL) and significant liver necroinflammation and rapid progression of fibrosis. This phase has variable outcomes; 90% of patients achieve seroconversion by losing hepatitis B e antigen and developing anti-HBe antibodies. Seventy to ninety percent of patients who seroconvert enter the inactive carrier state (HBe negative, chronic HBV infection). The others progress to become HBe negative chronic hepatitis B.

Phase 3—HBe negative chronic HBV infection. Known previously as the inactive carrier state is characterized by anti-HBe antibodies with low or undetectable levels of HBV DNA (<2000 IU/mL) and anti-HBc antibodies, normal ALT levels. Of those who remain in this phase over a long time, HBs antigen loss and/or seroconversion can occur spontaneously in 1–3% of cases annually.

Phase 4—HBe negative chronic Hepatitis B. This phase is characterized by the absence of HBe antigen, detectable anti-HBe antibodies, moderate to high levels of serum HBV DNA, elevated ALT levels and necroinflammation and fibrosis in the liver.

Phase 5—HBsAg negative phase—previously called the recovery phase. This is characterized by negative serum HBs antigen, positive anti-HBc with or without positive anti-HBs antibodies. This is also known as occult HBV infection. ALT levels are normal. Serum levels of HBV DNA may be undetectable. HBV DNA can be detected in the liver [12, 14].

In patients who have a resolution of acute or chronic HBV infection either spontaneously or after treatment (negative HBs antigen, positive anti-HBc antibodies, and positive anti-HBs antibodies), the immune system inhibits the general expression and the replication of HBV. Hence immunosuppression may lead to reactivation in these patients.

19.4.2 HBV Reactivation

- In a person, known to have inactive HBsAg carrier state or resolved hepatitis B infection, the reappearance of active hepatic inflammation and necrosis leading to elevated transaminases, an increase in serum HBV DNA levels from baseline by greater than 1-log10, or a change in HBV DNA detection from negative to positive, is defined as HBV reactivation. HBV reactivation has been reported in 20–50% of HBV carriers who receive immunosuppressive treatment [12, 13].

- Data has also shown that in patients with autoimmune rheumatic disease and resolved HBV infection, after commencing anti-TNF therapy, the rate of HBV reactivation is around 5%. In order to reduce the risk of HBV reactivation and its associated morbidity and mortality, identifying the patients at risk by screening and initiating prophylactic antiviral treatment is advisable.

19.4.3 Screening Recommendations

- Guidelines universally recommend that all patients undergoing treatment with biologicals and immunosuppressive medications should be screened for HBV serological markers (HBsAg, anti-HBc, anti-HBs) followed by a sensitive HBV DNA test and liver function tests if either HBsAg or anti-HBc is positive. HBe and anti-HBe should be checked for as well, in conjunction with hepatology (If both HBsAg and anti-HBc are positive) [5].
- At present, it is not known if different TNFI affect HBV reactivation to different extents. For instance, as Etanercept has a lower affinity for TNF-α, this risk may be lower. Infliximab appears to be associated with a much higher risk, perhaps due to a cytokine washout resulting from the 8 week intervals in the administration that could result in an 'immune -reconstitution' effect [15].
- In HBsAg positive patients and those who are HBsAg negative and anti-HBc positive receiving biologicals, the risk of reactivation of HBV is high. The risk of reactivation of HBV can be categorized as high risk (greater than 10% that is where the incidence of HBV reactivation is anticipated to be greater than 10%), moderate risk (1–10%) and low risk (less than 1%).
- Data from RCTs evaluating antiviral prophylaxis in HBs antigen-positive or anti-HBc positive patients versus on-demand rescue treatment in the presence of HBV reactivation showed that prophylaxis was associated with an 84% relative risk reduction of HBV associated flares of hepatitis and 87% relative risk reduction in reactivation of the hepatitis B infection [16].

19.4.4 In HBsAg Positive Patients

- All candidates who are to receive immunosuppressive therapy should be referred to a specialist for further assessment and diagnosis of the phase of HBV infection, and all should receive a nucleotide analog either as prophylaxis or as treatment [14].
- The patients with chronic hepatitis B who are untreated and developed concomitant rheumatological disorders needing biologicals have to be referred for appropriate antiviral therapy prior to immunosuppressive treatment [8].
- These patients should be treated with entecavir or tenofovir, similar to patients who are immunocompetent, with the monitoring and stopping rules of nucleoside analogs being the same.

- The treatment of patients with chronic HBV infection but without chronic hepatitis is not without controversy. They have to receive antiviral prophylaxis with entecavir or tenofovir. Lamivudine has also been used successfully as prophylaxis, but there is a risk of HBV reactivation.
- For rituximab-based regimens, the prophylaxis should continue for 18 months after stopping immunosuppressive treatment and 12 months in the case of other regimens. Viral prophylaxis should be discontinued only if the underlying disease is in remission. It is recommended that liver function tests and HBV DNA be checked every 3–6 months during the period of prophylaxis. This should be continued for at least 12 months after the withdrawal of antivirals.

19.4.5 In HBsAg Negative, anti-HBC Positive Subjects (Occult HBV Infection)

- It is recommended that serum HBV DNA be tested. If HBV DNA is detected in the serum, then management is similar to patients who are HBsAg positive before starting immunosuppression.
- In the high-risk group, (greater than 10% incidence of HBV reactivation), antiviral prophylaxis is recommended. The duration of the prophylaxis should be 18 months after stopping immunosuppression, and monitoring of LFTs and viral DNA should continue for at least 12 months after withdrawal of prophylaxis. The prophylactic agents that can be used are lamivudine, entecavir, or tenofovir. The latter two are preferred if the duration of the immunosuppressive regimen is likely to be a long one.
- If the risk of reactivation is moderate (less than 10%) or low (less 1%), the recommendation is preemptive therapy, not prophylaxis. Preemptive therapy is based upon monitoring HBsAg and/or HBV DNA every 1–3 months during and after immunosuppression. In case of detection of HBV DNA or HBsAg seroconversion, entecavir or tenofovir treatment is commenced. If there is likely to be a long duration of immunosuppression, patients are unlikely to be compliant with monitoring, or if the risk of viral reactivation for new biologicals is unknown, then universal prophylaxis is recommended over preemptive therapy [14].
- Thus immunosuppressive therapy can be safely used when concomitant prophylactic antiviral therapy is also prescribed under specialist guidance [8].
- It is recommended that HBV sero-negative patients receive vaccination [14].

19.5 Hepatitis C

19.5.1 Natural Course

- Sixty–eighty five percent of patients after acute hepatitis C infection remains chronically and persistently infected. Of those with chronic HCV infection, 20% are estimated to develop end-stage liver disease with liver-related complications leading to mortality. This progression takes place over several decades. Thus 75–85% of patients chronically infected will not die of HCV infection [12].

- Hepatitis C reactivation following immunosuppressive therapy, in contrast to HBV reactivation, is rare, though when reactivation occurs, the mortality and morbidity rates are the same. The pathogenesis of HCV reactivation following immunosuppressive therapy is believed to be due to an increase in HCV replication, a rise in viral load to at least 1-log10 IU/mL above baseline, leading to direct hepatotoxicity and cell death.
- HCV reactivation can vary from being asymptomatic to an increase in aminotransferases up to three times normal. They have been cases reported of severe hepatic failure [13].
- Pompili et al. undertook a comprehensive literature review between January 2000 and August 2013 in which 216 patients with HCV were observed for a cumulative total of 260 patients per year of anti-TNF treatment. Of the 216 patients, there were only 3 cases of withdrawal of the drugs due to suspected worsening of HCV liver disease. One hundred fifty-three patients received etanercept. Three cases had elevated transaminases. In 5 cases, there was an increase in HCV RNA, and two cases were withdrawn due to drug toxicity. Forty patients received infliximab of whom there were 2 cases with elevated transaminases and 4 cases with elevated HCV RNA. The 23 patients receiving adalimumab had no complications [17].
- Though studies continue to demonstrate that anti-TNF therapy has no detrimental effect on HCV infection, it remains advisable to aim for viral control before commencing immunosuppression. Data from a small study comparing safety profiles of TNF alpha inhibitors and rituximab therapy in patients with rheumatoid arthritis and chronic hepatitisC has shown that the viral load of hepatitisC is increased after treatment with rituximab as compared with anti-TNF therapy.
- Data to recommend the use of tocilizumab, abatacept, secukinumab, and ustekinumab in patients with chronic hepatitis C infection is insufficient, though small studies have not shown an increase in viral load or increased risk of hepatitis C reactivation with these agents in those who had received antiviral prophylaxis.

19.5.2 Screening Recommendations

- Guidelines recommend screening of all patients for HCV infection prior to commencing immunosuppression. Screening should include testing for anti-HCV antibodies in the serum or plasma. If anti-HCV antibodies are detected, HCV RNA should be determined by a sensitive molecular assay. If HCV RNA assays are not available, then HCV core antigen should be detected in the serum or plasma [5].
- All patients with evidence of HCV infection should be referred to a hepatologist for consideration of treatment with the highly effective direct-acting antiviral agents (DAA). This includes those with HCV-related mixed cryoglobulinemic vasculitis and HCV immune complex-mediated nephropathy. Rituximab has

been used along with interferon-free DAA (direct-acting antiviral agents) based anti-HCV combination in the treatment of these manifestations [18].

- Though studies have not demonstrated a detrimental effect of biologic therapies (especially anti-TNF) on HCV infections, working closely with a hepatologist with close monitoring of serum aminotransferases and HCV RNA during therapy is recommended in all patients with HCV infections and coexisting rheumatic disorder being treated with a biologic [5].
- Anti-TNF drugs should be used very cautiously in the presence of compensated cirrhosis and the benefit-risk ratio evaluated at the individual level. They are contraindicated in patients with decompensated liver disease.

19.6 HIV Infection

- Patients with HIV infections are at a higher risk of developing rheumatic diseases at any stage of the illness [19]. Greater than 5% of HIV-infected patients experience arthralgias or arthritis, and the prevalence for HIV arthritis can be up to 12%.
- In treating a rheumatic disorder in an HIV-infected patient, the treating clinician faces multiple challenges. These could range from choosing the appropriate medication that strikes the right balance between efficacy and safety to reducing the effects of chronic inflammation [20].
- In HIV-infected patients, biological DMARDs have been used fairly successfully and with a reasonably good safety profile [19]. Most information about the use of biologic agents in HIV-infected patients is limited to case series and case reports and mostly pertains to the use of TNFI.
- In 2007, a case report by Kaur et al. reported the successful use of etanercept in the treatment of RA in a patient with HIV infection. There was a significant decrease in the swollen and tender joint counts after 3 months of treatment, and there were no other adverse events noted. During therapy with etanercept, HIV RNA remained stable at 115 copies/mL, and CD4 T-cell count at the lowest was 236 cells/mm.
- Cepeda et al. described two HIV-infected patients with rheumatoid arthritis treated with etanercept for a year. Both patients had very low HIV RNA levels and CD4 counts greater than 600 cells/mm^3 and had a good clinical response to treatment with no complications from therapy with etanercept.
- The safety and efficacy of TNF inhibitors in HIV-infected patients with other rheumatic disorders such as psoriatic arthritis (etanercept, adalimumab, infliximab), HIV-related arthritis (etanercept, adalimumab), reactive arthritis (infliximab) have been demonstrated in many case reports [20].
- In a case series of 8 American HIV-positive patients, treatment with anti-TNF was administered for different rheumatic disorders. (2 with RA, 1 with AS, 1 with reactive arthritis, 1 with undifferentiated SPA, and 3 with psoriatic arthritis). All patients had a viral load less than 60,000 copies/mm^3 and CD4 count of more than 200 cells/mm^3 at the onset of therapy. There was a good response to treat-

ment over a mean follow-up of 28.1 months. There were no adverse effects to treatment with CD4 counts and HIV viral load remaining stable [21].

- The clinical outcomes have been good in most patients who have been receiving concomitant HAART [5].
- However, there is a case report by Aboulafia et al. of a patient with HIV infection on HAART and psoriatic arthritis treated with etanercept in whom, despite good clinical response, treatment had to be discontinued due to recurrent polymicrobial infections. His CD4 count of 20 and an HIV load of 14,000 copies/ml despite HAART may be an explanation of the negative outcome [20].
- Ustekinumab has been used successfully in a case report of a patient with HIV infection on HAART with refractive psoriasis and psoriatic arthritis with significant improvement in skin and joints after two years of treatment. The patient did not suffer any opportunistic infection and had an undetectable viral load and stable CD4 count [19].
- Gaylis (2012) reported successfully treating an HIV patient on HAART with reactive arthritis with infliximab. The duration of therapy was 10 years and with an improvement in patient symptoms, an undetectable viral load and CD4 count within normal range.
- Adalimumab has been used by Almoallen et al. in 2013 in successfully treating three cases with HIV infection on HAART with co-existent inflammatory arthritis. All patients had clinical improvement with stable CD4 counts and HIV viral load [22].
- A systematic review in 2016 on efficacy and safety of biological therapy for inflammatory conditions in individuals with HIV identified 37 treatment episodes encompassing ten different inflammatory conditions with 6 different biological agents and was limited to case reports and case series only. The rheumatological disorders were psoriatic arthritis (8 patients), RA (4 patients), reactive arthritis (2 patients), AS (1 patient), undifferentiated SpA (1 patient), and AAV (1 patient). All patients, except the one with AAV who received rituximab, were treated with anti-TNF. Treatment responses were broadly comparable to HIV uninfected patients receiving biological therapy. No significant negative effects on ART therapy were identified. In the minority of patients not receiving HAART at the time of biologic therapy, HIV control was not affected adversely. However, details concerning immunological and virological parameters of follow-up and ART regimens were limited [23].
- Risk factors for HIV infection should be documented, and if present, an HIV test should be done before commencing biologicals. If biologic therapy is being considered in HIV-positive patients, an HIV specialist should be involved. If HIV infection is controlled (CD4 count more than 200 cells/mm^3 and viral load undetectable) and anti-TNF is administered in combination with HAART, there is believed to be a reasonable benefit to risk ratio for HIV patients. Evidence to recommend the use of rituximab, tocilizumab, abatacept, or ustekinumab in patients with HIV infection is insufficient.

While anti-TNF therapy is ongoing in patients infected with HIV, close monitoring of viral load and CD 4 count is essential [5].

19.7 Other Infections

Legionella pneumophila—Tubach et al. have reported a series of pneumonia caused by *Legionella pneumophila* in 11 patients treated with anti-TNF. ARDS developed in 5 out of the 11 cases, but there was complete recovery in all patients with appropriate antibiotic therapy.

Listeria monocytogenes—Listeriosis has been reported in patients with infliximab, etanercept, and adalimumab. It can present as meningitis, arthritis, or sepsis. There is evidence that TNF signaling plays a significant role in complex host resistance to infection with *Listeria monocytogenes*. There are no reports linking golimumab, certolizumab, or abatacept with Listeria infection. As Listeria infections in immunocompromised patients run a severe course, it is recommended to advise patients receiving immunosuppressive therapy, including anti-TNF agents, to adequately heat or avoid foods that could be potential sources of Listeria monocytogenes infection.

Visceral Leishmaniasis—This should be suspected in patients from endemic areas presenting with fever, splenomegaly, and pancytopenia. It is a rare complication of biological treatments.

Salmonella Infection—Several case reports have indicated that patients treated with TNF inhibitors are susceptible to infection with different species of Salmonella, and the infection can run a severe course [1].

SARS-CoV-2 Infection—Due to the constantly evolving nature of the pandemic, EULAR has come up with a few provisional recommendations as a 'living document' and a starting point. It is recommended that patients with RMD (rheumatic and musculoskeletal disease) who do not have suspected or confirmed COVID 19 infection should be advised to continue their treatment unchanged, including bDMARDs, among others. In cases of mild symptoms of Covid, treatment alteration should be considered on a case-to-case basis and a careful watch kept for potential aggravation of the initial mild disease. RMD patients with moderate to severe Covid 19 infection should be referred to an expert in treating Covid 19, and local Covid treatment guidelines to be followed [24].

19.8 Conclusion

- Biologic DMARDs, both TNFI and non TNFI, according to existing literature, are associated with an increased risk of infection compared to patients on csDMARDs.
- Screening for TB and other serious infections is universally advocated before initiating biologic therapy.
- In the presence of any serious active infection (requiring IV antibiotics or hospitalization), biological therapy should not be initiated.
- In patients, who developed a serious infection while on biologics, the biological agent should be discontinued. It can be recommenced after the resolution of infection [5].

References

1. De Keyser F. Choice of biologic therapy for patients with rheumatoid arthritis: the infection perspective. Curr Rheumatol Rev. 2011;7:77–87.
2. Handa R, Upadhyaya S, Kapoor S, et al. Tuberculosis and biologics in rheumatology: a special situation. Int J Rheum Dis. 2017;20:1313–25.
3. Cantini F, Prignano F, Goletti D. Restarting biologics and Management of Patients with flares of inflammatory rheumatic disorders or psoriasis during active tuberculosis treatment. J Rheumatol. 2014;91:78–82.
4. Cantini F, Nannini C, Niccoli L, et al. Guidance for the management of patients with latent tuberculosis infection requiring biologic therapy in rheumatology and dermatology clinical practice. Autoimmune Rev. 2015;14(7):503–9.
5. Holroyd CR, Seth R, Bukhari M, et al. The British Society of Rheumatology biologic DMARD safety guidelines in inflammatory arthritis. Rheumatology. 2019;58:e3–e42.
6. WHO Tuberculosis Research Office. The 5TU versus the 10TU intradermal tuberculin test. Bull World Health Organ. 1955;12(1–2):169–77.
7. Malaviya AN, Thakaran R, Rawat R, et al. Real life experience of a screening strategy for latent tuberculosis before treatment with biologicals in Indian patients with rheumatic diseases. Indian J Rheumatol. 2018;13(4):233–9.
8. Singh JA, Saag KG, Bridges SLJR, et al. American College of Rheumatology Guideline for the treatment of rheumatoid arthritis. Arthritis Rheumatol. 2016 Jan;68(1):1–26.
9. Sterling RS, Njie G, Zenner D, et al. Guidelines for the treatment of latent tuberculosis infection: recommendations from the National Tuberculosis Controllers Association and CDC. MMWR. 2020 Feb;69(1):1–11.
10. Deodhar A, Mease PJ, McInnes IB, et al. Long-term safety of secukinumab in patients with moderate-to-severe plaque psoriasis, psoriatic arthritis, and ankylosing spondylitis: integrated pooled clinical trial and post-marketing surveillance data. Arthritis Res Ther. 2019;21:111.
11. Kammüller M, Tsai T, Griffiths CEM, et al. Inhibition of IL-17A by secukinumab shows no evidence of increased *Mycobacterium tuberculosis* infections. Clin Transl Immunol. 2017 Aug;6(8):e152.
12. Vassilopoulos D, Calabrese LH. Management of rheumatic disease with comorbid HBV or HCV infection. Nat Rev Rheumatol. 2012;8:348–57.
13. Bojito-Marrero L, Pyrsopoulos N. Hepatitis B and hepatitis C reactivation in the biologic era. J Clin Transl Hepatol. 2014;2:240–6.
14. Lampertico P, Agarwal K, Berg T, et al. EASL 2017 clinical practice guidelines on the management of hepatitis B virus infection. J Hepatol. 2017;67:370–98.
15. De Nard F, Todoerti M, Grosso V, et al. Risk of hepatitis B reactivation in rheumatoid arthritis patients undergoing biological treatment: extending perspectives from old to new. World J Hepatol. 2015 Mar 27;7(3):344–61.
16. Reddy RK, Beavers KL, Hammond PS, Lim KJ, Falck-Ytter YT. American gastroenterology association institute guideline on the prevention and treatment of hepatitis B virus reactivation during immunosuppressive drug therapy. Gastroenterology. 2015;148:215–9.
17. Abdulaziz S, Halabi H, Omair MA, et al. Biological therapy in arthritis patients with hepatitis B or C infection: a multicenter retrospective case series. Eur J Rheumatol. 2017;4:194–9.
18. Pawlotsky JM, Negro F, Aghimo A, et al. EASL recommendations on the treatment of hepatitis C 2018. J Hepatol. 2018;69(2):461–511.
19. Adizie T, Moots RJ, Hodkinson B, French N, Adebajo AO. Inflammatort arthritis in HIV positive patients: a practical guide. BMC Infect Dis. 2016;16:100. pp 1–7
20. Carroll MB, Fields JH, Clerc PG. Rheumatoid arthritis in patients with HIV: management challenges. Open Access Rheumatol Res Rev. 2016;8:51–9.
21. Cepeda EJ, Williams FM, Ishimori ML, Weisman MH. Use of anti -tumour necrosis factor therapy in HIV -positive individuals with rheumatic disease. Ann Rheum Dis. June 2008;67(5):210–2.

22. Weider S, Routt E, Levitt J, Lebwohl M. Treatment of refractory psoriasis with Ustekinumab in HIV -positive patient: a case presentation and review of biologic literature. Psoriasis Forum. 2014;20(3):96–102.
23. Fink DL, Hedley L, Miller RF. Systematic review of the efficacy and safety of biological therapy for inflammatory conditions in HIV – infected individuals. Int J STD AIDS. 2017 Feb;28(2):110–9.
24. Landewé RBM, Machado PM, Kroon F, et al. EULAR provisional recommendations for the management of rheumatic and musculoskeletal diseases in the context of SARS-CoV-2. Ann Rheum Dis. 2020;79:851–8.

Biologics in Rheumatologic Conditions with Malignancy

20

Lata Bichile, Dipti Patel, and Tanmayee Bichile

20.1 Introduction

A familiar association exists between various rheumatologic conditions and increased risk of different malignancies. Malignancy can be a presenting feature of, develop during, or years after the diagnosis of rheumatologic disease (Table 20.1).

Clinical presentations of malignancy in relation to rheumatologic diseases include:

1. Paraneoplastic syndromes—malignancy presenting as a rheumatologic disease
   - Dermatomyositis/polymyositis.
   - Hypertrophic osteoarthropathy.
   - Palmar fibromatosis with polyarthritis.
   - Remitting seronegative symmetrical synovitis with pitting edema (RS3PE).
   - Carcinomatous polyarthritis.
   - Paraneoplastic vasculitides.
   - Lambert–Eaton syndrome.
   - Multicentric reticulohistiocytosis.
   - Amyloidosis and others.

L. Bichile (✉)
Formerly Head Department of Medicine, Rheumatology Services Seth G.S Medical College, KEM Hospital, Mumbai, India

Centre for Arthritis and Rheumatic Diseases, Mumbai, India

D. Patel
Wockhardt Hospital, Mumbai, India

T. Bichile
Drexel University School of Medicine, Rheumatologist, Allegheny Health Network, Autoimmunity Institute, West Penn Hospital, Pittsburgh, PA, USA

N. Jain, L. Duggal (eds.), *Handbook of Biologics for Rheumatological Disorders*,
https://doi.org/10.1007/978-981-16-7200-2_20

Table 20.1 Common malignancies in Rheumatic diseases

Disease	Common associated malignancies	Option of biologics
Rheumatoid arthritis	Lymphoma, breast cancer, lung cancer, Colon cancer	High-grade cancer- avoid anti-TNF for at least 5 years Rituximab can be given Tocilizumab, Tofacitinib, Baricitinib, Abatacept—Sparse data available regarding cancer recurrence so to be used with clinical discretion on case-to-case basis
Ankylosying spondylitis	Bone and prostate cancer (more in males) Colon cancer (females predominantly)	Anti TNF does not increase risk of cancer development in AS. Use anti TNF taking into consideration the nature and grade of cancer.
Primary Sjogrens	Non-Hodgkin's lymphoma MALT Lung, salivary, ovarian, and pancreatic adenocarcinomas Basal cell and squamous cell carcinomas	Rituximab is a treatment option but vigilance to be observed for indolent lymphomas
Scleroderma	Breast cancer Lung cancer	Rituximab can be offered if clinical need
Myositis—Dermatomyositis/polymyositis	Ovarian, lung, pancreas, stomach and colon cancers	The treatment of active cancer usually improves the symptoms of myositis. Corticosteroids and IVIG can be administered
Psoriasis	Hodgkin's lymphoma and cutaneous T cell lymphoma	Anti TNF therapy to be used in caution with patients who received PUVA therapy
SLE	Large B cell lymphoma	Rituximab can be used if clinical need
Vasculitis	Leucocytoclastic vasculitis could be a paraneoplastic presentation	

2. Patients with pre-existing rheumatologic disease can develop malignancy early or late after diagnosis as seen in
   - Dermatomyositis/polymyositis.
   - Rheumatoid arthritis (RA).
   - Systemic lupus erythematosus (SLE).
   - Sjogren's syndrome (SS).
   - Scleroderma/systemic sclerosis (SSc) and others.
3. Certain treatments for rheumatologic diseases can increase the risk of malignancy. For example, cyclophosphamide use is linked to bladder and hematologic cancers particularly leukemia.
4. With the advent of immunotherapy for the treatment of malignancies, autoimmune and rheumatologic immune-related adverse events (iRAes) are increasingly recognized.

Therefore, physicians should be suspicious of, recognize early, evaluate, and treat rheumatologic diseases that occur in close relationship to malignancies [1].

20.2 Rheumatic Diseases and Cancer: A Possible Link

Chronic inflammation and carcinogenesis share a close link due to chronic immune dysregulation occurring in rheumatologic diseases. Following factors play a pivotal role in the development of malignancy:

- A lead role played is by inflammatory cells and mediators in initiation, promotion, and progression of cancer by the transition of epithelial to mesenchymal cells and metastases.
- Chronic inflammation creates a protumor genic environment via the production of proinflammatory mediators- such as cytokines, chemokines, reactive O2, cyclooxygenase-II (COX 2), 5-lipoxygenase (5-LOX), and Matrix metalloproteinases (MMPs).
- Proinflammatory transcription factors such as NF-kB promote tumor cell proliferation, transformation metastases, survival, invasion angiogenesis, chemoresistance, and radio-resistance.
- The activated inflammasomes play varied and contrasting roles in tumor promotion and therapy depending on the microenvironment in addition to producing cytokines.
- Autophagy is a process where intracellular degradation occurs to maintain cellular homeostasis and to inactivate inflammasomes. Also, it is observed that autophagy is involved in the progression of cancer to metastases. Hence, inflammasomes and autophagy are the key players in inflammation and thereby labeled as a two-edged sword for tumoregenesis [2].

Triggers for carcinogenesis include factors such as infectious agents, smoking, tobacco, stress, diet, obesity, and alcohol which drive 90% of the cancers. They are also linked to the pathogenesis of rheumatologic diseases.

20.3 The Possible Association Between Biologics and Malignancy

The current approach for the treatment of RD is early and persistent suppression of inflammation with targeted therapies to prevent long-term complications.

- Treatment of RD has evolved from conventional disease-modifying antirheumatic drugs (cDMARDS) to biologic DMARDs, targeted synthetic DMARDs, and biosimilars.
- Anti-TNF therapy and some non-TNF biologics that treat RD have raised concerns regarding their association with certain cancers.

- The role of TNF is pleiotropic and not restricted only to immune cells. It can be a tumor-promoting cytokine affecting tumor immunity.
- There is also a possibility that TNF blockers may abolish a TNF-driven mechanism that keeps indolent cancer such as lymphoma in check.

20.3.1 Rheumatoid Arthritis (RA)

RA is a chronic systemic immunoinflammatory disease predominantly affecting joints. Its worldwide prevalence is 1% with a male to female ratio of 1:4.

- RA is progressive and erosive in nature within 2 years of disease onset.
- It is hypothesized that tumorigenesis in RA may occur from sustained exposure to inflammatory mediators leading to increased cell proliferation, mutagenesis, oncogene activation, and angiogenesis.
- This persistent inflammatory state leads to higher disease activity and that in turn acts as a major risk factor for cancer development.
- The risk of some site-specific malignancies is increased in comparison to other cancers. A large meta-analysis reviewing incidence of malignancy in adults with RA found a high standardized incidence ratio (SIR) of:
  - Lymphoma (SIR-2.08).
  - Breast cancer (SIR-0.84).
  - Lung cancer (SIR-1.63).
  - Colorectal cancer (SIR-0.77) [3–5].

20.3.1.1 Lymphoma in RA

- A noticeable twofold increase in lymphoma risk is seen in RA patients as compared to the general population. This risk is pronounced in the first 10 years of RA diagnosis irrespective of treatment received. Following factors are hypothesized to contribute to the development of lymphoma in RA:
  - Genetic predisposition.
  - Persistence of longstanding disease activity.
  - Continued immune stimulation by infections like EBV.
  - Treatment with methotrexate, anti-TNF agents, cyclophosphamide.
- Most studies have revealed mixed data in this regard largely indicating high disease activity contributes to malignancy development rather than the treatment itself.
- In a large data obtained from 12 European Biologic registries analyzing the use of anti-TNF, abatacept, tocilizumab concluded that the risk of developing lymphoma with RA was related to disease activity rather than the treatment received. This data reassures that lymphoma risk can be reduced by reducing the burden of inflammation.

- It was found that treatment with adalimumab, etanercept, infliximab did not influence the development of lymphoma up to 8 years of therapy. This study ruled out the association of lymphoma in patients with RA on anti-TNF therapy over a period of 5 years.
- No significant difference in risk was found between malignancies and treatment with conventional DMARDs, targeted synthetic DMARDs (tofacitinib), and other biologic DMARDs [6].

20.3.1.2 Breast Cancer in RA

- Breast cancer is common in female patients with RA. There is a reported borderline increased risk of developing breast cancer even before RA manifests, for unknown reasons.
- The prognosis of breast cancer in women with RA is worse as compared to the general population.
- In patients with RA and history of breast cancer, no significant difference was noted in the risk of recurrence within 5 years in TNF-treated patients as compared to biologic naïve patients.
- Some clinical data link high levels of TNF with disease-free survival in patients with metastatic breast cancer, indicating adverse effects of anti-TNF treatment in these patients.
- In clinical practice, anti-TNF treatment is not recommended in RA patients with high-grade tumors.
- As stated by clinical guidelines, anti-TNF treatment in a patient with active breast cancer should be given with utmost prudence [7].

20.3.1.3 Lung Cancer in RA

- A high incidence of lung cancers in RA compared to the general population is observed in:
  - Men.
  - ≥ 55 years
  - Smokers.
  - Felty's syndrome.
- The survival for patients with RA and concomitant lung cancer is worse [8].

20.3.1.4 Other Cancers in RA

- A decrease in the concomitant incidence of RA with stomach, liver, and colon cancer is noted as compared to the general population along with a less favorable prognosis.
- The progression of pre-cancerous cervical lesions is accelerated in women with RA, with studies showing no consistent trend in cervical cancer risk [8].
- The majority of studies have detected an increased risk of non-melanoma skin cancer (NMSC) and possibly melanoma with anti-TNF use in RA patients.

- TNF may play a protective role in the growth or recurrence risk of melanoma since high doses of locally administered TNF display a powerful anti-neoplastic effect.
- This raised concern regarding the use of anti-TNF agents and the increased risk of developing melanoma.
- However, no study till date has noted an increased risk of melanoma in biologic naïve patients with RA while few studies have shown mixed results

20.4 Conclusions

- TNF inhibitors exert pleiotropic effects on carcinogenesis and tumor progression. Their impact is incompletely understood for different cancers that affect various sites at different stages of carcinogenesis.
- The consequences of anti-TNF therapy on short-term (6 months) and long-term occurrence of cancer remain a concern.
- The majority of studies have shown no increased incidence or relative risk of cancer increase with time and cumulative duration of active anti-TNF therapy with the 5 FDA-approved TNF inhibitors as shown in Table 20.2.
- Rituximab (RTX) is a B cell depleting antibody against CD 20 that can be effectively used in the treatment of B cell lymphoma in patients with RA without affecting the malignancy risk in such patients. RTX can be the biologic of choice in the treatment of RA patients with prior malignancy.
- Scant cancer risk information is noted for the following drugs. Although reports indicate no association with increased malignancy risk, anti-TNF therapies are more commonly used than these drugs:
  - Tocilizumab (IL6 inhibitor.
  - Tofacitinib (JAK inhibitor).
  - Baricitinib (JAK inhibitor).
  - Abatacept (Fusion immunoglobulin targeting CTLA-4).

20.4.1 Ankylosing Spondylitis (AS)

- An immune disorder characterized by chronic inflammation in large joints particularly sacroiliac (SI) joints.
- Pathologically chemokines, cytokines, prostaglandins can shift the microenvironment of a healthy organ to a dysplastic state causing malignant changes in the affected cells.

Table 20.2 FDA approved TNF inhibitors

Monoclonal antibodies	Adalimumab, Golimumab, Infliximab
Pegylated fab fragment	Certolizumab
Soluble receptor fusion protein	Etanercept

- The potential association of AS and cancer is controversial.
- As noted in a large study, male patients with AS had an increased risk of bone and prostate cancer, whereas females had an increased risk of colon cancer.
- Presence of HLA-B27 is linked to an increased risk of developing hematological malignancies in patients with AS.
- Overall, anti-TNF therapy does not affect the risk of cancer development in AS patients [9].

Clinical Tip

A lady with longstanding RA currently stable on Methotrexate (MTX) and adalimumab develops early stage breast cancer.

Treatment considerations—The treatment of breast cancer takes precedence over RA.The existing treatment of MTX and adalimumab should be ceased.

If RA is symptomatic—corticosteroids, pain relief and DMARDS like sulfasalazine, Hydroxychloroquine can be initiated.

Once the cancer treatment is completed—discuss with the oncologist regarding the nature, extent, recurrence risk, and prognosis of the tumor before considering the treatment agent for RA.

If RA is active and warrants biologic treatment—agents like Rituximab can be offered. If the breast cancer is high grade with high risk of recurrence, anti-TNF agents would be reasonable to avoid for until at least 5 years of the cancer.

Agents like JAK inhibitor, abatacept, Tocilizumab could be offered with counselling regarding sparse data on their use and risk of cancer recurrence.

This approach can be applied to all malignancies encountered during RA treatment.

20.4.2 Primary Sjogren's Syndrome

Primary Sjogren's syndrome (SS) is associated with increased risk for cancer, particularly lymphoma.

- The incidence of lymphoma is 37.5 times higher and incidence of non-Hodgkin's lymphoma is 13.76 times higher than that in the general population.
- There is a 11-fold increased risk of hematological cancers such as non-Hodgkin's lymphoma, MALT (in parotid, palate, stomach, bone marrow, plasma cell myeloma.
- Non-hematological malignancies frequently seen in SS include lung adenocarcinoma, salivary adenocarcinoma, ovarian adenocarcinoma, pancreatic adenocarcinoma.
- Non-melanoma skin cancer such as basal cell and squamous cell carcinoma is associated with increased risk in patients with SS.

- Hydroxychloroquine is commonly prescribed for patients with SS. It is neither associated with the development of nor does it offer any protection against the development of lymphoma.
- Methotrexate is often used for managing extraglandular manifestations of SS. Although the use of MTX is linked with the development of lymphoma, the causal relationship is not well established and could correlate with the severity and complications of the disease itself.
- Rituximab is used in patients with SS with no increased risk of cancer development.
- Rituximab is a treatment option for B cell lymphoma, which is a common association in patients with SS. The indolent lymphomas in these patients may not manifest clinically, hence high vigilance should be observed during the treatment with Rituximab [10–12].

20.4.3 Scleroderma

- Breast and lung cancers are prevalent in scleroderma patients.
- In a recent study by the Johns Hopkins Scleroderma Center, certain auto-antibodies and scleroderma subtypes had an increased risk of developing cancer, as shown in Table 20.3.
- Although there was no increased risk seen in overall cancers in scleroderma patients, an increased risk was observed in certain phenotypes at the onset of the disease.
- Patients presenting with late-onset diffuse cutaneous scleroderma irrespective of anti-RNAP3 antibody status frequently have synchronous malignancy [13, 14].

20.4.4 Myositis

- Although the overall risk of malignancy is high in myositis patients as compared to general population, the risk is especially high in dermatomyositis (DM) in the first 5 years of diagnosis.
- Anti-Jo1 antibody patients are at low risk of developing cancers.
- Anti-TIF1-γ and anti-NXP2 antibodies in DM have been associated with an increased risk of cancer.
- DM-associated cancers are mostly of ovarian, lung, pancreas, stomach, and colon.

Table 20.3 Risk of cancer development in scleroderma patients

Presentation	Auto-antibodies	Increase in risk of type of cancer
Diffuse scleroderma	Anti-RNA polymerase III antibodies (anti-RNAP3)	Breast cancer (within 2 years of diagnosis)
Limited cutaneous	Anti-topoisomerase, anti-centromere, and RNAP 3	Breast cancer
Limited cutaneous	Anti-RNAP3	Lung cancer

- Polymyositis is associated with NHL and cancers of lung and bladder.
- Treatment of underlying cancer usually improves the symptoms of myositis.
- Corticosteroids and IVIG are frequently used to treat myositis in cancer.
- The standard treatment should be continued throughout the course of primary cancer to prevent relapses [15].

20.4.5 Psoriasis

- Psoriasis patients are likely susceptible to lymphoproliferative malignancies and non-melanoma skin cancers (NMSC) due to its inflammatory nature, past immunosuppressive therapies, or ultraviolet (UV) exposure. The risk is directly proportional to the severity of the disease.
- A severe form of psoriasis is strongly linked to Hodgkin's lymphoma and cutaneous T-cell lymphoma.
- Anti-TNF therapy is relatively contraindicated in patients who have had prior treatment with >150 psoralens and ultraviolet A (PUVA) and/or >350 ultraviolet B (UVB) phototherapy. Such patients should be discussed with a dermatologist prior to commencing anti-TNF therapy.
- In clinical trial data of secukinumab (IL 17 inhibitor), the incidence rates of malignancy by week 52 were similar to etanercept, basal cell carcinoma (BCC), and squamous cell carcinoma (SCC) were commonly reported, particularly BCC occurring in patients with previous phototherapy exposure.
- The other malignancies reported for secukinumab were melanoma, bladder cancer, and thyroid cancer [16].

20.4.6 Systemic Lupus Erythematosus (SLE)

- SLE is a chronic multisystem autoimmune disease characterized by the production of auto-antibodies, immune complex deposition, and complement activation that results in organ inflammation and when untreated organ damage.
- SLE patients are at an increased risk of cancer particularly lymphoma compared to the general population.
- There is a four- to sevenfold increased risk of lymphoma in SLE compared to the general population.
- Diffuse large B cell lymphoma is the most common lymphoma seen.
- Pathogenesis of lymphoma in SLE remains unclear and there is sparse data regarding survival and outcomes [17].

20.4.7 Vasculitis

- Vasculitis in cancer is a true paraneoplastic syndrome of an underlying solid or hematological cancer.
- The commonest type is leukocytoclastic vasculitis that antedates, appears after cancer, or simultaneously.

- Vasculitis flares with tumor recurrence or progression supporting the concept it is a paraneoplastic syndrome.
- Effective therapy of cancer resolves vasculitis [18].

20.5 Summary

- According to British Society Guidelines, biologic therapies should not be commenced in patients with clinical signs of, or under investigation for malignancy (basal cell carcinoma excluded).
- Patients should be advised that there is no conclusive evidence for an increased risk of solid tumors or lymphoproliferative disease linked with biologic therapy, but that ongoing vigilance is required.
- There is an increased risk of NMSC with anti-TNF therapy (primarily in Caucasians); patients should be educated regarding sun protection techniques, surveillance, and prompt reporting of new persistent skin lesions.
- Caution should be exercised in the use of biologics in patients with previous malignancy. The timing of commencement of biologic therapy post-malignancy is not fixed and will depend on the type, stage of malignancy, risk of metastasis, and patient views.
- The effect of biologics on pre-malignant conditions remains unclear and the use of biologics in such patients should be of utmost care.
- RTX may be considered as a first-line biologic option in patients with malignancy.

References

1. Violeta Bojinca I. Rheumatic diseases and malignancies. [Online] PubMed central (PMC). Available at: https://www.ncbi.nlm.nih.gov/pmc/articles/PMC3593292/ (2019). Accessed 26 Aug 2019.
2. International Journal of Molecular Sciences. [Online] Mdpi.com. Available at: https://www.mdpi.com/journal/ijms/special_issues/Inflammation_Cancer Accessed 26 Aug 2019.
3. Malaviya AN, e. Prevalence of rheumatoid arthritis in the adult Indian population. - PubMed - NCBI. [Online] Ncbi.nlm.nih.gov. Available at: https://www.ncbi.nlm.nih.gov/pubmed/8310203 (2019). Accessed 26 Aug 2019.
4. Smitten A, Simon T, Hochberg M, Suisse S. A meta-analysis of the incidence of malignancy in adult patients with rheumatoid arthritis; 2019.
5. Mercer L, Regierer A, Mariette X, Dixon W, Baecklund E, Hellgren K, Dreyer L, Hetland M, Cordtz R, Hyrich K, Strangfeld A, Zink A, Canhao H, Hernandez M, Tubach F, Gottenberg J, Morel J, Zavada J, Iannone F, Askling J, Listing J. Spectrum of lymphomas across different drug treatment groups in rheumatoid arthritis: a European registries collaborative project; 2019.
6. Mercer L, Galloway J, Lunt M, Davies R, Low A, Dixon W, Watson K, Symmons D, Hyrich K. Risk of lymphoma in patients exposed to antitumor necrosis factor therapy: results from the British Society for Rheumatology Biologics Register for Rheumatoid Arthritis; 2019. https://doi.org/10.1136/annrheumdis-2016-209389

7. Raaschou P, Frisell T, Askling J. FRI0261 TNF inhibitor therapy and risk of breast cancer recurrence in patients with rheumatoid arthritis – a Nationwide cohort study. Ann Rheum Dis. 2014;73(Suppl 2):478.1–478.
8. Wilton K, Matteson E. Malignancy incidence, management, and prevention in patients with rheumatoid arthritis. Rheumatol Therapy. 2017;4(2):333–47.
9. Chang C, Chang C, Nguyen P, Chang T, Shih Y, Chang W, Horng J, Lee O, Ho J. Ankylosing spondylitis and the risk of cancer; 2019.
10. Liang Y, Yang Z, Qin B, Zhong R. Primary Sjögren's syndrome and malignancy risk: a systematic review and meta-analysis. Ann Rheum Dis. 2013;73(6):1151–6.
11. Brito-Zerón P, Kostov B, Fraile G, Caravia-Durán D, Maure B, Rascón F, Zamora M, Casanovas A, Lopez-Dupla M, Ripoll M, Pinilla B, Fonseca E, Akasbi M, de la Red G, Duarte-Millán M, Fanlo P, Guisado-Vasco P, Pérez-Alvarez R, Chamorro A, Morcillo C, Jiménez-Heredia I, Sánchez-Berná I, López-Guillermo A, Ramos-Casals M. Characterization and risk estimate of cancer in patients with primary Sjögren syndrome; 2019.
12. Lazarus M, Robinson D, Mak V, Møller H, Isenberg D. Incidence of cancer in a cohort of patients with primary Sjögren's syndrome; 2019.
13. Lazzaroni MG, e. Malignancies in Patients with Anti-RNA Polymerase III Antibodies and Systemic Sclerosis: Analysis of the EULAR Scleroderma Trials and Research Coho... - PubMed - NCBI. [Online] Ncbi.nlm.nih.gov. Available at: https://www.ncbi.nlm.nih.gov/pubmed/28089973 (2019). Accessed 26 Aug 2019.
14. Igusa T, Hummers L, Visvanathan K, Richardson C, Wigley F, Casciola-Rosen L, Rosen A, Shah A. Autoantibodies and scleroderma phenotype define subgroups at high-risk and low-risk for cancer. Ann Rheumatic Dis; 2018. pp. annrheumdis-2018-212999.
15. Stuhlmüller B, Schneider U, González-González J, Feist E. Disease specific autoantibodies in idiopathic inflammatory myopathies; 2019.
16. Anon. Biologic therapy and the risk of malignancy in psoriasis. [online] Available at: https://journals.sagepub.com/doi/abs/10.1177/247553031117a00401 (2019). Accessed 30 Aug 2019.
17. Choi M, Flood K, Bernatsky S, Ramsey-Goldman R, Clarke A. A review on SLE and malignancy; 2019.
18. Kermani T, Warrington K, Amin S. Malignancy risk in Vasculitis; 2019.

Biologics in Uveitis

21

Sirichai Pasadhika and James T. Rosenbaum

21.1 Introduction

Uveitis is one of the most common causes of blindness worldwide. The patients may present with eye pain, redness, light sensitivity, floaters, and decreased vision:

- It may arise in patients of any age group, but most commonly affects the working population (20–59 years old).
- Some subtypes, such as uveitis associated with juvenile idiopathic arthritis (JIA), occur in younger population and may cause lifelong visual sequelae. Therefore, treatment burden of uveitis is substantial.
- Uveitis can be categorized by anatomical involvement of the inflammation, into anterior (iritis, iridocyclitis), intermediate (vitritis), and posterior (retinitis, choroiditis) uveitis; or panuveitis (anterior + intermediate + posterior uveitis).
- It may also cause retinal vasculitis, cystoid macular edema (CME), and other secondary complications such as cataract and glaucoma.
- HLA-B27-related uveitis most frequently presents with acute, unilateral, alternating, recurrent, anterior uveitis, while JIA uveitis most commonly causes bilateral chronic anterior uveitis. Behçet's uveitis may cause panuveitis with retinal vasculitis.

S. Pasadhika (✉)
Legacy Devers Eye Institute, Oregon, USA
e-mail: spasadhi@LHS.ORG

J. T. Rosenbaum
Legacy Devers Eye Institute, Oregon, USA

Departments of Ophthalmology, Medicine and Cell Biology, Oregon Health & Science University, Oregon, USA

N. Jain, L. Duggal (eds.), *Handbook of Biologics for Rheumatological Disorders*,
https://doi.org/10.1007/978-981-16-7200-2_21

21.2 Conventional Treatment for Noninfectious Uveitis

- Uveitis may be caused by bacterial, fungal, viral, or parasitic infections. In rare occasions, neoplastic conditions such as intraocular lymphoma may masquerade as ocular inflammation. Additional eye conditions that can mimic or masquerade as uveitis include pigment dispersion syndrome, retinal detachment, and retinal degeneration. Precise diagnosis is crucial for appropriate therapy. Once malignant, masquerade, or infectious causes are excluded, the control of ocular inflammation is the key to the treatment of noninfectious uveitis.
  - We typically use a stepladder treatment approach, starting with topical, local (e.g., periocular or intravitreal injections), and/or systemic corticosteroids. Some patients may require systemic immunomodulators if they are unable to taper or are intolerant to steroids, or if the condition becomes recalcitrant to treatment.
  - Most commonly used systemic immunomodulating agents are methotrexate, azathioprine, and mycophenolate mofetil.

21.3 Systemic Biologic Therapy for Noninfectious Uveitis

- Biologic response modifiers are emerging therapy for uveitis. Biologics have been developed and approved to treat many systemic inflammatory diseases, such as JIA, ankylosing spondylitis (AS), psoriatic arthritis (PsA), psoriasis (PSO), inflammatory bowel disease (IBD) (ulcerative colitis (UC), and Crohn's disease (CD)), Behçet's disease (BD), and rheumatoid arthritis (RA).
  - Frequently, uveitis may be associated with systemic conditions.
  - Many observational reports initially showed that biologics may be effective for uveitis if the patients required therapy for their systemic conditions.
  - Over the past decade, more and more studies subsequently demonstrated the potential efficacy of various biologics for the treatment of uveitis (either related or unrelated to systemic conditions).
  - Tumor necrosis factor (TNF) antagonists (mainly infliximab and adalimumab) are the most common biologics studied and used for uveitis.
  - We generally reserve biologics as second-line therapy if the patients failed or are intolerant to conventional immunosuppression. Exceptions are applied to those with severe uveitis related to BD or other sight-threatening conditions.

21.3.1 Tumor Necrosis Factor Inhibitors (TNFi)

21.3.1.1 Infliximab (Remicade®, Janssen Biotech, Inc) [6, 10, 24]

- A chimeric monoclonal antibody that binds both circulating and membrane-bound TNF-α.

- Infliximab is approved in the US for RA, UC, CD, AS, PsA, and PSO.
- Route of administration: intravenous infusion (IV).
- Initial studies showed that infliximab can be a particularly rapid and very effective therapy for BD-related panuveitis and retinal vasculitis and JIA uveitis.
- Besides BD and JIA, infliximab has been reported as an effective therapy for various forms of uveitis such as HLA-B27-related anterior uveitis, birdshot chorioretinopathy (BSCR), pars planitis, intermediate uveitis, multifocal choroiditis, serpiginous choroidopathy, sympathetic ophthalmia, diffuse subretinal fibrosis, idiopathic uveitis, recalcitrant uveitic CME, and uveitis associated with sarcoidosis, AS, IBD, PSO, Takayasu disease and Vogt–Koyanagi–Harada (VKH) syndrome.
- Pediatric patients may require more frequent infusions or greater doses based on mg/kg compared to adults.
- A prospective trial for various types of refractory uveitis demonstrated initial benefit in approximately 3 of 4 patients. There was a 60% retention rate in both the first and second years.
- Infliximab is especially effective for BD-related uveitis. Fabiani et al. showed that the drug retention rates at 2-, 5-, and 10-year follow-up were 86%, 76%, and 47%, respectively.
- A few cases of recurrent inflammation after switching from original infliximab to biosimilar infliximab have been reported.

21.3.1.2 Adalimumab (Humira®, AbbVie Inc) [8, 16, 27, 28]

- A fully humanized monoclonal antibody against TNF-α.
- Adalimumab is approved in the US for uveitis, RA, UC, CD, AS, PsA, PSO, JIA, and hidradenitis suppurativa.
- Adalimumab is the *only* FDA approved biologic for noninfectious intermediate, posterior, and panuveitis.
- Route of administration: subcutaneous injection (SC).
- Recommended dosage.
  - Adult uveitis: 80 mg loading, followed by 40 mg at week 1, then 40 mg every 2 weeks.
  - Pediatric uveitis: 10–15 kg (10 mg every 2 weeks), 15–30 kg (20 mg every 2 weeks), ≥ 30 kg (40 mg every 2 weeks).
- It is highly effective for the treatment of BD and JIA-related uveitis.
- Like infliximab, adalimumab has been shown to reduce anterior uveitis flares in AS patients, to resolve uveitic CME, and to control various subsets of uveitis such as idiopathic, sarcoidosis, VKH, CD, BSCR, multifocal choroiditis with panuveitis, and Blau syndrome.
- Large clinical trials showed that adalimumab can be effective to control inflammation in patients with active (VISUAL I) and inactive (VISUAL II) intermediate, posterior, and panuveitis. The extension study of VISUAL I&II also confirmed its safety and efficacy (VISUAL III).

21.3.1.3 Golimumab (Simponi®, Janssen Biotech, Inc) [30]

- Subcutaneous golimumab (Simponi®) is approved for RA, PsA, AS, and UC, and intravenous golimumab (Simponi Aria® is indicated in RA, PsA, AS, and JIA.
- Case reports and series showed that it may be a successful treatment for uveitis associated with AS, JIA, BD, and idiopathic retinal vasculitis.
- The GO-EASY Study (multi-center, prospective, 93 patients with AS) showed that golimumab reduced acute uveitis attack rate from 11.1 to 2.2 per 100 patient-years.
- Miserocchi et al. retrospectively studied 34 eyes of 17 patients with severe recalcitrant uveitis (13 with JIA, 4 with HLA-B27 uveitis), with a mean follow-up of 21.9 months. Visual acuity was stable in 26 eyes, improved in 7, and worsened in 1.
- It can be effective in both TNFi-naïve and -experienced patients.
- Most commonly used dose: 50 mg every 4 weeks, subcutaneous injection.
- In some reports, more frequent injections (50 mg every 3 weeks), or higher doses (100 mg every 4 weeks) were used to control uveitis.

21.3.1.4 Certolizumab (Cimzia®, UBC, Inc) [18, 21]

- Certolizumab is approved for RA, PsA, AS, CD, PSO, and non-radiographic axial spondylitis.
- It differs from other TNFi in that it contains the Fab fragment which is bound to polyethylene glycol instead of the Fc fragment. This results in an increased half-life and less likelihood to cross the placenta.
- Case reports and series supported that it may be a successful treatment for uveitis associated with AS, BD, IBD, PsA, relapsing polychondritis, and psoriasis vulgaris.
- The RAPID-axSpA trial demonstrated a lower rate of uveitis flares for patients with axial spondyloarthritis treated with certolizumab compared to placebo.
- Llorenç et al. (retrospective case series, 14 eyes of 7 patients) showed that 71% (5/7 patients with chronic-relapsing uveitis who previously failed other TNFi) achieved quiescence with certolizumab therapy. Significant visual improvement was noted at 1 month.
- Prieto-Peña et al. reported efficacy and safety of certolizumab to control uveitis during pregnancy.
- Dose: 400 mg SC at weeks 0, 2, 4; then 200 mg every 2 weeks (400 mg every 4 weeks can be considered).

21.3.1.5 Etanercept (Enbrel®, Immunex Corporation) [7, 23]

- A fusion protein of a human Fc molecule and two p75 TNF receptors which binds free TNF-α and -β.
- Etanercept is approved for RA, polyarticular JIA, AS, PsA, and PSO.
- It is *NOT* as effective as other TNF inhibitors to treat ocular inflammatory diseases, including uveitis.
- Compared to infliximab and adalimumab, etanercept is more likely to paradoxically trigger inflammatory disease (e.g., psoriasis, uveitis, or sarcoidosis).

21.3.2 Lymphocyte Inhibitors and Lympho-Cytotoxic Medications

21.3.2.1 Rituximab (Rituxan®, Genentech, Inc) [11, 25, 26]

- B-cell inhibitor (cytotoxic to B cells).
- Rituximab is approved in the US for RA, granulomatosis with polyangiitis (GPA) and microscopic polyangiitis (MPA), pemphigus vulgaris, non-Hodgkin's lymphoma, and chronic lymphocytic leukemia (CLL).
- Rituximab can be a potent treatment for scleritis, ocular cicatricial pemphigoid, orbital inflammatory disease, retinal vasculitis, non-paraneoplastic autoimmune retinopathy, and recalcitrant uveitis, although randomized controlled trials are lacking to support these indications.
- Case reports and series demonstrated that it may be effective for the treatment of birdshot chorioretinopathy, refractory posterior uveitis, diffuse subretinal fibrosis, and uveitis associated with JIA, BD, GPA, and essential cryoglobulinemia.
- Most commonly used dose: 1000 mg (2 intravenous infusions at 2 weeks interval), followed by repeated infusions every 6–18 months.
- Uveitis inactivity is typically observed 4–5 months after the first infusion, and approximately half of the patients may need more infusions due to uveitic flares.
- Lasave et al. suggested an extended dosing regimen of 375 mg/m^2 intravenous weekly for 8 consecutive weeks, and thereafter, monthly for 4 consecutive months for long-term uveitis control.
- Intravitreal rituximab (1 mg/0.1 mL) (± intravitreal methotrexate) injections may be effective method to treat vitreoretinal lymphoma.
- To date, there are no reports on the use of Rituxan HYCELA®, a novel subcutaneous form, for ocular indications.

21.3.2.2 Abatacept (Orencia®, Bristol-Myers Squibb Company) [2, 29]

- T-cell inhibitor by blocking accessory molecules involved in antigen presentation.
- Abatacept is approved for RA, PsA and JIA.
- Uveitis studies, to date, are based on the intravenous route of administration in children and young adults.
- Case reports showed its promising efficacy to control or improve refractory JIA-uveitis.
- A sustained response from abatacept for refractory uveitis is uncommon.
- Tappeiner et al. retrospectively studied 21 patients with active refractory JIA-uveitis. Of 21 patients, uveitis inactivity was achieved in 11 patients (8 of 11 had recurrent uveitis) and remained active in another 10 patients.
- It offers comparable efficacy in severe JIA-uveitis either as first-line or after ≥1 TNFi.

21.3.2.3 Alemtuzumab (Lemtrada®, Genzyme Corporation) [4, 20, 32]

- A CD52-directed cytolytic antibody; CD52 is present on the surface of mature B and T lymphocytes, monocytes, and dendritic cells.

- Alemtuzumab is approved for multiple sclerosis (MS).
- Previously available brand, Campath® (approved for CLL), was withdrawn in 2012.
- Case reports and series showed its potential benefit in controlling uveitis related to various underlying conditions such as BD, sympathetic ophthalmia, and MS.
- It may cause secondary autoimmune diseases in 30–50% of treated patients, and Graves' disease is the most common. Cases of secondary thyroid orbitopathy have been reported.

21.3.3 Interleukin (IL) Inhibitors

21.3.3.1 Anakinra (Kineret®, Swedish Orphan Biovitrum AB [Publ]) and Canakinumab (Ilaris®, Novartis) [5]

- Anakinra is a competitive IL-1 receptor antagonist, and canakinumab is a selective anti-IL-1β antibody.
- Anakinra is approved for RA and neonatal-onset multisystem inflammatory disease.
- Canakinumab is approved for systemic JIA and periodic fever syndromes.
- A multicenter retrospective observational study showed that IL-1 inhibitors (anakinra or canakinumab) were effective to treat BD uveitis. At 12 months, uveitis flares significantly decreased from 200 to 49 episodes/100 patients/year, with significant improvement of retinal vasculitis on fluorescein angiogram.
- Interestingly, the rate of ocular inflammatory flares was significantly higher in patients co-administered with modifying anti-rheumatic drugs (DMARDs) than those using IL-1 inhibitor monotherapy (82 vs 0 episodes/100 patients/year).
- Studies on other types of uveitis are limited to a few case reports of rare uveitis syndromes.

21.3.3.2 Gevokizumab (XOMA 052, XOMA Corporation)

- A selective IL-1β blocker.
- Several clinical trials on noninfectious uveitis including one specifically on Behçet's disease were terminated as the primary efficacy endpoint was not met.
- A case series on the treatment of anterior scleritis demonstrated improvement of scleritis in 7 of 9 patients; however, 2 patients experienced new scleritis in previously uninvolved quadrants.

21.3.3.3 Tocilizumab (Actemra®, Genentech, Inc) [14, 19, 22, 31]

- An anti-IL-6 receptor monoclonal antibody.
- Tocilizumab is approved for RA, giant cell arteritis (GCA), polyarticular and systemic JIA, cytokine release syndrome (CRS), and systemic sclerosis-associated interstitial lung disease (SSc-ILD).
- Several case reports and series showed that it might be effective to treat uveitis associated with JIA, BD, sarcoidosis, Blau syndrome, and AS, other types of uveitis, such as BSCR, sympathetic ophthalmia, and idiopathic panuveitis.

- A randomized, controlled, multicenter trial (STOP-Uveitis) of 37 patients shows that tocilizumab (both 4 and 8 mg/kg IV every 4 weeks) is well tolerated and is effective to improve vision, decrease vitreous haze and central macular thickness in noninfectious, intermediate, posterior and panuveitis during 6-month follow up.
- It also has demonstrated efficacy, particularly on uveitic CME.
- The multicenter, single-arm, phase 2 trial on tocilizumab for patients (2–18 years old) with active JIA-associated uveitis was completed with only one-third (7 of 21 patients) responding to treatment. Therefore, the results did not support a phase 3 trial for JIA uveitis.
- A clinical trial, "Tocilizumab for the Treatment of Refractory Behçet's Uveitis" is recruiting participants.

21.3.3.4 Secukinumab (Cosentyx®, Novartis) [3, 12]

- An anti-IL-17A monoclonal antibody.
- It is approved for psoriasis, AS, and PsA.
- Although it failed to achieve the primary endpoint in 3 randomized clinical trials, a multicenter, randomized, double-blinded, phase 2 clinical trial of noninfectious uveitis compared secukinumab 300 mg SC every 2 weeks for 4 doses, 10 mg/kg IV every 2 weeks for 4 doses, and 30 mg/kg IV every 4 weeks for 2 doses. The response rates (at 2–4 weeks after last dose) were 33% vs 62% vs 73%, and the remission rates were 17% vs 39% vs 27%, respectively.
- High-dose IV secukinumab may be necessary to achieve therapeutic benefits.
- Retrospective data from ankylosing spondylitis trials suggest that secukinumab might reduce the rate of flares of anterior uveitis.

21.3.3.5 Ustekinumab (Stelara®, Janssen Biotech, Inc)

- An anti-IL-12 and -23 monoclonal antibody.
- It is approved for psoriasis, CD, and PsA.
- A 64-year-old with severe psoriasis, PSA and anterior uveitis, failed adalimumab, and was successfully treated with ustekinumab injections with complete remission of psoriasis and uveitis.
- It has also had some efficacy in children with uveitis associated with psoriatic arthritis.
- A clinical trial of ustekinumab for the treatment of active sight-threatening uveitis (STAR Study) is underway.

21.3.4 Janus Kinase (JAK) and Tyrosine Kinase (TYK) Inhibitors

21.3.4.1 Tofacitinib (Xeljanz®, Pfizer) [13, 17]

- Inhibits JAK 1, 2, and 3 and TYK2.
- Tofacitinib is approved for RA, UC, and PsA.
- Oral form (5 mg twice daily or extended-release 11 mg daily).

- A few case reports showed that it may be effective to control refractory HLA-B27-related and JIA-uveitis, as well as scleritis.
- A phase I/II randomized trial demonstrated that it may improve signs and symptoms of dry eye.
- A clinical trial for inflammatory eye disease (uveitis and scleritis) is underway.

21.3.4.2 Filgotinib (GLPG0634, Galapagos NV/Gilead)

- Selectively inhibits JAK 1.
- Filgotinib was studied for RA, AS, PsA, and IBD.
- Oral form.
- Phase 2 trials showed efficacy in RA (DARWIN 1 (as combination therapy with methotrexate) and DARWIN 2 trials (as a second-line monotherapy)), AS (TORTUGA trial), and PsA (EQUATOR trial).
- No reports on treatment for ocular conditions.
- A phase 2 clinical trial evaluating the efficacy and safety of filgotinib in subjects with active noninfectious uveitis was started but has ceased due to toxicity concerns.

21.3.4.3 Baricitinib (Olumiant®, Eli Lilly and Company) [15]

- A small case series suggested that baricitinib could be effective for the uveitis associated with JIA.
- Other JAK inhibitors including upacitinib have demonstrated efficacy in other immune-mediated diseases.

21.3.5 Interferons (IFN) [1, 9]

- IFN-α2a, −α2b, and -β1a have been reported to effectively treat refractory uveitic CME, especially in patients with MS and BD; however, uveitic CME frequently recurs after stopping treatment.
- IFN-α has been shown to control intraocular inflammation with sustained efficacy after discontinuing therapy.
- IFNs may induce sarcoidosis with or without uveitis. Depression and flu-like symptoms are fairly common toxicities.

21.4 Special Consideration

- Some biologics may be designed to be organ specific, thus this may limit efficacy in other organs.

21.4.1 Vedolizumab (Entyvio®, Takeda)

– Blocking the $\alpha_4\beta_7$ integrin resulting in gut-selective anti-inflammatory activity.
– Vedolizumab is approved for adult UC and CD.
– May increase the likelihood of scleritis and uveitis as it is not as effective as TNF inhibitors for extraintestinal manifestations.

Other biologics such as those that target IL-23 selectively or those that target granulocyte-macrophage colony-stimulating factor (GM-CSF) are being actively studied for other immune-mediated diseases and might ultimately be tested for efficacy in treating uveitis as well. The role of biologics delivered locally inside the eye either as proteins or via gene therapy is incompletely studied.

Acknowledgment This work was supported by NIH Grant EY026572, the Grandmaison Fund for Autoimmunity Research, the William and Mary Bauman Foundation, the Stan and Madelle Rosenfeld Family Trust, and Research to Prevent Blindness.

Both authors are investigators for Santen and for Gilead. Dr. Rosenbaum receives financial support from Abbvie, Gilead, Santen, UCB, Novartis, Eyevensys, Celldex, Corvus, Kyverna, Revolo, Affibody, and Roche. Pfizer and Horizon provide clinical trial support to OHSU. He receives royalties from UpToDate.

References

1. Becker MD, Heiligenhaus A, Hudde T, et al. Interferon as a treatment for uveitis associated with multiple sclerosis. Br J Ophthalmol. 2005;89(10):1254–7.
2. Birolo C, Zannin ME, Arsenyeva S, et al. Comparable efficacy of Abatacept used as first-line or second-line biological agent for severe juvenile idiopathic arthritis-related uveitis. J Rheumatol. 2016;43(11):2068–73.
3. Deodhar AA, Miceli-Richard C, Baraliakos X, et al. Incidence of uveitis in Secukinumab-treated patients with ankylosing spondylitis: pooled data analysis from three phase 3 studies. ACR Open Rheumatol. 2020;2(5):294–9.
4. Dick AD, Meyer P, James T, et al. Campath-1H therapy in refractory ocular inflammatory disease. Br J Ophthalmol. 2000;84(1):107–9.
5. Fabiani C, Vitale A, Emmi G, et al. Interleukin (IL)-1 inhibition with Anakinra and Canakinumab in Behçet's disease-related uveitis: a multicenter retrospective observational study. Clin Rheumatol. 2017;36(1):191–7.
6. Fabiani C, Sota J, Vitale A, et al. Ten-year retention rate of infliximab in patients with Behçet's disease-related uveitis. Ocul Immunol Inflamm. 2019;27(1):34–9.
7. Galor A, Perez VL, Hammel JP, Lowder CY. Differential effectiveness of Etanercept and infliximab in the treatment of ocular inflammation. Ophthalmology. 2006;113(12):2317–23.
8. Jaffe GJ, Dick AD, Brézin AP, et al. Adalimumab in patients with active noninfectious uveitis. N Engl J Med. 2016;375(10):932–43.

9. Kötter I, Günaydin I, Zierhut M, Stübiger N. The use of interferon alpha in Behçet disease: review of the literature. Semin Arthritis Rheum. 2004;33(5):320–35.
10. Kruh JN, Yang P, Suelves AM, Foster CS. Infliximab for the treatment of refractory non-infectious uveitis: a study of 88 patients with long-term follow-up. Ophthalmology. 2014;121(1):358–64.
11. Lasave AF, You C, Ma L, et al. Long-term outcomes of rituximab therapy in patients with noninfectious posterior uveitis refractory to conventional immunosuppressive therapy. Retina. 2018;38(2):395–402.
12. Letko E, Yeh S, Foster CS, et al. Efficacy and safety of intravenous Secukinumab in non-infectious uveitis requiring steroid-sparing immunosuppressive therapy. Ophthalmology. 2015;122(5):939–48.
13. Liew SH, Nichols KK, Klamerus KJ, Li JZ, Zhang M, Foulks GN. Tofacitinib (CP-690,550), a Janus kinase inhibitor for dry eye disease: results from a phase I/II trial. Ophthalmology. 2012;119(7):1328–35.
14. Mesquida M, Molins B, Llorenç V, et al. Twenty-four month follow-up of tocilizumab therapy for refractory uveitis-related macular edema. Retina. 2018;38(7):1361–70.
15. Miserocchi E, Giuffrè C, Cornalba M, et al. JAK inhibitors in refractory juvenile idiopathic arthritis-associated uveitis. Clin Rheumatol. 2020;39(3):847–51.
16. Nguyen QD, Merrill PT, Jaffe GJ, et al. Adalimumab for prevention of Uveitic flare in patients with inactive non-infectious uveitis controlled by corticosteroids (VISUAL II): a multicentre, double-masked, randomised, placebo-controlled phase 3 trial. Lancet. 2016;388(10050):1183–92.
17. Paley MA, Karacal H, Rao PK, Margolis TP, Miner JJ. Tofacitinib for refractory uveitis and Scleritis. Am J Ophthalmol Case Rep. 2018;13:53–5.
18. Prieto-Peña D, Calderón-Goercke M, Adán A, et al. Efficacy and safety of Certolizumab Pegol in pregnant women with uveitis. Recommendations on the management with immunosuppressive and biologic therapies in uveitis during pregnancy. Clin Exp Rheumatol. 2021;39(1):105–14.
19. Ramanan AV, Dick AD, Guly C, et al. Tocilizumab in patients with anti-TNF refractory juvenile idiopathic arthritis-associated uveitis (APTITUDE): a multicentre, single-arm, phase 2 trial. Lancet Rheumatol. 2020;2(3):e135–41.
20. Roos JCP, Moran C, Chatterjee VK, Jones J, Coles A, Murthy R. Immune reconstruction after Alemtuzumab therapy for multiple sclerosis triggering graves' Orbitopathy: a case series. Eye (Lond). 2019;33(2):223–9.
21. Rudwaleit M, Rosenbaum JT, Landewé R, et al. Observed incidence of uveitis following Certolizumab Pegol treatment in patients with axial Spondyloarthritis (the RAPID-axSpA study). Arthritis Care Res (Hoboken). 2016;68(6):838–44.
22. Sepah YJ, Sadiq MA, Chu DS, et al. Primary (Month-6) outcomes of the STOP-uveitis study: evaluating the safety, tolerability, and efficacy of tocilizumab in patients with noninfectious uveitis. Am J Ophthalmol. 2017;183:71–80.
23. Smith JA, Thompson DJ, Whitcup SM, et al. A randomized, placebo-controlled, double-masked clinical trial of Etanercept for the treatment of uveitis associated with juvenile idiopathic arthritis. Arthritis Rheum. 2005;53(1):18–23.
24. Suhler EB, Smith JR, Giles TR, et al. Infliximab therapy for refractory uveitis: 2-year results of a prospective trial. Arch Ophthalmol. 2009;127(6):819–22.
25. Suhler EB, Lim LL, Beardsley RM, et al. Rituximab therapy for refractory orbital inflammation: results of a phase 1/2, dose-ranging, Randomized. Clin Trial JAMA Ophthalmol. 2014a;132(5):572–8.
26. Suhler EB, Lim LL, Beardsley RM, et al. Rituximab therapy for refractory Scleritis: results of a phase I/II dose-ranging, randomized. Clin Trial Ophthalmol. 2014b;121(10):1885–91.

27. Suhler EB, Adán A, Brézin AP, et al. Safety and efficacy of adalimumab in patients with noninfectious uveitis in an ongoing open-label study: VISUAL III. Ophthalmology. 2018;125(7):1075–87.
28. Suhler EB, Jaffe GJ, Fortin E, et al. Long-term safety and efficacy of adalimumab in patients with noninfectious intermediate uveitis, posterior uveitis, or Panuveitis. Ophthalmology 2021;128(6):899–909.
29. Tappeiner C, Miserocchi E, Bodaghi B, et al. Abatacept in the treatment of severe, long-standing, and refractory uveitis associated with juvenile idiopathic arthritis. J Rheumatol. 2015;42(4):706–11.
30. van Bentum RE, Heslinga SC, Nurmohamed MT, et al. Reduced occurrence rate of acute anterior uveitis in ankylosing spondylitis treated with Golimumab – the GO-EASY study. J Rheumatol. 2019;46(2):153–9.
31. Vegas-Revenga N, Calvo-Río V, Mesquida M, et al. Anti-IL6-receptor tocilizumab in refractory and noninfectious Uveitic cystoid macular edema: multicenter study of 25 patients. Am J Ophthalmol. 2019;200:85–94.
32. Willis MD, Pickersgill TP, Robertson NP, Lee RWJ, Dick AD, Carreño E. Alemtuzumab-induced remission of multiple sclerosis-associated uveitis. Int Ophthalmol. 2017;37(5):1229–33.

Biologics in Sarcoidosis

22

Ved Chaturvedi and Mayank Gupta

22.1 Introduction

- Sarcoidosis is a multisystem granulomatous disorder of chronic nature that commonly involves the lungs and lymph nodes [1], but can also involve other organ systems. Sarcoidosis derives from the Greek word "sarco," meaning "flesh"; "eidos," meaning "like"; and "osis," meaning "condition." [2]
- Sarcoidosis occurs worldwide [3]. It has been reported in all races and ethnic groups with marked variations. In most series females were affected more than males. People of all ages can be affected, but it particularly occurs in young adults 20–40 years of age with a second peak in women in the seventh decade.
- Approximately 80% of patients will require treatment, and those who need systemic treatment may continue for another 5 years. Corticosteroids are the mainstay for treatment but their side effect profile and inability to change the course of disease has led to its limited uses [4].

22.2 Immunopathogenesis

- Alveolar macrophages play a key part in the pathogenesis of sarcoidosis. Once they increase, they lead to increase production of TNF which is considered to be a granuloma promoting factor in Sarcoidosis [5].

V. Chaturvedi (✉)
Senior Consultant, Department of Rheumatology & Clinical Immunology, Sir Gangaram Hospital, New Delhi, India

M. Gupta
DNB Resident, Department of Rheumatology & Clinical Immunology, Sir Gangaram Hospital, New Delhi, India

N. Jain, L. Duggal (eds.), *Handbook of Biologics for Rheumatological Disorders*, https://doi.org/10.1007/978-981-16-7200-2_22

22.3 Management

22.3.1 Glucocorticoids

- Corticosteroids are the mainstay in treatment.
- Corticosteroids act by reducing gene transcription of inflammatory genes, such as IL-1 and TNF-α, adhesion molecules and receptors, by interaction with pro-inflammatory transcription factors nuclear factor-κB (NF-κB) [6].
- Starting dose is 0.3–0.6 mg/kg (20–40 mg/day) for 4–6 weeks. If disease parameters are stable or improved, then the dose is tapered by 5–10 mg decrements every 4–8 weeks down to 10–20 mg/day.
- Acute respiratory failure or cardiac, neurologic, ocular or upper airway disease may need higher doses (80–100 mg/day). Maintenance dose is 10–20 mg for 6–8 months.

22.3.2 Methotrexate

- Immunosuppressive drugs are used in corticosteroids refractory disease or in those who require high doses of steroids for prolonged periods. Efficacy of around 40–60% is found in lungs, skin, eyes, and neurological disease [7].
- Methotrexate (MTX) dose administration and monitoring is similar to those in rheumatoid arthritis. However, MTX-associated liver fibrosis may occur in up to 10% of sarcoidosis patients, especially those who received long-term treatment.
- MTX-associated interstitial pneumonitis should be kept in mind in rare cases [8].

22.3.3 Azathioprine

- Azathioprine is used in patients who have failed MTX [9]. Often used along with combination with glucocorticoids although data is limited.

22.3.4 Leflunomide

- It has been shown equally effective as MTX in ocular and pulmonary disease when used alone or in combination with methotrexate in some case series [10].

22.3.5 Mycophenolate

- Mycophenolate does not appear to provide extra benefit in sarcoidosis patients that are unresponsive to previous corticosteroid-sparing agents. In neurosarcoidosis, its role has been studied in very few studies [11].

22.3.6 Antimalarial Agents

- In cutaneous sarcoidosis, it has a good role [12].

22.3.7 Biological Therapy

Tumor necrosis factor-alpha (TNF-α) plays a pivotal role in the maintenance of granulomas formation in sarcoidosis and can be a potential therapeutic target. However, data is limited and results in pulmonary sarcoidosis have been disappointing.

22.3.7.1 Infliximab

- Infliximab has been used in patients with pulmonary and extrapulmonary sarcoidosis refractory to corticosteroids in case reports and small case series with success. It has been studied with good results in active pulmonary sarcoidosis resistant to corticosteroids [13].
- Infliximab did not demonstrate any significant benefit in lung function. In 24 month follow-up period, the efficacy was not maintained [14]. It has been seen that peripheral blood CD4 T cell lymphopenia may be more likely to respond to infliximab [15].

22.3.7.2 Etanercept

- Its efficacy in sarcoidosis is not been proven. On the contrary, there are case reports in which sarcoidosis developed during etanercept treatment [16]. The pathogenesis for this is unclear.

22.3.7.3 Adalimumab

- Adalimumab therapy in extrapulmonary sarcoidosis in case reports have shown some improvement [17].

22.3.7.4 Non Targeted TNF Inhibitors

- The third line drugs Thalidomide, pentoxifylline, and apremilast have disappointing data on efficacy and side effects [18, 19].

22.3.7.5 Cytotoxic T-lymphocyte Associated Blockade

- Abatacept is a fusion protein composed of the Fc region of the IgG1 fused to the extracellular domain of CTLA-4 that binds to the CD80 and CD86 molecule and results in T cell downregulation. In sarcoidosis, it can be a useful immunosuppressant [20].

22.3.7.6 IL-12/IL-23P40 and Th17 Pathways

- IL-12/IL-23 is a heterodimeric cytokine composed of the IL-12 p40 minor subunit and the IL-23 p19 major subunit. IL-12p40 and IL23 receptor and Th1 and Th17 pathways have a role in sarcoidosis [21].

- Ustekinumab was studied recently in patients with chronic pulmonary sarcoidosis and/or skin sarcoidosis was found not much effective in patients with sarcoidosis [22].

22.3.7.7 Other Therapies

- Cyclophosphamide, chlorambucil, and thalidomide [23] were used in the past.
- Rituximab has been used in refractory pulmonary disease with an inconsistent response [24].

22.3.7.8 Novel Therapeutics

- Recent studies have shown that Targeting p38 MAP kinases may have a potential role as it plays [25]. p38 MAP kinase inhibitors are BIRB 796 and Semapimodbut neither has been studied in sarcoidosis [26].
- NLRP3 inflammasome is the most studied inflammasome; they are newly recognized pattern-recognition receptors.
- They are involved in both acute and chronic inflammatory responses in a variety of inflammatory diseases including sarcoidosis [27].
- The ubiquitin-proteasome system (UPS) regulates many cellular activities and functions [28, 29]. In sarcoidosis, these can be potential novel therapies [30].

Future: In recent years lots of newer understanding of disease has taken place and to reduce morbidity and mortality, a need for effective "disease-modifying therapies" is required [31]. Many advances in other autoimmune diseases also offer a hope that novel therapies will be available in sarcoidosis also.

References

1. Valeyre D, Prasse A, Nunes H, et al. Sarcoidosis Lancet. 2014;383:1155–67.
2. James DG, Sharma OP. From Hutchinson to now: a historical glimpse. Curr Opin Pulm Med. 2002;8:416–23.
3. Sharma OP. Sarcoidosis around the world. Clin Chest Med. 2008;29:357–63.
4. Baughman RP, Grutters JC. New treatment strategies for pulmonary sarcoidosis: antimetabolites, biological drugs, and other treatment approaches. Lancet Respir Med. 2015;3:813–23.
5. Zissel G, Prasse A, Müller-Quernheim J. Immunologic response of sarcoidosis. Semin Respir Crit Care Med. 2010;31:390–403.
6. Grutters JC, Van den Bosch JM. Corticosteroid treatment in sarcoidosis. Eur Respir J. 2006;28:627–36.
7. Baughman RP, Winget DB, Lower EE. Methotrexate is steroid sparing in acute sarcoidosis: results of a double blind, randomized trial. Sarcoidosis Vasc Diffuse Lung Dis. 2000;17:60–6.
8. Baughman RP, Lower EE. A clinical approach to the use of methotrexate for sarcoidosis. Thorax. 1999;54:742–6.
9. Baughman RP, Lower EE. Medical therapy of sarcoidosis. Semin Respir Crit Care Med. 2014;35:391–406.
10. Baughman RP, Lower EE. Leflunomide for chronic sarcoidosis. Sarcoidosis Vasc Diffuse Lung Dis. 2004;21:43–8.
11. Androdias G, Maillet D, Marignier R. Mycophenolate mofetil may be effective in CNS sarcoidosis but not in sarcoid myopathy. Neurology. 2011;76:1168–72.

12. Doherty CB, Rosen T. Evidence-based therapy for cutaneous sarcoidosis. Drugs. 2008;68:1361–83.
13. Baughman RP, Lower EE. Infliximab for refractory sarcoidosis. Sarcoidosis Vasc Diffuse Lung Dis. 2001;18:70–4.
14. Baughman RP, Drent M, Kavuru M. Infliximab therapy in patients with chronic sarcoidosis and pulmonary involvement. Am J Respir Crit Care Med. 2006;174:795–802.
15. Crouser ED, Lozanski G, Fox CC, et al. The CD4+ lymphopenic sarcoidosis phenotype is highly responsive to anti-tumor necrosis factor-{alpha} therapy. Chest. 2010;137:1432–5.
16. Field S, Regan AO, Sheahan K, at al. Recalcitrant cutaneous sarcoidosis responding to adalimumab but not to etanercept. Clin Exp Dermatol. 2010;35:795–6.
17. Sweiss NJ, Noth I, Mirsaeidi M, et al. Efficacy results of a 52-week trial of adalimumab in the treatment of refractory sarcoidosis. Sarcoidosis Vasc Diffuse Lung Dis. 2014;31:46–54.
18. Baughman RP, Judson MA, Ingledue R, et al. Efficacy and safety of apremilast in chronic cutaneous sarcoidosis. Arch Dermatol. 2012;148:262–4.
19. Park MK, Fontana BH, et al. Steroid-sparing effects of pentoxifylline in pulmonary sarcoidosis. Sarcoidosis Vasc Diffuse Lung Dis. 2009;26:121–31.
20. Sandborn WJ, Colombel J-F, Sands BE, et al. Abatacept for Crohn's disease and ulcerative colitis. Gastroenterology. 2012;143:62e4–69.e4.
21. Moller DR, Forman JD, Liu MC, et al. Enhanced expression of IL-12 associated with Th1 cytokine profiles in active pulmonary sarcoidosis. J Immunol. 1996;156:4952–60.
22. Judson MA, Baughman RP, Costabel U, et al. Safety and efficacy of ustekinumab or golimumab in patients with chronic sarcoidosis. Eur Respir J. 2014;44:1296–307.
23. Fazzi P, Manni E, Cristofani R, et al. Thalidomide for improving cutaneous and pulmonary sarcoidosis in patients resistant or with contraindications to corticosteroids. Biomed Pharmacother. 2012;66:300–7.
24. Bomprezzi R, Pati S, Chansakul C, et al. A case of neurosarcoidosis successfully treated with rituximab. Neurology. 2010;75:568–70.
25. Schreiber S, Feagan B, D'Haens G, et al. Oral p38 mitogen-activated protein kinase inhibition with BIRB 796 for active Crohn's disease: a randomized, double-blind, placebo-controlled trial. Clin Gastroenterol Hepatol. 2006;4:325–34.
26. Dotan I, Rachmilewitz D, Schreiber S, et al. A randomised placebo-controlled multicentre trial of intravenous semapimod HCl for moderate to severe Crohn's disease. Gut. 2010;59:760–6.
27. Shao BZ, Xu ZQ, Han BZ, et al. NLRP3 inflammasome and its inhibitors: a review. Front Pharmacol. 2015;6:262.
28. Weathington NM, Sznajder JI, Mallampalli RK. The emerging role of the ubiquitin proteasome in pulmonary biology and disease. Am J Respir Crit Care Med. 2013;188:530–7.
29. Lohr NJ, Molleston JP, Strauss KA, et al. Human ITCH E3 ubiquitin ligase deficiency causes syndromic multisystem autoimmune disease. Am J Hum Genet. 2010;86:447–53.
30. Teicher BA, Tomaszewski JE. Proteasome inhibitors. Biochem Pharmacol. 2015;96:1–9.
31. Cremers JP, Drent M, Bast A, et al. Multinational evidence-based world association of sarcoidosis and other granulomatous disorders recommendations for the use of methotrexate in sarcoidosis. Curr Opin Pulm Med. 2013;19:545–61.

Biologics in IgG4-Related Disease 23

Amit Dua, Neeraj Jain, Lalit Duggal, and Bhavya Chintala

23.1 Case Vignette

A 49-year-old male with no co-morbidities and with right-sided orbital myositis was diagnosed with IgG4-related disease on the basis of clinical picture, serology imaging, and biopsy. He was started on a combination of prednisolone (0.6 mg/kg/day) and escalating doses of methotrexate. Tapering the steroid to less than 10 mg per day after three months of treatment led to a recurrence of symptoms. Prednisolone was increased to 30 mg per day and methotrexate was switched to azathioprine (2 mg/kg/day). The patient improved symptomatically and his IgG4 levels came down to within normal range. However, on reducing the steroid dose and despite increasing azathioprine, pain and swelling of the eye and proptosis returned. A repeat MRI of orbits showed an increase in the right orbital myositis, from that of the beginning of the disease.

Rituximab was administered, two injections of 1 g each, 15 days apart. At 6 months, the patient was better clinically and by way of investigations and prednisolone was tapered to 5 mg per day [1].

A. Dua
Consultant, Dua's Clinic, Rheumatology and Arthritis Care,
Bilaspur, Chhattisgarh, India

N. Jain · L. Duggal (✉)
Department of Rheumatology & Clinical Immunology, Sir Ganga Ram Hospital,
New Delhi, India

B. Chintala
DNB Resident, Department of Rheumatology & Clinical Immunology,
Sir Ganga Ram Hospital, New Delhi, India

N. Jain, L. Duggal (eds.), *Handbook of Biologics for Rheumatological Disorders*,
https://doi.org/10.1007/978-981-16-7200-2_23

23.2 Introduction

IgG4-Related Disease (IgG4-RD) is a chronic immune-mediated fibro-inflammatory condition that can affect multiple organs either in a synchronous or metachronous fashion [2].

It can affect nearly every structure of the body but the most frequently involved organs are lacrimal and salivary glands, thyroid gland, pancreas, bile ducts, retroperitoneum, kidney aorta, meninges, and lymph nodes [3, 4]. It can present as mass forming lesions which can lead to permanent organ damage and can be fatal if left untreated [4]. This disease is a great mimicker of many malignant, infectious and inflammatory conditions [3, 4].

Histopathologically, it is characterized by lymphoplasmacytic infiltrate rich in IgG4 plasma cells with simultaneous development of storiform fibrosis and presence of obliterative phlebitis [3]. Patient may often, but not always have elevated serum IgG4 levels [5].

The goal of treatment is to reduce inflammation and to achieve and maintain remission so as to prevent organ damage. Glucocorticoids (GCs) remain the mainstay of treatment. Starting dose of GCs is 0.6 mg/kg/day of prednisolone equivalent which is tapered slowly to maintain remission [6]. In view of the adverse effects associated with the chronic use of GCs, especially in patients with substantial co-morbidities (e.g., hypertension, diabetes mellitus, osteoporosis), immunomodulatory agents like Methotrexate, azathioprine, mycophenolate mofetil, cyclosporine, cyclophosphamide are used as steroid-sparing agents. However, definitive evidence showing their steroid-sparing effect in preventing relapses in long run is limited [7].

Consequently, there is an unmet need for drugs with a better efficacy and safety profile. A range of different biologic agents have been proposed and subjected to clinical trials, particularly dedicated to this subset of patients whose disease is inadequately controlled by conventional treatment regimes. Rituximab being the most commonly used targeted therapy for IgG4-RD, several novel biologic agents targeting B cells, T cells, or cytokines are constantly being evaluated. It seems that they may enhance the therapeutic efficacy when combined with standard therapies. This article reviews the current biological therapies being used and being tested in the treatment of IgG4-RD.

23.3 Biologics

- These are a new class of disease-modifying agents engineered to target specific chemicals, cytokines, and immune cells responsible for the disease.
- These are designed to reduce the disease, slow down the disease progression and improve the quality of life of the patients.
- They are fast-acting as compared to conventional disease-modifying drugs.

- Although biologics are expensive; but in long run, they are cost-effective because of major clinical benefits.
- Major infections and infusion reactions are some of the side effects seen with their use, so proper and periodic monitoring is needed.

23.4 Understanding the Targets of Biological Therapies in IgG4-RD

- Antigen-driven B and T cells collaboration plays a central role in the pathophysiology of IgG4-RD at various levels.
- Follicular T helper cells (T_{FH}) secrete IL4, which stimulates the maturation of naive B cells into IgG4 secreting plasmablasts.
- CD4 cytotoxic T lymphocytes (CTLs) and plasmablasts, express a surface transmembrane molecule called SLAMF-7 (signaling lymphocytic activation molecule F7) that has been involved in cell–cell interaction and chronic lymphocytic activation [7, 8].
- Plasmablasts at inflamed site sustain the activation of CD4 and CD8 cytotoxic T lymphocytic cells (CTLs) via antigen presentation, SLAMF-7 (signaling lymphocytic activation molecule F7) mediated homodimer interaction, and CD80/86 interaction of CD28.
- These cytotoxic T cells secrete cytotoxic and profibrotic molecules like TGF-B, INF-Y, IL-IB, IL6, etc. and cause tissue damage.
- Plasmablasts produce lyoyl oxidase homolog 2(LOXL2) which leads to fibroblasts activation and extracellular matrix deposition.
- Plasmablast also secretes IgG4 and IgG1 antibodies which form immune complexes and thus activate complement pathways and further cause tissue damage [7, 8].
- There has been growing interest in the role of innate immunity in IgG4-RD. Type 2 macrophage, eosinophils, and plasmacytoid dendritic cells are involved in the pathophysiology of the disease. Although it is much less studied, it seems to be associated with transiting the disease from inflammatory to fibrotic phase [7].

  Several targets have been identified to halt this ongoing disease pathophysiology. These include:
- B cell depletion.
- T cell inhibition.
- B and T cell costimulation inhibition.
- Inhibition of complement activation.
- Cytokine blockage.
- Inhibition of extracellular matrix organization.

Table 23.1 shows a concise summery of potential therapeutic agents which are used in IgG4-RD and their targets.

Table 23.1 A concise summary of the potential therapeutic agents for IgG4RD

Biological agent	Target	Mechanism of action	Evidence/trial	Status of trial
Rituximab	B cell	Anti CD20 + B cell depletion	Open-label prospective clinical trial of 30 patients	Completed
XmAb5871	B cell	CD 19 directed B cell inhibition	Open-label prospective clinical trial of 21 patients	Completed
Inebilizumab	B cell	CD 19 + B cell depletion	Phase ii b, prospective, randomized, blinded trial	Recruiting 160 patients. Expected to be completed in June 2024
Bortezomib	B cells	Inhibits autoreactive plasma cells by targeting proteasome depletion	Case report	
Abatacept	T cells	Co stimulation blockage	Phase 2, single-center, proof-of-concept clinical trial	Results recently submitted
			Case report	
Elotuzumab	B and T cells	Inhibits SLAMF7	Proof-of-concept trial	Under development
Infliximab	Cytokine	TNF a inhibition	Case report	
Dupilumab	Cytokines	IL4 and IL13 inhibition	Case report	

23.5 Screening Before Starting Biologics

- Viral markers (HbsAg, Anti HCV, and HIV).
- Screening for latent Tuberculosis (Mantoux, IGRA, X-ray Chest).

23.6 Use of Biological Agents in IgG4 RD

The emergence of biological agents has increased the therapeutic armamentarium for the treatment of IgG4 RD, especially the severe and refractory cases.

23.6.1 B Cell-Targeted Therapies

23.6.1.1 Rituximab

- *Mechanism of action*—It is a Chimeric CD 20 monoclonal antibody which acts by depleting B cells and hence disrupts B–T cell interaction and antigen presentation to CD4 CTLs and therefore chronic activation of CD4 CTLs [9].
- B cell depletion also reduces tissue fibrosis by decreasing the number of B lymphocyte subsets with profibrotic properties thereby reducing the number of infiltrating activated myofibroblasts [10, 11].

- B cell reduction also decreases serum IgG4 levels, which are generally associated with striking clinical improvement [8].

23.6.1.2 Dose Protocol

- Rituximab was administered either as two 1 gm infusions 15 days apart or in four weekly doses of 375 mg/m^2 infusions.
- In some cases, a lower dose of rituximab (single 1 gm infusion) was used [12, 13].
- The best dose and timing of the administration are yet to be defined.

23.6.1.3 Use of Rituximab in IgG4 RD

- Evidence to suggest the role of Rituximab in IgG4-RD was obtained in a study of 30 patients of the disease. Response was seen in 97% of patients. Seventy-seven percent of patients achieved remission. Forty percent of patients remained in complete remission at 1 year although rituximab dose was not repeated on follow-up [14].
- It is usually used in combination with Glucocorticoids but studies have shown it to be effective even in the absence of GCs [14, 15].
- It is commonly administered as a rescue therapy in patients who failed to achieve sustained remission with the use of GCs or are refractory to GCs therapy. Less commonly it is also used as induction therapy.
- Patients with multiorgan or organ threatening involvement and very high baseline IgG4 levels may form the subset where upfront Rituximab could be indicated [1].
- In a French multicentric nationwide study, 42% of patients with IgG4-RD treated with rituximab relapsed [16].
- In a French multicentric nationwide study, 42% of patients with IgG4-RD treated with rituximab relapsed [16].
- Relapses are common after B cell reconstitution. So, maintenance therapy (i.e., before occurrence of relapse) with systematic Rituximab infusion (doses in the range of 300 mg to 1 gm, at fixed interval, usually every 6 months to 30 months) prolongs remission and decreases chances of relapse [16, 17].
- Rituximab maintenance therapy is even found to be better than combination of GCs and other immunosuppressants agents used for IgG4 RD [18].
- In a retrospective study from India (2020), Rituximab was administered (2–4 doses) in 12 patients who had disease relapse on steroids and immunomodulator therapy. All 12 patients responded well and achieved disease remission [1].

23.6.1.4 Side Effects

- Hypoalbuminemia or serious infections was seen in 33% of cases in a French nationwide study [16].
- Allergic reactions to the drug and reduced response with Rituximab are also noticed in some studies [13, 19, 20].

Consequently, there is an unmet need for drugs with a better efficacy and safety profile. Other therapies targeting B cells also appear promising.

23.6.2 Other Therapies Targeting B Cells

The apparent success of Rituximab by B cell depletion in IgG4-RD has generated interest in other agents targeting b cell lineage.

23.6.2.1 XmAb5871

- A phase II trial of XmAb5871, homodimer monoclonal antibodies which inhibit B cell by binding simultaneously to FcyRIIb and CD 19 is recently completed. Its preliminary results are promising.
- It can decrease the disease activity by suppressing B cell activation and proliferation [21, 22].

23.6.2.2 Bortezomib

- It inhibits auto-reactive plasma cells by targeting proteasome depletion and has proven to be successful in the treatment of multiple myeloma.
- A case report shows that it was effective in a patient with recurrent pulmonary infiltration with IgG4 plasma cells, consistent with IgG-RD [23].

23.6.2.3 Inebilizumab

- It depletes B cells by targeting CD19+ cells.
- A phase II b prospective, randomized trial studying the Efficacy and Safety of Inebilizumab in IgG4-Related Disease (clinicaltrials.gov:NCT04540497) is recruiting 160 patients and is expected to be completed in June 2024 [24].

23.6.3 T Cells Targeted Therapy

23.6.3.1 Abatacept

- It is an anti-cytotoxic T lymphocyte-associated protein 4 (CTLA 4) antibody and acts by preventing CD28 mediated T cell activation by targeting CD 80 and CD86 costimulatory molecules on antigen-presenting cells.
- Abatacept was reported to be effective in inducing and maintaining remission in one anecdotal report of a patient of rituximab resistant Mikulicz's disease and autoimmune pancreatitis [20, 21].
- Abatacept is recently being tested in Phase 2, single-center, proof-of-concept clinical trial [25].

23.6.4 B and T Cells Targeted Therapy

23.6.4.1 Elotuzumab

- It is an immuno-*stimulatory* monoclonal antibody directed against SLAMF7, is approved for the treatment of refractory multiple myeloma.

- SLAMF7 is a highly appealing therapeutic target as it is present in both B cells and CD4 CTLs.
- Depletion of activated cells that express this surface molecule will interfere with the interaction of CD4 CTLs and Antigen-presenting B cells and thus interfere with the pathogenesis of IgG4-RD.
- A proof-of-concept trial with Elumtuzumab is under development [8, 21].

23.6.5 Cytokine Inhibitors

Anecdotal case reports are also available on the use of *infliximab* and *dupilimab*.

23.6.5.1 Infliximab

- It is a chimeric anti-TNF agent that was successfully used in a patient with orbital pseudo-tumor refractory to other agents [26].

23.6.5.2 Dupilimab

- It is a monoclonal anti-interleukin 4 (IL-4) and IL-13 antibody.
- IL-4 causes isotype switching from IgM to IgG4 and IL-13 is implicated in fibrosis.
- It was successfully used in a patient with IgG4-RD with retroperitoneal fibrosis [27–29].

23.6.6 Other Possible Cytokine Targets

23.6.6.1 IL6 Inhibitor Tocilizumab

- IgG4RD with multiorgan involvement has raised serum Interleukin 6 levels.
- IL6 inhibitor *tocilizumab* was found to be useful in a patient with Multicentric Castleman's disease with pulmonary eosinophilic infiltrate.
- It is pathologically difficult to differentiate sometimes between Castleman's disease and IgG4RD, especially if there is an eosinophilic infiltrate, which is more common in IgG4RD.
- Successful use of tocilizumab in this case also indicates that IL6 inhibitors can be used in IgG4RD. Further studies are still needed to prove this [30, 31].

23.6.6.2 Anakinra and Canakinumab

- Increased levels of soluble Interleukin 1 receptors (IL1R) are seen in IgG4RD which is responsible for IL1 mediated tissue inflammation.
- So conceptually IL1R antagonists like *anakinra* and *canakinumab* may be used to dampen the IL1 mediated inflammation.
- But as yet studies and case reports are not available to support this theory [32].

23.6.7 Other Targets

23.6.7.1 Omalizumab

- *It* is a biological agent that acts by inhibiting the binding of IgE to the high-affinity IgE receptor (FCER1) on the surface of mast cells and Eosinophils.
- It may be of use in patients of IgG4 RD with atopic disease or asthma and elevated IgE levels.
- Omalizumab is also tried in some patients with IgG4-related eosinophilic esophagitis by Clayton et al. [33]

23.6.7.2 Eculizumab and Simtuzumab

- Inhibitors of complement activation targeting C5 and C5a (eculizumab), and disrupting extracellular matrix by targeting LOXL2 (Simtuzumab), theoretically are some other appealing targets to be studied in IgG4-RD [7].

23.7 Conclusion

Conventional treatment (GCs and immunomodulator) of IgG4-RD is associated with many long-term adverse effects and frequent relapses of this disease. With the growing understanding of the pathophysiology of the disease, targeted therapies are needed to achieve the unmet needs of these patients.

The pathogenesis of IgG4-RD involves abnormalities in multiple components of the immune system including B cells, T cells, and cytokines. Therapeutic agents targeting these mediators selectively are being tested for the treatment of IgG-RD. The growing understanding of the pathophysiology of IgG4-RD is leading to the identification of promising novel therapeutic targets and a new era of biological treatments. Some of the agents are already in use (e.g., Rituximab) and others are in clinical trials. Biological therapies hold much promise in IgG4-RD and as we become wiser about the disease and apply the lessons learned from recent trials, we will be able to develop more and more useful targeted drugs in future for this disease.

References

1. Duggal L, Singh B, Patel J, Gupta M, Grover A, Jain N. IgG4-related disease. JCR: J Clin Rheumatol. 2020; Publish Ahead of Print.
2. Stone J, Zen Y, Deshpande V. IgG4-related disease. N Engl J Med. 2012;366(6):539–51.
3. Kamisawa T, Zen Y, Pillai S, Stone J. IgG4-related disease. Lancet. 2015;385(9976):1460–71.
4. Khosroshahi A, Wallace Z, Crowe J, Akamizu T, Azumi A, Carruthers M, et al. International consensus guidance statement on the management and treatment of IgG4-related disease. Arthritis Rheumatol. 2015;67(7):1688–99.
5. Deheragoda M, Church N, Rodriguez-Justo M, Munson P, Sandanayake N, Seward E, et al. The use of immunoglobulin G4 immunostaining in diagnosing pancreatic and Extrapancreatic involvement in autoimmune pancreatitis. Clin Gastroenterol Hepatol. 2007;5(10):1229–34.

6. Kamisawa T, Okazaki K, Kawa S, Ito T, Inui K, Irie H, et al. Amendment of the Japanese consensus guidelines for autoimmune pancreatitis, 2013 III. Treatment and prognosis of autoimmune pancreatitis. J Gastroenterol. 2014;49(6):961–70.
7. Lanzillotta M, Mancuso G, Della-Torre E. Advances in the diagnosis and management of IgG4 related disease. BMJ. 2020;369:m1067.
8. Zhang W, Stone J. Management of IgG4-related disease. Lancet Rheumatol. 2019;1(1):e55–65.
9. Mattoo H, Mahajan V, Maehara T, Deshpande V, Della-Torre E, Wallace Z, et al. Clonal expansion of CD4+ cytotoxic T lymphocytes in patients with IgG4-related disease. J Allergy Clin Immunol. 2016;138(3):825–38.
10. Della-Torre E, Feeney E, Deshpande V, Mattoo H, Mahajan V, Kulikova M, et al. B-cell depletion attenuates serological biomarkers of fibrosis and myofibroblast activation in IgG4-related disease. Ann Rheum Dis. 2014;74(12):2236–43.
11. Della-Torre E, Rigamonti E, Perugino C, Baghai-Sain S, Sun N, Kaneko N, et al. B lymphocytes directly contribute to tissue fibrosis in patients with IgG4-related disease. J Allergy Clin Immunol. 2020;145(3):968–981.e14.
12. Della-Torre E, Campochiaro C, Cassione E, Albano L, Gerevini S, Bianchi-Marzoli S, et al. Intrathecal rituximab for IgG4-related hypertrophic pachymeningitis. J Neurol Neurosurg Psychiatry. 2017;89(4):441–4.
13. Della-Torre E, Conti A, Berti A, Yacoub M, Alessio M. Rituximab hypersensitivity in IgG4-related disease: successful desensitization in a patient with IgG4 rheumatoid factor. Int J Rheum Dis. 2016;20(2):276–9.
14. Carruthers M, Topazian M, Khosroshahi A, Witzig T, Wallace Z, Hart P, et al. Rituximab for IgG4-related disease: a prospective, open-label trial. Ann Rheum Dis. 2015;74(6):1171–7.
15. Wallwork R, Wallace Z, Perugino C, Sharma A, Stone J. Rituximab for idiopathic and IgG4-related retroperitoneal fibrosis. Medicine. 2018;97(42):e12631.
16. Ebbo M, Grados A, Samson M, Groh M, Loundou A, Rigolet A, et al. Long-term efficacy and safety of rituximab in IgG4-related disease: data from a French nationwide study of thirty-three patients. PLoS One. 2017;12(9):e0183844.
17. Majumder S, Mohapatra S, Lennon R, Piovezani Ramos G, Postier N, Gleeson F, et al. Rituximab maintenance therapy reduces rate of relapse of Pancreaticobiliary immunoglobulin G4-related disease. Clin Gastroenterol Hepatol. 2018;16(12):1947–53.
18. Omar D, Chen Y, Cong Y, Dong L. Glucocorticoids and steroid sparing medications monotherapies or in combination for IgG4-RD: a systematic review and network meta-analysis. Rheumatology. 2019;59(4):718–26.
19. Yamamoto M, Awakawa T, Takahashi H. Is rituximab effective for IgG4-related disease in the long term? Experience of cases treated with rituximab for 4 years. Ann Rheum Dis. 2015;74(8):e46.
20. Yamamoto M, Takahashi H, Takano K, Shimizu Y, Sakurai N, Suzuki C, et al. Efficacy of abatacept for IgG4-related disease over 8 months. Ann Rheum Dis. 2016;75(8):1576–8.
21. Perugino C, Mattoo H, Mahajan V, Maehara T, Wallace Z, Pillai S, et al. Emerging treatment models in rheumatology: IgG4-related disease: insights into human immunology and targeted therapies. Arthritis Rheumatol. 2017;69(9):1722–32.
22. Stone JH, Wallace ZS, Perugino CA, Fernandes AD, Patel P, Foster PA Zack DJ. Final results of an open label phase 2 study of a reversible B cell inhibitor, XmAb5871, in IgG4-related disease [abstract]. Arthritis Rheumatol 2017; 69(Suppl 10).
23. Khan M, Colby T, Viggiano R, Fonseca R. Treatment with Bortezomib of a patient having hyper IgG4 disease. Clin Lymphoma Myeloma Leuk. 2010;10(3):217–9.
24. A study of Inebilizumab efficacy and safety in IgG4- related disease – full text view - ClinicalTrials.gov [internet]. Clinicaltrialsgov 2021 [cited 20 June 2021]. Available from: https://clinicaltrials.gov/ct2/show/NCT04540497
25. Safety and efficacy of Abatacept in IgG4-related disease - full text view - ClinicalTrials.gov [internet]. Clinicaltrials.gov. 2021 [cited 20 June 2021]. Available from: https://clinicaltrials.gov/ct2/show/study/NCT03669861

26. Karim F, Paridaens D, Westenberg L, Guenoun J, Verdijk R, van Hagen P, et al. Infliximab for IgG4-related orbital disease. Ophthalmic Plast Reconstr Surg. 2017;33(3S):S162–5.
27. Simpson R, Lau S, Lee J. Dupilumab as a novel steroid-sparing treatment for IgG4-related disease. Ann Rheum Dis. 2019;79(4):549–50.
28. Ebbo M, De Sainte-Marie B, Muller R, Piperoglou C, Grados A, Vély F, et al. Comment on article: 'Dupilumab as a novel steroid-sparing treatment for IgG4-related disease' by Simpson et al. Ann Rheum Dis. 2020; https://doi.org/10.1136/annrheumdis-2020-217010.
29. Della-Torre E, Lanzillotta M, Yacoub M. Dupilumab as a potential steroid-sparing treatment for IgG4-related disease. Ann Rheum Dis. 2020; https://doi.org/10.1136/annrheumdis-2020-216945.
30. Ikeura T, Horitani S, Masuda M, Kasai T, Yanagawa M, Miyoshi H, et al. IgG4-related disease involving multiple organs with elevated serum Interleukin-6 levels. Intern Med. 2016;55(18):2623–8.
31. Katsumata Y, Ikari J, Tanaka N, Abe M, Tsushima K, Yonemori Y, et al. Tocilizumab-effective multicentric Castleman's disease with infiltration of eosinophil and IgG4-positive plasma cells: a case report. Respir Med Case Rep. 2018;25:25–9.
32. Capecchi R, Italiani P, Puxeddu I, Pratesi F, Tavoni A, Boraschi D, et al. IL-1 family cytokines and receptors in IgG4-related disease. Cytokine. 2018;102:145–8.
33. Clayton F, Fang J, Gleich G, Lucendo A, Olalla J, Vinson L, et al. Eosinophilic esophagitis in adults is associated with IgG4 and not mediated by IgE. Gastroenterology. 2014;147(3):602–9.

Biosimilars in Rheumatology 24

Mohit Goyal and Vinod Ravindran

24.1 Introduction

Biologic disease-modifying antirheumatic drugs (bDMARDs) although proven efficacious, have remained inaccessible for many people in large parts of the world owing to their high costs. The high cost has been a hindrance to their use even where conventional synthetic DMARDs (csDMARDs) have failed to suffice. After the expiration of patents of the originator bDMARDs, biosimilars have arrived as options with substantially lower costs. Cost reductions to the tune of 30–60% have been estimated with the use of biosimilars in USA, Denmark, and Norway [1].

Biosimilars by definition are molecules that are similar to the originator bDMARD taken as reference. They may not be identical to the reference product but exhibit a high degree of similarity in efficacy and safety and do not have any relevant differences with respect to the said parameters [2]. These agents are rigorously tested to ensure that they have the same primary amino acid sequence.

Declaration: The table included in the manuscript is original.

M. Goyal (✉)
Division of Rheumatology, CARE Pain & Arthritis Centre, Goyal Hospital, Udaipur, Rajasthan, India

V. Ravindran
Centre for Rheumatology, Calicut, Kerala, India

N. Jain, L. Duggal (eds.), *Handbook of Biologics for Rheumatological Disorders*,
https://doi.org/10.1007/978-981-16-7200-2_24

24.2 Biomimics and Biocopies

- Biosimilars differ from biomimics and biocopies in having to adhere to stringent regulations regarding their production process. The terms biocopies or intended copies are also used for products that were available in the market before regulations regarding biosimilars were put in place.
- Regulations vary from country to country but ensure a high degree of similarity before a product is labeled as a biosimilar. Two biocopies of etanercept marketed in China were found to have higher rates of adverse events, and a biomimic of rituximab marketed in Mexico was recalled after reports of anaphylactic reactions [3].
- Biosimilars available in the market have demonstrated efficacy and safety comparable to the originator bDMARDs [4].
- Biosimilars differ from generic drugs in that the latter are chemicals identical to the reference drug and have to only demonstrate similar pharmacokinetics in vitro for approval.

24.3 Development of Biosimilars

- For determining biosimilarity the products undergo a rigorous analysis of their pharmacokinetics and pharmacodynamics followed by assessment of the clinical data so as to demonstrate equivalent quality, biological activity, efficacy, and safety and to have no clinically significant difference when compared to the reference product [5].
- Biotherapeutic agents are proteins produced in living cells and are thus generally not identical to the reference product. However, biosimilars bear the same primary amino acid sequence and are usually produced in similar cell lines.
- Differences in secondary, tertiary, and quaternary structure as well as glycosylation and post-translational changes due to choices of host are permissible if it could be demonstrated that they do not cause significantly raised immunogenicity.
- Impurities that might creep in during the manufacturing process may however cause increased immunogenicity. Improved assays for detection of anti-drug antibodies have higher sensitivity and have led to reporting of a higher incidence of immunogenicity in more recent studies with biosimilars as well as originator bDMARDs [6].
- The process of producing a biosimilar drug starts with studying the amino acid sequence of the reference biologic agent and reverse-engineering the DNA sequence. The various factors that may lead to differences from the reference product are the choice of host cells and methods used for purification and stabilization of the product.
- Intentional as well as unintentional changes do occur in originator biologic products as well as biosimilars over a period of time.
- Certain changes are made by manufacturers; however, other unintentional changes may occur with changes in production processes and still others are attributable to drift and evolution.
- Even with drift and evolution, these products have shown continued efficacy and safety.

24.4 Evaluation of Proposed Biosimilars

- Equivalence approach for study designs to evaluate the efficacy and safety of biosimilars has been used in most countries. The approach focuses not on the proposed biosimilar being identical to the reference product but on it being within a predetermined range of the reference product.
- Meta-analyses of multiple placebo-controlled trials of the originator molecule may serve as a reference for determining the range for equivalence in studies designed to evaluate a potential biosimilar.
- A non-inferiority approach for comparing proposed biosimilars with reference products has been mentioned in the guideline on the evaluation of biosimilars by the World Health Organisation (WHO) [2].
- Compared to the equivalence approach, in the non-inferiority approach, the biosimilar product may even be superior to the reference product. The fault-line though lies in that a proposed biosimilar evaluated through a non-inferiority trial may be superior to the reference product in efficacy but at the same time be more toxic and thus end up being only a "bio-better" and not biosimilar.

24.5 Regulations for Biosimilars

- Regulations have been put in place by the European Medicines Agency (EMA), the US Food and Drug Administration (FDA), and similar authorities in various countries. The International Committee on Harmonisation (ICH) guidance for permissible variations in biological products has been extended to biosimilars [7].
- The regulatory process starts with a thorough structural and functional preclinical analysis of the proposed biosimilar. The product is then subjected to clinical assessment of its pharmacokinetic and pharmacodynamic properties.
- The US FDA mandates at least one clinical trial comparing the proposed biosimilar to the reference product in patients with the disease and demonstrating equivalent efficacy, adverse effect profile, and immunogenicity.
- Like the reference products, biosimilars also exhibit immunogenicity and regulations demand measurement of both binding as well as neutralizing anti-drug antibodies (ADAbs). The measure of immunogenicity is of utmost importance as high anti-drug antibodies lead to lower trough levels of the drug and reduced efficacy.
- Regulations in certain countries for certain biosimilars may also require studies involving switching from the originator bDMARD to the proposed biosimilar and measurement of consequent change if any in the immunogenicity.
- The current evidence suggests that antibodies to the reference drug cross-react with its biosimilars and thus switching to a biosimilar when a patient develops antibodies to the reference product is not advocated.
- The regulatory pathway outlined by the EMA requires a thorough in-vitro analysis of the proposed biosimilar's structure and function. In-vivo studies may not be necessary if there are no post-translational changes noted in the molecule.
- The EMA in 2013 allowed the use of CT-P13, biosimilar infliximab for all the indications of the reference product.

- In USA, biosimilars are named with the common non-proprietary name followed by a 4-letter suffix. CT-P13 or Infliximab-dyyb marketed by the proprietary name Inflectra was the first biosimilar used in rheumatology to be approved by the US FDA in 2016.

24.6 Switching, Substitution, Interchangeability, and Extrapolation

- Switching implies changing from one product to another by the treating doctor on account of loss of efficacy or side effects.
- Substitution on the other hand is done for non-medical reasons by somebody other than the prescribing doctor, for example by the pharmacist or by the payer and is in most cases governed by the cost.
- Studies have demonstrated that switching from an originator biologic molecule to its biosimilar is safe and there is no loss of efficacy.
- Decision to change to a biosimilar from the reference product may be taken by the doctor in view of cost.
- A reference product and its biosimilar are designated "interchangeable" when it has been established through data that switching between the two does not result in loss of efficacy or safety and these two parameters for the biosimilar are no different from when the reference product is used continuously without a switch.
- Extrapolation refers to extending the indications of biosimilars to other indications of the reference biologic agent (apart from that for which the biosimilar was studied).
- PLANETAS and PLANETRA studies demonstrated the similarity of Infliximab-dyyb to the reference product in patients with Ankylosing Spondylitis (AS) and Rheumatoid Arthritis (RA), respectively [8, 9]. There was an initial uneasiness about the extension of the indications of this biosimilar to Inflammatory Bowel Disease (IBD). NOR-SWITCH and some post-marketing studies however provided reassuring data regarding the use of this biosimilar in Crohn's disease [10].
- Most biosimilars have not been studied in childhood rheumatic conditions but have been used by extrapolation.

24.7 Clinical Experience with Biosimilars

While the Asian countries were quicker to embrace the biosimilars, with time, biosimilars of infliximab, etanercept, adalimumab as well as rituximab have been approved by the US FDA and the EMA.

24.7.1 Biosimilars of Infliximab

- PLANETRA and PLANETAS were landmark studies for evaluation of the infliximab biosimilar, CT-P13, which led to its approval later for treatment of RA and AS.
- PLANETAS found comparable ASAS20 and ASAS40 responses to the biosimilar and the reference product at 14, 30, and 54 weeks.

- PLANETRA, where the originator and biosimilar infliximab were used in combination with methotrexate, found similar ACR20, ACR50, and ACR70 responses in both groups and also similar safety profiles.
- Extrapolation of indications of CT-P13 was allowed in many countries to include psoriasis, psoriatic arthritis (PsA) and IBD. The extrapolation to IBD was not allowed in Canada on account of certain differences from the originator molecule in structure and antibody-dependant cell-mediated cytotoxicity (ADCC) assays.
- Monoclonal antibodies have a functionally active Fc region, that induces ADCC, which seems to play an important role in their efficacy in IBD. Support for the same comes from the inefficacy of etanercept and certolizumab, which lack the power to induce ADCC, in IBD.
- Studies conducted later though have shown the efficacy of CT-P13 in IBD [8–10].
- A double-blind, active comparator trial found an infliximab biosimilar, BOW015 to be equivalent to the originator product in patients with rheumatoid arthritis, which led to its approval in India. Its usage in the country has been extended to other indications of the originator molecule [11].

24.7.2 Biosimilars of Etanercept

- HERA, a South Korean study that compared HD203, an etanercept biosimilar with the originator molecule in patients with rheumatoid arthritis found the proposed biosimilar to be equivalent [12]. Here, researchers allocated 294 patients in a 1:1 proportion to be administered the reference drug or HD203. The primary endpoint of ACR20 response at 12 weeks as well as the secondary endpoints were met. There were no significant differences in the adverse event rates and the discontinuation rates, and both the reference product and HD203 exhibited low immunogenicity.
- Researchers from India shared their data on the use of two etanercept biosimilars in patients with spondyloarthritis and found both to be effective and safe [4].

24.7.3 Biosimilars of Adalimumab and Rituximab

- ZRC-3197, a biosimilar adalimumab used in India for RA, AS, and PsA is said to be identical to the originator molecule in terms of efficacy, adverse effect profile, purity, and immunogenicity [13]. It was later also approved for use in ulcerative colitis and Crohn's disease.
- Researchers from India have reported biosimilars of rituximab to be effective in patients with seropositive [14] as well as seronegative [15] RA.

24.8 Biosimilars in Other Fields

- The use of biosimilars in oncology started much before than in rheumatology in Europe. The availability of equivalent yet more cost-effective therapeutic agents enhanced reach and thus transformed cancer care [16].
- Availability of rituximab biosimilars at much lesser costs has been helpful toward improving oncology care in India.

A representative list of originator bDMARDs, date of expiration of their patents, and available biosimilars is given in Table 24.1.

Table 24.1 Originator biologic disease-modifying anti-rheumatic drugs and their currently approved biosimilars (as of March 2021)

Originator drug	Patent expired/expiring (Country)	Biosimilars in use (Country) (Since)
Remicade (infliximab)	February 2015 (Europe) September 2018 (US)	Infimab (India) (September 2014) Inflectra (Europe) (September 2013) Remsima (Europe) (September 2013) Flixabi (Europe) (May 2016) Zessly (Europe) (May 2018) Inflectra (USA) (April 2016) Renflexis (USA) (April 2017) Ixifi (USA) (December 2017) Avsola (USA) (December 2019)
Enbrel (etanercept)	August 2015 (Europe) November 2028 (USA)	Etacept (India) (April 2013) Intacept (India) (March 2015) Benepali (Europe) (January 2016) Erelzi (Europe) (June 2017) Nepexto (Europe) (May 2020) Erelzi (USA) (August 2016) Eticovo (USA) (April 2019)
Humira (adalimumab)	October 2018 (Europe) January 2023 (USA)	Exemptia (India) (December 2014) AdaliRel (India) (January 2016) Solymbic (Europe) (March 2017) Amgevita (Europe) (March 2017) Imraldi (Europe) (August 2017) Mabura (India) (January 2018) Halimatoz (Europe) (July 2018) Hefiya (Europe) (July 2018) Hyrimoz (Europe) (July 2018) Hulio (Europe) (September 2018) Idacio (Europe) (April 2019) Amsparity (Europe) (February 2020) Yuflyma (Europe) (February 2021) Amjevita (USA) (September 2016) Cyltezo (USA) (August 2017) Hyrimoz (USA) (October 2018) Hadlima (USA) (July 2019) Abrilada (USA) (November 2019) Hulio (USA) (July 2020)
MabThera (rituximab)	November 2013 (Europe) September 2016 (USA)	Reditux (India) (April 2007) MabTas (India) (February 2013) Maball (India) (February 2015) RituxiRel (India) (February 2015) Truxima (Europe) (February 2017) Rixathon (Europe) (June 2017) Riximyo (Europe) (June 2017) Blitzima (Europe) (July 2017) Ritemvia (Europe) (July 2017) Ruxience (Europe) (April 2020) Truxima (USA) (November 2018) Ruxience (USA) (July 2019) Riabni (USA) (December 2020)

24.9 Challenges

- Switching and extrapolation of indications still remain challenges in the field of biosimilars. Drift and evolution do occur continuously, but the product does not require additional testing until the variations are within prespecified limits.
- Due to the enhanced availability of biosimilars and continually declining costs, multiple switching is imminent in future and that mandates a better understanding of the process.
- Shared experiences have not found any major safety risks with switching but the lack of large studies involving multiple switching and consequent lack of guidelines for the same do pose a significant challenge to our understanding and predictability of response in such clinical settings.
- Head-to-head studies are not possible for all indications of any molecule but the use of correct molecular processes in the development of biosimilars can help predict its efficacy in all indications of the reference product.
- The regulations pertaining to extrapolation vary between countries.
- The EMA looks at biosimilars on a case-to-case basis and allows extrapolation after looking at the totality of evidence.
- The US FDA looks at the scientific justification and the totality of evidence.
- CT-P13 when marketed had the same US FDA and EMA label as the reference product, whereas Canada which has more stringent regulations even for minor variations did not initially approve its use for IBD owing to structural and functional differences with reference product.
- Studies have found that ADAbs are more frequent in individuals with RA than those with AS. Theoretically, this could be a potential reason to not extrapolate the use of a biosimilar (studied for AS) to RA even when the originator product is licensed for RA.
- But a majority of these factors are hypothetical and robust registries and post-marketing data collection should help dispel the fears if any.

24.10 Summary

- Biosimilars are molecules produced in confirmation with stringent regulatory processes such that they are equivalent in efficacy, safety, and purity to the reference product.
- With proper regulations in place, a high degree of similarity with the reference products can be ascertained before a proposed biosimilar is licensed for use.
- Biosimilars have enhanced the reach and use of biotherapeutic agents by substantially lowering the cost of therapy. These agents are beginning to be embraced by markets and healthcare regulators across the world.
- With more experience likely to be gained from post-marketing data, extrapolation would be done with higher confidence, which would further enhance the switching from an originator to a biosimilar.

References

1. Doheny K. Biosimilars and Rheumatology: how popular will they be? Practical Pain Management. https://www.practicalpainmanagement.com/pain/myofascial/biosimilars-rheumatology-how-popular-will-they-be. Accessed 21 November 2021.
2. WHO | GUIDELINES ON EVALUATION OF SIMILAR BIOTHERAPEUTIC PRODUCTS, WHO. https://www.who.int/biologicals/areas/biological_therapeutics/BIOTHERAPEUTICS_FOR_WEB_22APRIL2010.pdf. Accessed 21 November 2021.
3. Dörner T, Kay J. Biosimilars in rheumatology: current perspectives and lessons learnt. Nat Rev Rheumatol. 2015;11(12):713–24. https://doi.org/10.1038/nrrheum.2015.110.
4. Kumar A, Goel A, Lapsiwala M, Goyal M, Dembla G. Clinical experience with two etanercept biosimilars in Indian patients with spondyloarthritis. Indian J Rheumatol. 2017;12(3):139. https://doi.org/10.4103/injr.injr_40_17.
5. Biosimilar Development, Review, and Approval | FDA. https://www.fda.gov/drugs/biosimilars/biosimilar-developmentreview-and-approval. Accessed 21 November 2021.
6. Biosimilars for prescribers - GaBI Journal. http://gabi-journal.net/biosimilars-for-prescribers.html. Accessed 21 November 2021.
7. Abraham J. International Conference on Harmonisation of technical requirements for registration of pharmaceuticals for human use. In: Brouder A, Tietje C, eds. Handbook of transnational economic governance regimes. Brill; 2009:1041–1054. https://doi.org/10.1163/ej.9789004163300.i-1081.897.
8. Park W, Hrycaj P, Jeka S, et al. A randomised, double-blind, multicentre, parallel-group, prospective study comparing the pharmacokinetics, safety, and efficacy of CT-P13 and innovator infliximab in patients with ankylosing spondylitis: the PLANETAS study. Ann Rheum Dis. 2013;72(10):1605–12. https://doi.org/10.1136/annrheumdis-2012-203091.
9. Yoo DH, Hrycaj P, Miranda P, et al. A randomised, double-blind, parallel-group study to demonstrate equivalence in efficacy and safety of CT-P13 compared with innovator infliximab when coadministered with methotrexate in patients with active rheumatoid arthritis: the PLANETRA study. Ann Rheum Dis. 2013;72(10):1613–20. https://doi.org/10.1136/annrheumdis-2012-203090.
10. Jørgensen KK, Olsen IC, Goll GL, et al. Switching from originator infliximab to biosimilar CT-P13 compared with maintained treatment with originator infliximab (NOR-SWITCH): a 52-week, randomised, double-blind, non-inferiority trial. Lancet Lond Engl. 2017;389(10086):2304–16. https://doi.org/10.1016/S0140-6736(17)30068-5.
11. Kay J, Chopra A, Chandrashekara S, et al. OP0012 a phase 3, randomized, double-blind, active comparator study of the efficacy and safety of Bow015, a biosimilar infliximab, in patients with active rheumatoid arthritis on stable methotrexate doses. Ann Rheum Dis. 2014;73(Suppl 2):64. https://doi.org/10.1136/annrheumdis-2014-eular.1595.
12. Bae S-C, Kim J, Choe J-Y, et al. A phase III, multicentre, randomised, double-blind, active-controlled, parallel-group trial comparing safety and efficacy of HD203, with innovator etanercept, in combination with methotrexate, in patients with rheumatoid arthritis: the HERA study. Ann Rheum Dis. 2017;76(1):65–71. https://doi.org/10.1136/annrheumdis-2015-207613.
13. Adalimumab similar biologic launched in India/News/Biosimilars/Home - GaBI Online - Generics and Biosimilars Initiative. http://gabionline.net/Biosimilars/News/Adalimumab-similar-biologic-launched-in-India. Accessed 21 November 2021.
14. Roshique KK, Ravindran V. Efficacy and safety of a biosimilar rituximab in biologic naïve patients with active rheumatoid arthritis. Clin Rheumatol. 2015;34(7):1289–92. https://doi.org/10.1007/s10067-015-2980-4.
15. Jamshid N, Ravindran V. No impact of seronegativity on the efficacy of a biosimilar rituximab in biologic-naïve patients with active rheumatoid arthritis. Indian J Rheumatol. 2019;14(1):77. https://doi.org/10.4103/injr.injr_158_18.
16. Gascón P, Tesch H, Verpoort K, et al. Clinical experience with Zarzio® in Europe: what have we learned? Support Care Cancer. 2013;21(10):2925–32. https://doi.org/10.1007/s00520-013-1911-7.

Off-Label Use of Biologics in Rheumatological Disorders

25

Sumantro Mondal and Alakendu Ghosh

25.1 Introduction

Biologic drugs are produced from human, animal, or living organisms. Currently, biologics are widely used to treat different diseases. In rheumatic diseases, licensed use of biologic started more than 20 years back for the treatment of Rheumatoid arthritis (RA). European medicines agency (EMA) and the United States food and drug administration (USFDA) are the regulatory agencies for the approval of b-DMARDs in the European Union and the US, respectively. Off-label indication means using a drug to treat a disease or certain manifestation of a disease for which that particular drug is not officially approved. At present, biologics are approved for use in RA, Ankylosing spondylitis (AS), Psoriatic arthritis (PsA), anti-neutrophilic cytoplasmic antibody (ANCA) associated vasculitis, giant cell arteritis (GCA), etc. Interestingly, biologics are also used as an off-label drug to treat various other rheumatic diseases, and these off-label uses of biologics will be reviewed in this chapter.

25.2 Commonly Used Biological DMARDs in Rheumatic Diseases

Most of the b-DAMRDs target various pro-inflammatory cytokines. b-DMARDs targeting, IL-6 (Tocilizumab), Rituximab (anti-CD 20 monoclonal antibody), Anti-tumor necrosis factor-α (TNF-α) agents, anti-IL-1 agents (Anakinra, Rilonacept, Canakinumab), anti-IL-17A (secukinumab, ixekizumab), or anti-IL-17 receptor (brodalumab) are commonly used for the management of various rheumatic diseases.

S. Mondal · A. Ghosh (✉)
Department of Rheumatology, IPGME&R, Kolkata, India

N. Jain, L. Duggal (eds.), *Handbook of Biologics for Rheumatological Disorders*,
https://doi.org/10.1007/978-981-16-7200-2_25

25.2.1 Tocilizumab

- Tocilizumab is a humanized monoclonal antibody, which targets both membrane-bound and soluble IL-6 receptor alpha subunit, thereby preventing the binding of IL-6 with its receptor with subsequent inhibition of downstream signalling of IL-6 [1].
- It is approved for use in RA (moderate to severe) and also in systemic-onset and polyarticular Juvenile Idiopathic Arthritis (JIA).

In 2017 it was approved in both US and EU for the treatment of Giant cell arteritis, the first b-DMARD to get approval for this large vessel vasculitis (LVV). In addition to the approved indications, Tocilizumab has shown promising results in some other rheumatic conditions.

25.2.1.1 Takayasu Arteritis (TA)

- TA is an LVV that classically affects the aorta and its major branches and is associated with significant morbidity. The beneficial role of Tocilizumab, especially in the refractory cases of TA, has been documented in some recent studies [2, 3].
- Apart from symptomatic improvement in TA patients, Tocilizumab therapy can reduce the mean prednisolone dose, ESR value, and Indian Takayasu Arteritis Activity Score (ITAS2010). In some of the patients, there was an improvement of disease status as evaluated by MRI.
- Tocilizumab is more efficacious and has a better safety profile in comparison to the Cyclophosphamide. Few case reports and small case series showed the efficacy and safety of Tocilizumab in pediatric patient with TA as well [4].
- The recently published French TOCITAKA trial concluded that Tocilizumab may be an effective steroid-sparing agent in TA [5]. According to the 2018 EULAR recommendation for the management of LVV, Tocilizumab may be used in relapsing and refractory TA.

25.2.1.2 Adult-Onset Still Disease (AOSD)

- Though any prospective study is still lacking, case reports and series have shown a promising role of Tocilizumab in this disease. Tocilizumab can improve clinical features and reduction in acute phase reactants in AOSD [6].
- Tocilizumab may be more effective for the management of the chronic articular symptoms of AOSD. Importantly, it has been shown that Tocilizumab increases the probability of corticosteroid withdrawal in patients with AOSD [7].
- Tocilizumab is currently used as an off-label drug in steroid-refractory AOSD patients and is a promising drug for the management of conventional treatment-resistant AOSD.

25.2.1.3 Systemic Sclerosis (SSc)

It has been found that serum level of IL 6 correlates with the disease activity and internal organ involvement in SSc.

- In phase 2, randomized, placebo-controlled trial (faSScinate), the efficacy and safety of subcutaneous Tocilizumab were assessed in SSc patients. There was some evidence of less reduction of forced vital capacity (FVC) in the Tocilizumab group; however, reduction in the skin thickening did not show statistical significance.
- In the open-label extension of the same trial, improvement in the skin score and FVC stabilization were maintained. Improvements of both these parameters were also observed among placebo-treated patients who were shifted to the Tocilizumab group in the open-label extension phase [8, 9]. Subsequently, one multicenter, phase 3 trial with subcutaneous tocilizumab 162 mg/week for 48 weeks failed to meet the primary endpoint of improvement of the skin fibrosis; however, it may have some role in preserving the lung function in early SSC [10]. So, it is evident that Tocilizumab may have some role in preventing pulmonary fibrosis in SSC, but not on skin fibrosis. Further studies are required to come to a definite conclusion regarding the utility of Tocilizumab in SSc.

25.2.1.4 Behcet's Disease (BD)

- BD is a multi-organ disease, predominantly affecting skin, mucous membrane, vascular system, eye, and nervous system. Uveitis is commonly seen in BD.
- In a small study, Tocilizumab was used in 11 patients with BD-associated uveitis. There was an improvement in visual acuity, retinal vasculitis, and vitritis in Tocilizumab-treated patients along with a reduction of the number of blood cells in the anterior chamber of the eye. Reduction of steroid dose was also observed [11].

A recent systematic literature review concluded that Tocilizumab could be an alternative treatment option for the refractory ocular, neuro, and vascular symptoms of BD, and also for secondary amyloidosis [12].

25.2.1.5 Polymyalgia Rheumatica (PMR)

- It is a disease of the elderly, characterized by pain and stiffness, especially of shoulder and hip girdles. This condition shows good response to corticosteroid, but adverse effects of steroids is a major concern. Sometimes the disease may be recurring.
- Currently, Tocilizumab is used as a second-line treatment for PMR. A recently published, prospective, open-label study with twenty new-onset PMR patients, Tocilizumab was used as first-line therapy. Results showed good efficacy and steroid-sparing action of Tocilizumab in PMR, indicating a promising role of Tocilizumab in this disease [13]. The large GiACTA trial with 250 patients with GCA received either TCZ weekly or every other week.
- The result showed that TCZ improved clinical outcomes in patients who presented with PMR or cranial symptoms only or both, and another trial showed quick improvement of the inflammatory markers with Tocilizumab in early PMR [14, 15].

25.2.2 Rituximab

Rituximab is a chimeric (murine/human) monoclonal antibody of the IgG1 kappa subclass which is directed against the CD20 antigen expressed on the surface of pre-B cells and mature B cells. After binding with the CD 20, expressed on the cell surface, Rituximab induces apoptosis of these cells and depletion of peripheral B cell pool. It is approved by EMA for the treatment of adult RA patients who are intolerant to or inadequate responders to other DMARDs or anti-TNF therapy. It is also approved for ANCA-associated small-vessel vasculitis. This drug, though not approved, is still frequently used in some of the other rheumatic diseases.

25.2.2.1 Systemic Lupus Erythematosus (SLE)

- SLE is a multisystem autoimmune disease characterized by distinct clinical features and the presence of certain subsets of autoantibodies. The level of anti-ds-DNA antibody, one of the most specific autoantibodies of SLE, positively correlates with the disease activity of SLE.
- In the earlier trials (EXPLORER and LUNAR), Rituximab failed to meet the primary endpoints in SLE. In the EXPLORER trial with 257 SLE patients who had moderate to severe active extra-renal features, Rituximab did not show any difference compared to the placebo, however, a beneficial effect of rituximab was noted among the African American and Hispanic subgroups [16].
- In contrast to the EXPLORER trial, LUNAR was conducted to find the efficacy of Rituximab in class III/IV renal histology SLE patients but failed to achieve the primary outcome. The positive findings of this study were greater reductions in anti-dsDNA and C3/C4 levels and more responders in the Rituximab group [17]. In contrast to these trials, the beneficial role of Rituximab in SLE has been documented by other studies.
- In a retrospective, longitudinal study of lupus patients who were non-responders to standard therapy (LESIMAB), Rituximab therapy achieved response in 62.9% of patients at 6 months. This study highlighted the efficacy of Rituximab in refractory and life-threatening SLE [18].
- The efficacy of Rituximab in patients with active SLE, SLE with active nephritis, SLE with autoimmune cytopenia, biopsy-proven SLE nephropathy, and mild to moderately active SLE has been supported by various studies [19].
- In the study by Condon MB, et al. where 50 consecutive SLE nephritis patients were treated with two doses of rituximab (1 g) and methylprednisolone (500 mg) on days 1 and 15, and Mycophenolate mofetil as maintenance treatment, complete or partial remission was observed in 90% of patients. Among the 45 responders, only two required steroids for more than 2 weeks. In contrast to the EXPLORER and LUNAR trials, this study showed both the efficacy and steroid-sparing effect of Rituximab in SLE nephritis [20].
- It has been found that earlier initiation of Rituximab in SLE patients has good efficacy and steroid-sparing capacity. Long-term follow-up (up to 7 years) study by Gracia-Tello B et al. also supports this notion [21].

- Rituximab is currently not licensed for use in SLE, but it is used as an off-label drug in severe SLE nephritis and autoimmune cytopenia in SLE. Sequential therapy of Rituximab followed by Belimumab (BLyS inhibitor) is theoretically more attractive in the management of SLE.

25.2.2.2 Systemic Sclerosis (SSc)

- The role of the B cells in the pathogenesis of SSc has already been established, so B cell-targeted therapy may be effective in this multisystem disease. Some of the retrospective analyses, case reports, and uncontrolled trials have demonstrated the beneficial effect of Rituximab, especially for skin, lung, and articular involvement [22].
- A recently published open-label, randomized controlled trial from India showed the efficacy and safety of Rituximab as a primary treatment modality for the skin and lung manifestation (ILD) of SSc. In this comparative study between Rituximab and intravenous Cyclophosphamide, improvement in the forced vital capacity (FVC) was observed in the Rituximab group at 6 months, whereas FVC declined in the Cyclophosphamide group. There was a better improvement of the modified Rodnan skin score with Rituximab [23].
- Improvement in the FVC is a very promising finding of this study as lung involvement is one of the important causes of both morbidity and mortality in SSc patients. Further RCTs are required in this aspect, especially regarding the long-term outcome of Rituximab in lung manifestation of SSc before getting its approval.

25.2.2.3 Sjogren Syndrome (SS)

- SS is another autoimmune disease where B cells play an important role in pathogenesis.
- Currently, Rituximab is used for the extra glandular manifestations of SS, including vasculitis, nervous system manifestations, etc.
- An earlier trial showed that Rituximab could reduce fatigue in patients with SS [24]. This finding is, however, not supported by a recent multicenter, randomized, double-blind, placebo-controlled trial in which Rituximab failed to show any benefit in relieving fatigue and pain in SS patients. The unstimulated salivary flow rate was increased in the Rituximab group compared to the placebo, but it was not translated clinically to the improvement of oral dryness [25].
- It is important to note that the efficacy of Rituximab in SS-associated ILD was not assessed in this study, which may be as high as 78% among newly diagnosed SS patients [26].
- One retrospective study documented the efficacy of Rituximab in the improvement of pulmonary function in SS patients. Contrary to the findings of Bowman SJ et al. this study also showed that Rituximab therapy could cause a symptomatic improvement of dryness and fatigue in SS [27].

25.2.2.4 Idiopathic Inflammatory Myositis (IIM)

- IIM is a cluster of multisystem diseases predominantly characterized by the weakness of the proximal muscles. Myositis-specific or myositis-associated autoantibodies are seen in a large number of patients of IIM, suggesting a pathogenic role of B cells in this disease.
- Corticosteroids and second-line immunosuppressants like, Methotrexate, Azathioprine is currently used for the treatment of IIM.
- Considering the role of B cells in the pathogenesis of IIM, Rituximab is used as an off-label drug in this condition. In one RCT, where Rituximab was used in refractory IIM, including both adult and juvenile populations, improvement was seen in 83% of patients [28].
- In addition to the improvement of muscular symptoms, Rituximab may also be effective in the treatment of refractory ILD associated with anti-synthatase syndrome [29].
- Based on these observations, currently off-label use of Rituximab in IIM is restricted to refractory muscle, lung, or skin disease of Dermatomyositis.

25.2.3 Anti-TNF α Agents

TNF-α plays an important role in the pathogenesis of multiple rheumatic diseases, including RA and SpA. It also modulates the production of other cytokines during the process of inflammation, acting as a master regulator of the inflammatory process. Consequently, b-DMARDs targeting TNF-α were started almost three decades back for the treatment of RA, and Etanercept was the first b-DMARD that got approval for the treatment of RA. Anti-TNF-α agents are currently licensed for use in RA, AS, and Psoriatic arthritis. These drugs (except Infliximab) are approved by the EMA for the management of non-radiographic axial SpA, but not by USFDA, until March 2019, when Certolizumab pegol got USFDA approval for this condition. Anti-TNF agents are also used as an off-label drug in certain other rheumatic diseases.

25.2.3.1 Sarcoidosis

A chronic granulomatous disease with multisystem involvement. TNF-α is considered to play a role in the formation of sarcoid granuloma, justifying their off-label use in this disease. Interestingly, not all anti-TNF drugs showed efficacy in Sarcoidosis.

- Golimumab and Etanercept did not show any better efficacy than placebo, whereas Infliximab and Adalimumab were effective. Infliximab has a beneficial role in pulmonary Sarcoidosis, and it can increase FVC in patients with Sarcoidosis; however, improvement can be observed after 6 weeks. Improvement in chest imaging can also be observed after 6 weeks. A better response is seen in patients with elevated C reactive protein and who are on <20 mg of prednisone at the time of initiation of Infliximab [30, 31].

- Adalimumab can also improve FVC in Sarcoidosis, and both of these drugs can improve quality of life and symptom severity in patients. It is also reported that Infliximab may be effective for Sarcoidosis of other locations like ocular, hepatic, nervous system, etc. [32].
- At present, Infliximab is used as an off-label drug in the management of refractory pulmonary Sarcoidosis not responding to steroid and second-line drugs.

25.2.3.2 Uveitis in Rheumatic Diseases

- Uveitis is commonly associated with SpA, JIA (oligoarticular and enthesitis-related arthritis), Behcet's disease, Sarcoidosis. Recurrent uveitis can cause varying degrees of visual impairment, so timely intervention is very much necessary. Studies in animals and humans support the role of TNF-α in the pathogenesis of uveitis.
- Adalimumab is already approved by USFDA for non-infectious uveitis. Infliximab also showed its efficacy in the treatment of uveitis associated with Ankylosing spondylitis and JIA.
- Golimumab showed a favorable result in the management of refractory uveitis associated with SpA.
- The efficacy outcome with Etanercept is somewhat different with a high recurrence rate, and even new-onset uveitis in Etanercept treated patients has been reported [33].
- Infliximab is also useful in refractory posterior uveitis of Behcet's disease, and complete response was noted in 68% of patients in one study. Infliximab can also improve visual acuity in this group of patients [34]. The efficacy and safety of Infliximab for 10 years in refractory uveitis of BD have also been documented [35]. Based on these observations, Infliximab is used as an off-label drug in the management of refractory uveitis associated with certain rheumatic diseases.

25.2.3.3 Behcet's Disease (BD)

- In addition to the management of refractory uveitis, anti-TNF agents also seem to be effective in extraocular features of this variable vessel vasculitis. Few case series and case reports have demonstrated the efficacy of Infliximab in controlling gastrointestinal, central nervous system, and vascular manifestations of BD.
- In Methotrexate and steroid-resistant neuro BD, Infliximab therapy can cause both symptomatic and improvement and regression of parenchymal lesions [36].

25.2.3.4 Kawasaki Disease (KD)

- KD is a childhood-onset, medium vessel vasculitis. The most dreaded complication of KD is coronary artery aneurism (CAA) which can develop in 15–25% of patients without treatment.
- TNF-α again is implicated in the pathogenesis of KD and Infliximab has been used in various studies to find out its efficacy in this disease. Results of these studies are most promising, and one recent trial showed that Infliximab treatment could reduce the incidence of significant CAA, even in IVIG-resistant KD patients. Previously one large RCT showed that the addition of Infliximab as a

primary treatment of KD could reduce fever duration and the Z score of the left anterior descending coronary artery.

- Infliximab can achieve a significantly more defervescence rate than IV polyethylene glycol-treated human immunoglobulin in IVIG-resistant KD [37–39]. Based on these observations, Infliximab is used as an off-label drug in patients with refractory KD.

25.2.4 Anti IL-1 Agents

- Anakinra, an anti-IL 1 b-DMARD was initially approved for the treatment of RA. Based on the important role of IL 1 in the pathogenesis of various autoinflammatory diseases and the success of IL 1 targeted therapy in these diseases, EMA approved this drug for the management of the cryopyrin-associated periodic syndromes (CAPS) and AOSD.
- Canakinumab, another anti-IL 1 agent is approved for the CAPS, systemic-onset JIA, and acute gouty arthritis. The off-label uses of these drugs are much more than its approved indications.
- A retrospective analysis from Italy showed that off-label use of Anakinra and Canakinumab is as high as 86% and 56%, respectively. Anti-IL 1 agents, were used as an off-label drug in patients with BD, Chronic Recurrent Multifocal Osteomyelitis (CRMO), Familial Mediterranean Fever (FMF), and Tumor Necrosis Factor Receptor-Associated Periodic Syndrome (TRAPS) [40].
- One recently published open-label study showed partial efficacy of Anakinra in the treatment of resistant oral and genital ulcers in patients with BD [41]. In a single-center study from Turkey with 36 FMF patients, Anakinra showed its effectiveness in those who were inadequate responders to colchicine, and in FMF-associated amyloidosis [42]. Similarly, in addition to its licensed indications, Canakinumab may be useful in FMF and TRAPS [43, 44]. Anti-IL 1 agents are particularly useful for the primary treatment-resistant autoinflammatory syndromes.

25.2.5 Anti IL-17 Agents

Secukinumab, an IL-17A neutralizing antibody, is already approved for the management of AS, PsA. It is used as an off-label drug in patients with SAPHO syndrome to improve the skin lesion and osteitis seen in this disease [45].

25.3 Conclusion

It is evident from the above discussion is that the b-DMARDs are used as an off-label drug in numerous rheumatic diseases, and the numbers of these off-label uses are not less than their licensed indications. Adequate numbers of RCT s lack in this context, and the off-label uses of b-DMARDs are mostly based on the positive results of uncontrolled trials or case series. It is expected that the licensed indications of b-DMARDs will expand in the future (Table 25.1).

Table 25.1 Approved and off-label indications of different b-DMARDs

Name of b-DMARD	Approved indications (by EMA or USFDA)	Off-label indications
Tocilizumab	• Adults with moderate to severe active RA not responding to cs-DMARDs or TNF blockers. • Children with active SOJIA and pJIA not responding to conventional therapy. • Refractory GCA	• Refractory TA • AOSD • SSc • BD (for ocular disease) • PMR (second line treatment option)
Rituximab	• Adults with moderate to severe active RA not responding to cs-DMARDs or TNF blockers. (with methotrexate) • In severe, active GPA and MPA (for remission induction and follow-up treatment)	• Refractory SLE nephritis and autoimmune cytopenia in SLE • SSc (for skin and ILD), • Sjogren syndrome (ILD, and probably for fatigue/ dryness). • IIM (refractory myositis, skin disease and ILD of ASS)
Anti-TNF agents	• Active RA, • Severe, active AS and PSA (inadequate responders to conventional therapy), • Non-radiographic axial SpA,	• Refractory pulmonary sarcoidosis (IFN and ADA), • Uveitis associated with rheumatic diseases (IFN, ADA, GOL), • BD (resistant ocular, CNS, and GI symptoms), • IvIg refractory KD
Anti IL-1 agents	• RA (not responding to methotrexate), • CAPS • Still's disease	• BD (refractory skin and genital lesions), • FMF • TRAPS • CRMO
Anti IL-17 agents	• AS • PsA • Active Non-Radiographic Axial Spondyloarthritis	• SAPHO syndrome

Abbreviations: *b-DMARD* biological disease-modifying anti-rheumatic drug, *RA* Rheumatoid arthritis, *cs-DMARD* conventional synthetic DMARD, *SOJIA* Systemic-onset juvenile idiopathic arthritis, *pJIA* Polyarticular JIA, *GCA* Granulomatosis with polyangiitis, *TA* Takayasu arteritis, *AOSD* adult onset still disease, *SSc* systemic sclerosis, *BD* Behcet disease, *PMR* polymyalgia rheumatica, *MPA* microscopic polyangiitis, *ILD* interstitial lung disease, *IIM* idiopathic inflammatory myositis, *ASS* anti synthetase syndrome, *AS* ankylosing spondylitis, *PSA* psoriatic arthritis, *SpA* spondyloarthritis, *IFN* Infliximab, *ADA* Adalimumab, *GOL* Golimumab, *KD* Kawasaki disease, *CAPS* cryopyrin-associated periodic syndromes, *FMF* Familial Mediterranean Fever, *TRAPS* Tumor Necrosis Factor Receptor-Associated Periodic Syndrome, *CRMO* Chronic Recurrent Multifocal Osteomyelitis

References

1. Nishimoto N, Kanakura Y, Aozasa K, Johkoh T, Nakamura M, Nakano S, et al. Humanized anti-interleukin-6 receptor antibody treatment of multicentric Castleman disease. Blood. 2005;106(8):2627–32.
2. Liao H, Pan LL, Du J, Gao N, Wang T. Efficacy and safety of tocilizumab in patients with Takayasu arteritis. Zhonghua Nei Ke Za Zhi. 2019;58(6):444–8.
3. Decker P, Olivier P, Risse J, Zuily S, Wahl D. Tocilizumab and refractoryTakayasu disease: four case reports and systematic review. Autoimmun Rev. 2018;17(4):353–60.
4. Jung J-Y, Kim M-Y, Suh C-H, Kim H-A. Off-label use of tocilizumab to treat nonjuvenile idiopathic arthritis in pediatric rheumatic patients: a literature review. Paediatr Rheumatol. 2018;16:79.
5. Mekinian A, Saadoun D, Vicaut E, Thietart S, Lioger B, Jego P, et al. French Takayasu network. Tocilizumab in treatment-naïve patients with Takayasu arteritis: TOCITAKA French prospective multicenter open-labeled trial. Arthritis Res Ther. 2020;22(1):218.
6. Rubbert-Roth A, Furst DE, Nebesky JM, Jin A, Berber E. A review of recent advances using tocilizumab in the treatment of rheumatic diseases. Rheumatol Ther. 2018;5(1):21–42.
7. Vercruysse F, Barnetche T, Lazaro E, Shipley E, Lifermann F, Balageas A, et al. Adult-onset Still's disease biological treatment strategy may depend on the phenotypic dichotomy. Arthritis Res Ther. 2019;21(1):53.
8. Khanna D, Denton CP, Jahreis A, van Laar JM, Frech TM, Anderson ME, et al. Safety and efficacy of subcutaneous tocilizumab in adults with systemic sclerosis (faSScinate): a phase 2, randomised, controlled trial. Lancet. 2016;387(10038):2630–40.
9. Khanna D, Denton CP, Lin CJF, van Laar JM, Frech TM, Anderson ME, et al. Safety and efficacy of subcutaneous tocilizumab in systemic sclerosis: results from the open-label period of a phase II randomised controlled trial (faSScinate). Ann Rheum Dis. 2018;77(2):212–20.
10. Khanna D, Lin CJF, Furst DE, Goldin J, Kim G, Kuwana M, FocuSSced Investigators, et al. Tocilizumab in systemic sclerosis: a randomised, double-blind, placebo-controlled, phase 3 trial. Lancet Respir Med. 2020;8(10):963–74.
11. Domínguez-Casas LC, Calvo-Río V, Blanco R, Beltran E, Martinez-Costa L, Valls-Pascual E, et al. Anti-IL6-R tocilizumab in refractory uveitis associated with BehçEt's disease. Multicenter study of 11 patients [abstract]. Arthritis Rheumatol. 2016;68(suppl 10):2954.
12. Akiyama M, Kaneko Y, Takeuchi T. Effectiveness of tocilizumab in Behcet's disease: a systematic literature review. Semin Arthritis Rheum. 2020;50(4):797–804.
13. Devauchelle V, Saraux A, Berthelot JM, Cornec D, Renaudineau Y, Jousse-Joulin S, et al. Dramatic efficacy of tocilizumab as first line therapy in patients with recent polymyalgia rheumatica (PMR): results of the first longitudinal prospective study [abstract]. Arthritis Rheumatol. 2015;67(suppl 10):1987.
14. Spiera R, Unizony SH, Bao M, Luder Y, Han J, Pavlov A, et al. Tocilizumab vs placebo for the treatment of giant cell arteritis with polymyalgia rheumatica symptoms, cranial symptoms or both in a randomized trial. Semin Arthritis Rheum. 2021;51(2):469–76.
15. Carvajal Alegria G, Cornec DYK, Renaudineau Y, Saraux A, Devauchelle-Pensec V. Inflammatory markers are quickly improved by tocilizumab in early polymyalgia rheumatica and might predict early response to interleukin-6 blockade. Rheumatol Ther. 2021;21:1–10.
16. Merrill JT, Neuwelt CM, Wallace DJ, Shanahan JC, Latinis KM, Oates JC, et al. Efficacy and safety of rituximab in moderately-to-severely active systemic lupus erythematosus: the randomized, double-blind, phase II/III systemic lupus erythematosus evaluation of rituximab trial. Arthritis Rheum. 2010;62(1):222–33.
17. Rovin BH, Furie R, Latinis K, Looney RJ, Fervenza FC, Sanchez-Guerrero J, et al. LUNAR Investigator Group. Efficacy and safety of rituximab in patients with active proliferative lupus nephritis: the lupus nephritis assessment with rituximab study. Arthritis Rheum. 2012;64(4):1215–26.

18. Fernández-Nebro A, de la Fuente JL, Carreño L, Izquierdo MG, Tomero E, Rúa-Figueroa I, et al. Multicenter longitudinal study of B-lymphocyte depletion in refractory systemic lupus erythematosus: the LESIMAB study. Lupus. 2012;21(10):1063–76.
19. Schioppo T, Ingegnoli F. Current perspective on rituximab in rheumatic diseases. Drug Des Devel Ther. 2017;11:2891–904.
20. Condon MB, Ashby D, Pepper RJ, Cook HT, Levy JB, Griffith M, et al. Prospective observational single-centre cohort study to evaluate the effectiveness of treating lupus nephritis with rituximab and mycophenolate mofetil but no oral steroids. Ann Rheum Dis. 2013;72(8):1280–6.
21. Gracia-Tello B, Ezeonyeji A, Isenberg D. The use of rituximab in newly diagnosed patients with systemic lupus erythematosus: long-term steroid saving capacity and clinical effectiveness. Lupus Sci Med. 2017;4(1):e000182.
22. Jordan S, Distler JH, Maurer B, Huscher D, van Laar JM, Allanore Y, et al. EUSTAR rituximab study group. Effects and safety of rituximab in systemic sclerosis: an analysis from the European scleroderma trial and research (EUSTAR) group. Ann Rheum Dis. 2015;74(6):1188–94.
23. Sircar G, Goswami RP, Sircar D, Ghosh A, Ghosh P. Intravenous cyclophosphamide vs rituximab for the treatment of early diffuse scleroderma lung disease: open label, randomized, controlled trial. Rheumatology (Oxford). 2018;57(12):2106–13.
24. Dass S, Bowman SJ, Vital EM, Ikeda K, Pease CT, Hamburger J, et al. Reduction of fatigue in Sjögren syndrome with rituximab: results of a randomised, double-blind, placebo-controlled pilot study. Ann Rheum Dis. 2008;67(11):1541–4.
25. Bowman SJ, Everett CC, O'Dwyer JL, Emery P, Pitzalis C, Ng WF, et al. Randomized controlled trial of rituximab and cost-effectiveness analysis in treating fatigue and oral dryness in primary Sjögren's syndrome. Arthritis Rheumatol. 2017;69(7):1440–50.
26. Wang Y, Hou Z, Qiu M, Ye Q. Risk factors for primary Sjögren syndrome-associated interstitial lung disease. J Thorac Dis. 2018;10(4):2108–17.
27. Chen MH, Chen CK, Chou HP, Chen MH, Tsai CY, Chang DM. Rituximab therapy in primary Sjögren's syndrome with interstitial lung disease: a retrospective cohort study. Clin Exp Rheumatol. 2016;34(6):1077–84.
28. Oddis CV, Reed AM, Aggarwal R, Rider LG, Ascherman DP, Levesque MC, et al. RIM Study Group. Rituximab in the treatment of refractory adult and juve ile dermatomyositis and adult polymyositis: a randomized, placebo-phase trial. Arthritis Rheum. 2013;65(2):314–24.
29. Marie I, Dominique S, Janvresse A, Levesque H, Menard JF. Rituximab therapy for refractory interstitial lung disease related to antisynthetase syndrome. Respir Med. 2012;106(4):581–7.
30. Rossman MD, Newman LS, Baughman RP, Teirstein A, Weinberger SE, Miller W Jr, et al. A double-blinded, randomized, placebo-controlled trial of infliximab in subjects with active pulmonary sarcoidosis. Sarcoidosis Vasc Diffuse Lung Dis. 2006;23(3):201–8.
31. Baughman RP, Drent M, Kavuru M, Judson MA, Costabel U, du Bois R, et al. Sarcoidosis Investigators. Infliximab therapy in patients with chronic sarcoidosis and pulmonary involvement. Am J Respir Crit Care Med. 2006;174(7):795–802.
32. Sánchez-Cano D, Callejas-Rubio JL, Ruiz-Villaverde R, Ríos-Fernández R, Ortego-Centeno N. Off-label uses of anti-TNF therapy in three frequent disorders: Behçet's disease, sarcoidosis, and noninfectious uveitis. Mediat Inflamm. 2013;2013:286857.
33. Wendling D, Paccou J, Berthelot JM, Flipo RM, Guillaume-Czitrom S, Prati C, Dernis E, Direz G, Ferrazzi V, Ristori JM. New onset of uveitis during anti-tumor necrosis factor treatment for rheumatic diseases. Semin Arthritis Rheum. 2011;41(3):503–10.
34. Cantini F, Niccoli L, Nannini C, Kaloudi O, Cassarà E, Susini M, Lenzetti I. Efficacy of infliximab in refractory Behçet's disease-associated and idiopathic posterior segment uveitis: a prospective, follow-up study of 50 patients. Biologics. 2012;6:5–12.
35. Horiguchi N, Kamoi K, Horie S, Iwasaki Y, Kurozumi-Karube H, Takase H, Ohno-Matsui K. A 10-year follow-up of infliximab monotherapy for refractory uveitis in Behçet's syndrome. Sci Rep. 2020;10(1):22227.
36. Kikuchi H, Aramaki K, Hirohata S. Effect of infliximab in progressive neuro-Behçet's syndrome. J Neurol Sci. 2008;272(1–2):99–105.

37. Hur G, Song MS, Sohn S, Lee HD, Kim GB, Cho HJ, et al. Infliximab treatment for intravenous immunoglobulin-resistant Kawasaki disease: a multicenter study in Korea. Korean Circ J. 2019;49(2):183–91.
38. Tremoulet AH, Jain S, Jaggi P, Jimenez-Fernandez S, Pancheri JM, Sun X, et al. Infliximab for intensification of primary therapy for Kawasaki disease: a phase 3 randomised,double-blind, placebo-controlled trial. Lancet. 2014;383(9930):1731–8.
39. Mori M, Hara T, Kikuchi M, Shimizu H, Miyamoto T, Iwashima S, et al. Infliximab versus intravenous immunoglobulin for refractory Kawasaki disease: a phase 3, randomized, open-label, active-controlled, parallel-group, multicenter trial. Sci Rep. 2018;8(1):1994.
40. Vitale A, Insalaco A, Sfriso P, Lopalco G, Emmi G, Cattalini M, et al. A snapshot on the on-label and off-label use of the interleukin-1 inhibitors in Italy among rheumatologists and pediatric rheumatologists: a nationwide multi-center retrospective observational study. Front Pharmacol. 2016;7:380. eCollection 2016.
41. Grayson PC, Yazici Y, Merideth M, Sen HN, Davis M, Novakovich E, et al. Treatment of mucocutaneous manifestations in Behçet's disease with anakinra: a pilot open-label study. Arthritis Res Ther. 2017;19(1):69.
42. Ugurlu S, Ergezen B, Ozdogan H. Anakinra treatment in patients with familial Mediterranean fever: a single-center experience. Pediatr Rheumatol Online J. 2015;13(Suppl 1):P123.
43. Gül A, Ozdogan H, Erer B, Ugurlu S, Kasapcopur O, Davis N, Sevgi S. Efficacy and safety of canakinumab in adolescents and adults with colchicine-resistant familial Mediterranean fever. Arthritis Res Ther. 2015;17:243.
44. Brizi MG, Galeazzi M, Lucherini OM, Cantarini L, Cimaz R. Successful treatment of tumor necrosis factor receptor-associated periodic syndrome with canakinumab. Ann Intern Med. 2012;156(12):907–8.
45. Daoussis D, Konstantopoulou G, Kraniotis P, Sakkas L, Liossis SN. Biologics in SAPHO syndrome: a systematic review. Semin Arthritis Rheum. 2019;48(4):618–25.

Biologics and Ethical Issues in Rheumatology

26

Nibha Jain, Dhaiwat Shukla, Prashant Chotalia, and Sapan C. Pandya

26.1 Introduction: Ethical Issues in Rheumatology

- With a deeper understanding of the pathogenesis of rheumatic diseases, newer therapies have been developed or are in the process of being developed. These include biological therapies, now commonly used in rheumatology. However, many ethical issues arise with the use of these in day-to-day practice or research settings.
- Ethical issues in rheumatology are rampant, and in a survey, the investigators found more than half of the participants reported a lack of comprehension regarding these [1]. They reported ethical dilemmas both in practice and clinical research. Most frequent *practice-related concerns* were the cost of therapy to the patient (the newer therapies, e.g., biologics are costlier than traditional ones) and society, and limitations of time when interviewing patients due to sheer numbers, especially in a country like ours where the majority do not have proper insurance. Among some other ethical considerations are relationship of the healthcare giver with the Industry and the other challenges one faces when dealing with chronic ailments especially work disability related [2].
- One of the most preferred systems for following medical ethics has outlined 4 clusters of ethical principles, which include respect for autonomy, beneficence, non-maleficence and distributive justice [3].

N. Jain
Pune, India

D. Shukla
Ahmedabad, India

P. Chotalia
Musculoskeletal Medicine, NHL medical college, Ahmedabad, India

S. C. Pandya (✉)
Vedanta Institute of Medical Sciences, Ahmedabad, India

N. Jain, L. Duggal (eds.), *Handbook of Biologics for Rheumatological Disorders*, https://doi.org/10.1007/978-981-16-7200-2_26

- Despite such ethical dilemmas in rheumatology, literature related to the same is sparse. Not many have discussed these in medical literature, and a search for the same done earlier revealed only 0.026% of published articles addressing them [4]. The commonest and least common theme therein was found to be Non-maleficence and Justice, respectively.
- Issues related to our country as regards physician–industry relationships have been addressed [5].

26.2 Biologics/Biosimilars and their Cost-Effectiveness

- *Biologics* represent one of the fastest-growing segments of the pharmaceutical industry [6]. The DCGI (Drug Controller General of India) has come out with a special Dossier for biosimilar manufacture and sale, which is also updated regularly. It is through this that the majority of these drugs receive sanctions [7]. Since the biosimilars were approved and marketed in 2003, many followed the trail, including adalimumab, infliximab, rituximab [8]. One of the biggest problems in dealing with biosimilars and innovator drugs for use in patients is the lack of head-to-head trials between these and also patient-related issues like maintaining their autonomy in taking consent—explaining to them the possibility of adverse effects/efficacy especially comparative between the alternatives when data regarding these is suboptimal [9, 10].
- Autoimmune diseases, especially rheumatic, are still not covered under insurance and hence cost remains an issue with these agents. Even otherwise, as far as all of India's population is concerned, only a small segment opts for health insurance, more so from the rural sector. By the nature of the course of these diseases, which are often relapsing remitting and continue for years or decades, even for those who can afford, cost-effectiveness becomes an issue. *Put simply, even if a patient agrees to use biological therapy, how much benefit will it provide above conventional therapy and will the extra expenditure be worth it?*
- Pharmacoeconomics is that branch of therapeutic science that deals with the cost-effectiveness of a new drug, especially in the context of the disease it will be used for and the relevant population [11].. However, an ethical dilemma arises when the patient is unable to access the options and or make a decision.
- Cost-effectiveness analysis comes into relevance when costs justify benefit gained, e.g., in a situation where it prevents mortality, most would agree to use it, but if the perceived or actual gain is only marginal, its use in that disease and for that population would be difficult. Van der Velde et al. actually studied this willingness in patients of RA to pay extra for a unit of gain in their health [12].

26.3 Patient-Related Ethical Issues

26.3.1 Control Arms and Healthy Controls

- The safety studies for new drugs are normally done first in healthy volunteers. The problem with biologics is that they are designed to be very specific to their targets that are usually present in high number only in diseased states. They cannot be hence carried out in healthy volunteers, and this poses an ethical issue. The selection of these appropriate control arms leads to complex ethical issues.

- Clinical equipoise happens when in the designing of a clinical trial, both interventions are assumed to be equal and one not better than the other in efficacy [13]. When an investigator also feels the same, it becomes a personal equipoise. In an ethical scenario with clinical equipoise, patients should be assigned randomly to different study arms. In many trials, a placebo is a preferred comparator. And while placebo-controlled studies are essential to rule out chance as a confounder, an ethical issue does arise, especially in the context of biosimilars/biologics, as most of these are highly efficacious and do not have a comparator arm in studies. It would be important to use at least the standard of care or other disease-modifying drugs in the parallel arm so that the disease is not left to progress in that arm.

26.3.2 Treatment Naïve and Treated Patients

Two important issues in including treatment naïve patients into clinical trials are: (1) As discussed above, the possibility of disease progression in those where the standard of care is available and of proven efficacy and (2) Exclusion of patients with co-morbidities or those on some drugs to avoid drug interactions, especially in RCTs and controlled trials—and this is where observational studies or data from registries is gaining more importance these days as the latter more accurately reflect real-life situations which is not so in RCTs. It is therefore imperative to develop a safety database.

26.3.3 Beneficence and Non-Maleficence

- There are two aspects to ethical dilemmas in the use of newer drugs like biologics—in technical terms these are called Beneficence and non-maleficence. While the former deals with balancing costs versus risks involved in the usage of these, the latter is more about avoiding harm. When deciding on any therapeutic options, these two factors go hand in hand. As per various guidelines, anti-inflammatory compounds are still the first-line therapy for axial spondyloarthritis (axSpA), failing which biologic therapy is considered. There are a number of social and economic factors that a treating physician has to consider before finalizing the best treatment option for his/her patient—like age, sex (possibility of pregnancy and hence family planning), co-morbidities, allergies, etc. Treatment of inflammatory diseases is beyond just symptomatic control but also includes long-term continuous control of inflammation to prevent damage. One of the measures in assessing outcomes of diseases, e.g., Spondyloarthritis, involves patients' mental component for gaging improvement (patient global), and if the patient is depressed, it would affect the score. Depression is not uncommon in many of these patients who are young working males [14]. In using NSAIDs which are, as per the guidelines, the first drugs to be tried, the inflammation might be partly controlled but may not have the mental impact, e.g., that a biologic would have, even for fatigue.

- As we deal with chronic conditions, biologic therapies may be required for a longer period of time or sometimes lifelong. The safety data of long-term use of many biologics are not yet available. Important risks with the use of biologics are infections and the possibility of malignancy, among others.
- Amongst other exclusions in many clinical trials are also patients with extremes of age, Hep B, Hep C and or congestive cardiac failure—these would again be there in the real-life situation, and hence using the drugs in this subset of patients would raise ethical dilemmas.
- One of the paradoxes in drug usage has been that since systemic therapies like biologics might have more risks both in terms of adverse effects and costs, physicians will be more inclined to use conventional therapies. The trials that were done with the latter drugs earlier involved a much lesser number of patients and were poorly designed—most of them. Whereas with drugs like biologics, since the stakes are much higher and with the use of modern gadgets and techniques, the trials are more rigorous and hence the data more robust.
- When compared to drugs like corticosteroids, biologic therapies, in the long run, may be associated with lesser damage, systemic and organ based both due to better disease control and lack of such adverse effects. Although lymphomas have been reported with the use of anti-TNF therapies, which have resolved when these therapies were withdrawn [15]—it remains to be proven if the drugs caused these or the disease itself. Treating physicians should explicitly discuss even these remote possibilities with the patients choosing to use them and also both screen them initially and monitor for them on follow-up with whatever tests/investigations are needed.

A checklist prior to commencing biologic therapy in India has been proposed [16].

26.3.4 Patient Autonomy

- Another issue while adhering to the ethical principles of beneficence and non-maleficence is not respecting the patient's preference for treatment. In today's times, patient preferences and perspectives are becoming more and more important.
- In an ideal scenario, all possible alternatives available as treatment modalities must be discussed with the patients before helping them decide on one. With increasing access to social media and free access to websites, many patients are aware of available treatment options. They should be provided with all available options in a balanced manner, and clinicians must consider patient's preferences and guide them in decision-making. The field of biologic therapy is evolving every day with new data and molecules coming in, and it is only imperative that

patients must be apprised of all newer concepts. Adverse effects that have already been registered and also those likely to happen when used in the real-life scenario and in the long run also have to be discussed with them.

- The doctor-patient ratio in populous countries like India continues to be poor despite many advances in medical education and healthcare. Due to the same, the average time a doctor spends with a patient is abysmally less, and many healthcare givers do not explain in detail the efficacy and adverse/side effects of medicines prescribed. In fact, even details related to the diseases they suffer are not shared with them due to lack of time. They thus end up violating a fundamental right of these patients [17].

26.3.5 Distribution of Justice

- While it is only ideal that patients get the best possible treatments notwithstanding costs that do not happen in real life, and physicians prescribe medicines looking into the cost-effectiveness of these. The biologics/biosimilars are costly drugs especially taking into consideration the average incomes of most patients in countries like India whereas conventional DMARDs are much cheaper. Considering long-term or lifelong therapy, these might pose a significant financial burden. Treating physicians must have advocacy lobbies along with patient leaders that influence the insurance and government sectors to make these accessible for most patients.
- India poses a unique dilemma to the physician where many patients turn to private practitioners and often do not have medical insurance covering biologic therapy. Even when they do have, most insurance covering companies make it mandatory first to use DMARDs to full effects before biologics are offered to them. Even when they do agree to share the cost, a substantial part of the same is still borne by patients. There are NGOs and even other organizations, including waivers/discounts from the pharmaceutical companies themselves, to help such patients in need, but that is usually for a limited period which again may not be of much use in a chronic illness that, in most cases, is lifelong! Lack of extensive guidelines regarding the use of biologics in India has led to a muddy picture of the insurance companies reimbursing these costs.
- What is important to consider in such diseases is also the societal cost and not just the individual ones. When a patient suffers from a disease and has to resort to costly treatment, from the payer's point of view, he/she has to bear a higher cost. But when he/she gets better with this treatment, occupational or professional absence from work reduces and overall the society and community benefits. Often this aspect is not considered in cost-effectiveness. This was proven in a study on patients with axSpA where the patients on biologics benefitted in terms of presenteeism at work and improvement in activity and workmanship [18]. Ideally, this should be taken into account when deciding on the long-term benefits of apparently costly drugs.

26.4 Physician-Related Issues

26.4.1 Physician–Pharmaceutical Industry Relations

Physician–pharmaceutical industry relationship is a complex one. There are many ways the pharmaceutical industries influence a doctor's judgment about treatment. Many hospitals have also restricted access of pharmaceutical executives to clinicians. Even a small gift can compromise your objectivity in the long run. It has been studied that conflicts arise mainly in relation to prescribers being on the Board of directors in three-fourth of cases, talking to audiences without declaring conflicts in more than a half and consulting with the Industry in about the same numbers [1]. It was also soon that the industry influenced the decision-making and prescribing patterns of practitioners [19]. It is the moral and ethical obligation of the physician to avoid being influenced, however, at the same time, the contribution of the industry to healthcare cannot be ignored. Conflicts also arise when companies are trading costly drugs like biologics fund conferences/lunches/educational grants, etc. While not being directly at conflict at an individual level, health care givers have an indirect relationship by agreeing to grants/help from the industry for conferences, etc., where international and national speakers are sponsored as a trade-off.

26.4.2 Conflict of Interest

Clinicians must adhere to the principles of informed consent when explaining the potential risks of newer therapies while trialing. Conflict of interest can arise in multiple scenarios, right from biased inclusion of patients in drug development trials to unnecessary commencement of a medication in a patient. Ideally, the funding provided to the clinician should also be clearly stated to the subject being enrolled.

26.4.3 Medical Education and Bias

The healthcare system must cater to the human resources training policy in the country, thus ensuring the integration of young specialists into the society. This necessitates Medical postings in rheumatology and continued medical education to ensure correct decision-making on the part of treating physicians.

26.5 Industry-Related Issues

26.5.1 Fair Control Trials

- Head-to-head trials comparing biologics are very rare; approximately 90% of the trials so far are placebo-controlled trials [20]. Such trials require stringent regulatory requirements, and most of the pharma industry would not want to invest if there is the slightest doubt of inferiority of their product; comparator biologics drugs are expensive, and companies do not want to invest in their competitor's product, lack of such trials create a false impression that all biologics are equally efficacious and it promotes the sale of all of them instead of one which can be used judiciously over others because of superiority. The sample size requirement for head-to-head trial is also larger as compared to placebo-controlled trial [20].

- As discussed before, one of the biggest problems, especially as regards the trials of biologics, is the use of placebo in the control arm in most of them [21]). Since even standard of care is not included in the control arm, these trials are more designed to validate the superiority of these costly drugs to placebo. What is needed is ideally head-to-head comparison of these against one another OR at least against DMARDs or other standard of care depending on the illness being studied.
- An alternative way to remove bias that has been used is to continue treatment in the responders after a pre-decided duration of treatment and withdraw from the others the investigational drug (which is added on to some baseline drugs)—disease flares are documented as an outcome measure in these. While this may be able together some sound evidence of the efficacy of the investigational drug, such designs have problems of needing more power of the study, which will ultimately increase the costs.
- There are important differences between industry-sponsored trials and public-funded trials or trials funded through other sources. In fact, industry-sponsored trials have better study designs, and stringently follow-up of regulatory recommendations, but at the same time, they are usually for a short duration and are less likely to be published. These trials are more likely to show superiority of sponsor's product over comparator, and the reason for this is not the quality of methods in research but the selection of inappropriate comparator, by and large. Most of the time, the comparator is inactive placebo or the same drug in different strength or different formulation of the same drug or the other biologic of the same pharma company! [22].
- However, it is expected that in coming times, with the availability of more and more biosimilars which will be cheaper and with the expiry of originator biologic molecule patents, the operating cost for conducting trials would be reduced, and in future, we should see more head-to-head comparison trials [19].
- India has specific trial-related ethical issues: most of the time, our subjects do get enrolled in clinical trials because they cannot afford existing treatment. There are significant differences in the public and private health care setups and patients enrolled therein have different reasons for participation in trials. Most of these trials have to be registered under the DCGI and follow the ICMR guidelines. As of now, the infrastructure for ethics, regulation, and conduct of trials has many deficiencies [23].

26.5.2 Publication Biases

- Studies with positive results showing statistically significant treatment outcomes have higher chances of being published, and they also get published early as compared to ones that show neutral or negative results. There is also the problem of about half of these had changed the definition of their primary/secondary outcomes to suit publication—this leads to bias [24]. Industry-sponsored RCTs have a lesser publication chance despite being generally more robust in design [25].
- Amongst biologics, out of 212 registered clinical trials on anti-TNF therapies, only 82 (38.7%)have been published so far. So, we have a potential loss of information from 61.3% of studies. Some of them may get published in due course of time, but at least 56 have not got published even after 1 year of their completion [20] (Table 26.1).

26.6 Future and Conclusion

Small molecules are believed to be the future of rheumatology. Where in the therapeutic armamentarium will biologics be in that case? Only time will tell. Increasing biosimilars are bound to be manufactured as patents for innovators' ease, especially in countries like India, which might actually turn out to be a global giant in producing these. It will be more relevant then to lay out the rules for not only manufacturing in a standardized way but also testing them through proper trials. With the increasing availability of these, costs will come down—even innovators and patients might want to switch to a cheaper copy of the one they are taking, and ethical issues will arise at such times, and we will need to clarify those. Cost-effectiveness will be increasingly important in the long run, and more than that, safety as these very potent immunosuppressive drugs will be increasingly used. Physicians prescribing these will need to take time out or share

Table 26.1 Total and published RCTs of anti-TNF agents in each rheumatic disease indication [20]

	Infliximab		Etanercept		Adalimumab		Certolizumab pegol		Golimumab	
Disease indication	Total	Published (%)	Total	Published (%)	Total	Published (%)	Total	Published (%)	Total	Published (%)
RA	20	7 (35)	23	7 (30)	28	9 (32)	19	5 (26)	12	7 (58%)
Psoriasis	7	5 (71)	13	6 (46)	15	5 (30)	2	1 (50)	0	0
PsA	3	2 (67)	1	1 (100)	3	2 (67)	1	0 (0)	1	1 (100)
AS	4	2 (50)	7	4 (57)	3	2 (67)	1	0 (0)	3	1 (33)
JIA	2	2 (100)	3	2 (67)	2	1 (50)	0	0	1	0 (0)

RA rheumatoid arthritis, *PsA* psoriatic arthritis, *AS* ankylosing spondylitis, *JIA* juvenile idiopathic arthritis handouts that are comprehensive to explain side effects and efficacy. Pharmacogenomics may make it easier to shortlist which drug will work best in a given host. New biomarkers will make treatment response more objective, and there will be an increasing role of patients in decision-making—something not common in countries like ours but what we should promote. In conclusion, with ethical issues clearly outlined, defined, and elaborated, the consumer should be increasingly benefitted in the times to come.

References

1. Mackenzie CR, Meltzer M, Kitsis EA, Mancuso CA. Ethical challenges in rheumatology: a survey of the American college of rheumatology membership. Arthritis Rheum. 2013;65(10):2524–32. This article discusses the important ethical issues identified by American rheumatologists. These include costs related to treatments, profiting from infusions, relationships with industry, and conflict of interest. A commitment to ethics education was suggested
2. Mckeown EJ. The ethical challenges in rheumatology. Curr Rev Musculoskelet Med. 2015;8(2):107–12. https://doi.org/10.1007/s12178-015-9263-1.
3. Beauchamp TL, Childress JF. Principles of biomedical ethics. 3rd ed. Oxford: Oxford University; 1989.
4. Caplan L, Hoffecker L, Prochazka AV. Ethics in the rheumatology literature: a systematic review. Arthritis Rheum. 2008;59(6):81621.
5. Nagral S, Roy N. The medical council of India guidelines on industry-physician relationship: breaking the conspiracy of silence. Natl Med J India. 2010;23:69–71.
6. Revers L, Furczon E. An introduction to biologics and biosimilars. Part 1: biologics:what are they and where do they come from? CanpharmJ. 2010;143:134–9.
7. Guidelines on similar biologics: regulatory requirements for marketing authorization in India 2012. www.cdsco.in/bio%20similar%20guifeline.pdf.
8. GaBi online - Similar biologics approved and marketed in India (www.gabionline.net). http://www.gabionline.net/Biosimilars/General/Similar-biologics-spproved-and-marketed-in-india.
9. Sharma SK. Use of biologics and biosimilars in rheumatology. J Assoc Physicians India. 2017;65(5 Suppl):9–14.
10. Murdoch B, Caulfield T. The law and ethics of switching from biologic to biosimilar in Canada. J Can Assoc Gastroenterol. 2020;3(5):228–33. https://doi.org/10.1093/jcag/gwz043.
11. Bootman JL, Townsend RJ, McGhan WF. Introduction of Pharmacoeconomics. Principlrs of Pharmacoeconomics. 2nd ed. Cincinnati, OH: Harvey Whitney Books; 1996.
12. van der Velde G, Pham B, Machado M, Ieraci L, Witteman W, Bombardier C, et al. Cost-effectiveness of biologic response modifiers compared to disease-modifying antirheumatic drugs for rheumatoid arthritis: a systematic review. Arthritis Care Res (Hoboken). 2011;63(1):65–78.
13. Chad Cook & Charles Sheets. Clinical equipoise and personal equipoise: two necessary ingredients for reducing bias in manual therapy trials. J Man Manip Ther. 2011;19(1):55–7.
14. Zhao S, Thong D, Miller N, et al. The prevalence of depression in axial spondyloarthritis and its association with disease activity: a systematic review and meta-analysis. Arthritis Res Ther. 2018;20:140. https://doi.org/10.1186/s13075-018-1644-6.
15. Mariette X, Tubach F, Bagheri H, et al. Lymphoma in patients treate with anti-TNF: results of the 3-year prospective French RATIO registry. Ann Rheum Dis. 2010;69:400–8.
16. Dudam R, Gumdal N. Checklist prior to biologics: Indian perspective. Indian J Rheumatol. 2016;11:126–8.

17. Ghooi RB, Deshpande SR. Patients' rights in India: an ethical perspective. Indian J Med Ethics. 2012;9(4):277–81.
18. Shim J, et al. Impact of biological therapy on work outcomes in patients with axial spondyloarthritis: results from the British Society for Rheumatology Biologics Register (BSRBR-AS) and meta-analysis. Ann Rheum Dis. 2018;77:1578–84. https://doi.org/10.1136/annrheumdis-2018-213590.
19. Sah S. Conflicts of interest and your physician: psychological processes that cause unexpected changes in behavior. J Law Med Ethics. 2012;40(3):482–7.
20. Ioannidis JP, et al. Biologic agents in rheumatology: unmet issues after 200 trials and $200 billion sales. Nat Rev Rheumatol. 2013;9(11):665–73. https://doi.org/10.1038/nrrheum.2013.134.
21. Estellat C, Ravaud P. Lack of head-to-head trials and fair control arms: randomized controlled trials of biologic treatment for rheumatoid arthritis. Arch Intern Med. 2012;172(3):237–44.
22. Lexchin J, Bero LA, Djulbegovic B, Clark O. Pharmaceutical industry sponsorship and research outcome and quality: systematic review. BMJ. 2003;326:1167–70.
23. Sandhya Srinivasan, et al. Ethical concerns in clinical trials in India: an investigation. CSER report; Feb 2019.
24. Dwan K, et al. Systematic review of the empirical evidence of study publication bias and outcome reporting bias. PLoS One. 2008;3:e3081.
25. Khan NA, Lombeida JI, Singh M, Spencer HJ, Torralba KD. Association of industry funding with the outcome and quality of randomized controlled trials of drug therapy for rheumatoid arthritis. Arthritis Rheum. 2012;64:2059–67.

Patient Consent for Biologics

27

S. J. Gupta

27.1 Introduction

The advent and regular use of Biologics has revolutionised the management of patients with inflammatory joint disorders. Disease remission has now become a distinct reality and perhaps even drug-free remission, albeit in a small number of patients [1]. However, biologics, like most drugs, are not without their problems. These include: (1) common for all biologics- significantly increased cost of treatment which makes continuing treatment and even initiation, difficult if not impossible, for some patients; increased infection risk and infusion or local injection reactions; and (2) related to specific agents- cardiac failure, demyelinating disease and hyperlipidemia [2]. In recent times, a fresh dimension to the initiation and use of biologic agents has been added by the COVID-19 pandemic and a potential increased infection risk for patients on biologics. It is therefore important that prior to commencing a patient on a biologic agent detailed information about the drug(s) including indication for use, cost of treatment, potential risks and screening measures prior to treatment, is provided to the patient by the treating physician/rheumatologist. Treatment should be initiated, only after obtaining the consent of the patient.

27.2 Consent

- The evolution of Consent or more accurately, Informed Consent, from a patient has been influenced by advances in surgical procedures and medical research. Though there are some reports of written informed consent being taken as far back as 1539 [3] the development of written informed consent has really taken place since the twentieth century.

S. J. Gupta (✉)
Apollo Indraprastha & Sant Parmanand Hospitals, New Delhi, India

N. Jain, L. Duggal (eds.), *Handbook of Biologics for Rheumatological Disorders*,
https://doi.org/10.1007/978-981-16-7200-2_27

- Signed, informed consent from the patient is absolutely essential, prior to embarking on a surgical procedure or commencing a volunteer on an experimental or trial drug, or a novel medical intervention.
- Over the years, the patient–physician relationship has been one of awe and benevolence. Patients would accept the word and advice of the Physician, without demur. However, with changes in society and legal practices, written informed consent for surgical procedures and medical research is now accepted by all healthcare institutions and is enshrined in law.
- There are three fundamental criteria that must be fulfilled, for informed consent- the patient must be an adult and competent; complete and adequate information must be provided; and he/she must not be coaxed or persuaded [4]. However, signed written consent prior to commencing a patient on a therapeutic regime such as conventional DMARDs or a biologic agent, may not necessarily be required and is not mentioned as a requisite in published guidelines for the use of biologics [5–7].
- The patient must be adequately informed; however, before they can be expected to consent to the use of biologics and while providing this information, the same principles ought to be relevant and applicable as for written consent.

27.3 Consent for Biologics

- Prior to commencing a patient on a biologic, he/she needs to be provided the following information: (1) indications for use; (2) potential risks of treatment; (3) toxicity/side effects of the drug and any pre-treatment screening investigations required; (4) mode of administration; and (5) cost of therapy.
- In countries such as India, where most patients bear the cost of treatment themselves, cost of treatment might be the most important factor determining commencement or otherwise, of the biologic agent.

27.3.1 Indications

- There are now a fairly large number of biologic agents that are approved for the treatment of various auto-immune inflammatory disorders—Table 27.1 [8].
- In addition, there are some situations where non-approved or off-label use of a biologic may be required- such as Rituximab for refractory lupus nephritis.
- A patient being considered for a biologic must be adequately informed about the reason/indication for which a biologic is being considered and whether an alternative approach could also be tried. This could be a patient with rheumatoid arthritis (RA) who has failed DMARDs; or a patient of axial spondarthritis (axSpA) unresponsive to non-steroidal anti-inflammatory drugs (NSAIDs); or as

Table 27.1 Approved Biologics and their indications (and year of approval)

I. Anti-TNF inhibitors: 1. Etanercept: 1998- RA; 2003- Ank Spond; 2. Infliximab: 1999- RA; 2004- Ank Spond; 2005- PsA 3. Adalimumab: 2002- RA; 2005- PsA; 2006- Ank Spond 4. Certolizumab pegol: 2009- RA; 2013- PsA & Ank Spond 5. Golimumab: 2009- RA; 2017- PsA & Ank Spond	IV. Anti B Cell & Co stimulator blocker: 1. Abatacept: 2005- RA; 2008- PA JIA; 2017- PsA 2. Rituximab: 2006- RA; 2019- GPA; 3. Belilumab: 2011- SLE V. IL-6 inhibitors: 1. Tocilizumab: 2010- RA; 2011- SOJIA; 2013: PA JIA; 2017- GCA; 2019: AOSD (Japan)
II. IL-I inhibitors: 1. Anakinra: 2001- RA; 2013- CAPS 2. Rilonacept: 2008- CAPS 3. Canakinumab: 2009- CAPS; 2013- SOJIA; 2013- refractory gout (Europe) 2020- AOSD	VI. IL-12 inhibitors: 1. Ustekinumab: 2009- psoriasis 2013- PsA
III. IL-23 inhibitors: 1. Guselkumab: 2017- psoriasis 2. Risankizumab: 2019- psoriasis 3. Tildrakizumab: 2019- psoriasis	VII. IL-17 inhibitors: 1. Secukinumab: 2015- psoriasis; 2016- PsA; 2016- Ank Spond; 2020- nr-axSpA (Europe) 2. Ixekinumab: 2017- PsA; 2019- Ank Spond 2020- nr-axSpA 3. Broadulmab: 2017- psoriasis

RA rheumatoid arthritis, *Ank Spond* ankylosing spondylitis, *PsA* psoriatic arthritis, *CAPS* cryopyrin-associated autoinflammatory syndrome, *AOSD* adult-onset Still's disease, *JIA* juvenile idiopathic arthritis, GPA granulomatosis with polyangiitis, *SLE* systemic lupus erythematosus, SOJIA systemic onset juvenile idiopathic arthritis, *GCA* giant cell arteritis, *nr-ax SpA* non-radiographic axial spondarthritis

mentioned earlier, a patient with refractory lupus nephritis or another connective tissue disorder.

- In some situations the indication would be unequivocal; for a patient with active axSpA who has failed an adequate trial of NSAIDs, the only appropriate further treatment would be with a TNFα inhibitor (TNFi) or an anti-IL-17 agent [9].
- For a patient of RA failing to achieve remission or low disease activity despite an adequate DMARD regime (at least 2–3 drugs in combination, including Methotrexate up to 20–25 mg weekly preferably parenteral, for at least 3–6 months) a biologic agent along with csDMARD would be a logical choice (a tsDMARD could be another possibility) [10]; the biologic agent could be any of the following: (1) TNFi (Infliximab or Etanercept or Adalimimab or Golimumab or Certolizumab); (2) anti-B Cell agent (Rituximab); (3) co-stimulation blocker (Abatacept); (4) IL-6 inhibitor (Tocilizumab).
- It would be essential to discuss these options with the patient, providing adequate information to allow the patient to reach a decision. The final decision of the patient will also depend upon other considerations as outlined below.

27.3.2 Toxicity and Pre-Treatment Screening

27.3.2.1 Infection Risk

The most significant potential toxicity to consider is the risk of serious infection. Overall, data indicates a definite albeit small absolute increased risk of infection with most biologics; serious infections, however, being rather rare. One also needs to consider atypical, opportunistic and viral infections.

- TNFi has been associated with an increased risk of reactivation of latent tuberculosis (TB), other granulomatous infections and fungal infections. Amongst the TNFi the risk of TB appears to be greater with Infliximab and Adalimumab compared to Etanercept, though why this happens is not clear.
- Varicella-zoster virus (VZV) infections have been reported with the use of anakinra, abatacept, rituximab or tocilizumab; and reactivation of Hepatitis B (Hep B) has been reported with TNFi and Rituximab [2]. Progressive multifocal leukoencephalopathy (PML) due to reactivation of J C Virus (Human polyomavirus 2 or John Cunningham virus) has been reported with the use of Rituximab; however, out of 57 cases of PML reported in 2009 the majority received treatment as part of chemotherapy and only 5 patients received Rituximab for autoimmune conditions [11].

27.3.2.2 Pre-Treatment Counselling and Screening

- It would be important to inform the patient about the risk albeit small of infection including specific infections. The patient should be advised that in addition to clinical examination and 'routine' blood work-up to rule out infection, more specific tests to look for Hep B and Hep CV status and occult TB would also need to be carried out.
- The presence of co-morbidities such as diabetes (poorly controlled), severe obstructive pulmonary disease or renal dysfunction might alter the choice of biologic agent due to their increased risk of infection and this would need to be explained [7].
- In recent times an additional challenge in the management of patients with inflammatory joint disorders has been provided by the COVID-19 pandemic and this requires additional and careful counselling of the patient. Though it is not clear exactly how a biologic might influence the course of COVID-19 infection, it would be prudent to delay the introduction of a biologic agent as far as possible. However, if the clinical situation does not permit delay, then screening the patient for active COVID-19 infection by RT-PCR would be justified, even if asymptomatic [12].
- For patients continuing or starting biologic infusions in the present scenario, appropriate sanitisation of infusion rooms/chambers, physical distancing in the waiting areas and screening for COVID-19 symptoms prior to entering the facility, must be carried out [13].

27.3.3 Mode of Administration and Cost

- The frequency and route of administration would need to be explained to the patient allowing him/her to choose the most suitable agent. Some might prefer intravenous infusion and others might choose the freedom of self-injection with a pre-filled syringe or injection pen.
- The cost of treatment might be the most important factor for some patients, particularly if paying for the treatment themselves.

27.4 Conclusion

Biologics are an essential part of the management of many auto-immune inflammatory joint disorders. Though they pose certain specific problems such as the cost of treatment and potential toxicity, their utility is unquestionable. The final decision regarding initiation of biologic therapy and which agent to use should be a joint decision between physician and patient. However, an appropriate decision can be made only after complete and detailed information regarding the treatment has been provided to the patient and after seeking his/her consent.

References

1. Machold KP. Prevention and cure of rheumatoid arthritis- is it possible? Best Prac Res Clin Rheum. 2010;24:353–61.
2. Woodrick RS, et al. Safety of biologic therapy in rheumatoid arthritis. Nat Rev Rheumatol. 2011;7:639–52.
3. Selek S. A Written Consent 5 Centuries Ago. J Med Ethics. 2010;36:639.
4. Cocanour CS. Informed consent —It'ss more than a signature on a piece of paper. Am J Surg. 2017; https://doi.org/10.1016/j.amjsurg.2017.09.015.
5. NICE. Adalimumab, etanercept, infliximab, certolizumab pegol, golimumab, tocilizumab and abatacept for rheumatoid arthritis not previously treated with DMARDs or after treated with DMARDs or after conventional DMARDs only have failed- Technology appraisal guidance. Jan 2016. www.nice.org.uk/guidance/ta375
6. Smolen JS, Landewe R, et al. EULAR recommendations for the management of rheumatoid arthritis with synthetic and biological disease-modifying antirheumatic drugs: 2016 update. Ann Rheum Dis. 2017;0:1–18. https://doi.org/10.1136/annrheumdis-2016-210715.
7. Holroyd CR, Seth R, et al. The British Society for Rheumatology biologic DMARD safety guidelines in inflammatory arthritis. Rheumatology. 2019;58:e3e42. https://doi.org/10.1093/rheumatology/key208.
8. Kingsmore KM, et al. Drug repurposing to improve treatment of rheumatic autoimmune inflammatory diseases. Nat Rev Rheum. 2019; https://doi.org/10.1038/s41584-019-0337-0.
9. van der Heijde D, Ramiro S, et al. 2016 update of the ASAS-EULAR management recommendations for axial spondyloarthritis. Ann Rheum Dis. 2017;0:1–14. https://doi.org/10.1136/annrheumdis-2016-210770.
10. Smolen JS, Landewe RBM, et al. EULAR recommendations for the management of rheumatoid arthritis with synthetic and biological disease-modifying antirheumatic drugs: 2019 update. Ann Rheum Dis. 2020;0:1–15. https://doi.org/10.1136/annrheumdis-2019-216655.

11. Carson KR, et al. Progressive multifocal leukoencephalopathy after rituximab therapy in HIV-negative patients: a report of 57 cases from the research on adverse drug events and reports project. Blood. 2009;113:4834–40.
12. Zingone F, Buda A, et al. Screening for active COVID-19 infection and immunization status prior to biologic therapy in IBD patients at the time of the pandemic outbreak. Dig Liver Dis. 2020; https://doi.org/10.1016/j.dld.2020.04.004.
13. ACR Infusion Guidance During COVID-19 Crisis. American College of Rheumatology. Available at https://www.rheumatology.org/Portals/0/Files/ACR-Infusion-Guidance-COVID-19. 3/23/2020.

GPSR Compliance

The European Union's (EU) General Product Safety Regulation (GPSR) is a set of rules that requires consumer products to be safe and our obligations to ensure this.

If you have any concerns about our products, you can contact us on ProductSafety@springernature.com

In case Publisher is established outside the EU, the EU authorized representative is:

Springer Nature Customer Service Center GmbH
Europaplatz 3
69115 Heidelberg, Germany

Batch number: 10732090

Printed by Printforce, the Netherlands